DEMCO

Other Key Aspects Books

Key Aspects of Preventing and Managing Chronic Illness
Editors: Sandra G. Funk, PhD, Elizabeth M. Tornquist, MA, Jennifer Lee-man, DrPH, MDiv, Margaret S. Miles, PhD, RN, and Joanne S. Harrell, PhD, RN 2000

Key Aspects of Caring for the Acutely Ill: Technological Aspects, Patient Education, and Quality of Life
Sandra G. Funk, PhD, Elizabeth M. Tornquist, MA, Mary T. Champagne, PhD, RN, and Ruth Wiese, MSN, RN
1995 Winner, AJN Book of the Year Award

Key Aspects of Caring for the Chronically Ill: Hospital and Home
Sandra G. Funk, PhD, Elizabeth M. Tornquist, MA, Mary T. Champagne, PhD, RN, and Ruth Wiese, MSN, RN
1993 Winner, AJN Book of the Year Award

Key Aspects of Elder Care: Managing Falls, Incontinence, and Cognitive Impairment
Sandra G. Funk, PhD, Elizabeth M. Tornquist, MA, Mary T. Champagne, PhD, RN, and Ruth Wiese, MSN, RN
1992 Winner, AJN Book of the Year Award

Key Aspects of Recovery: Improving Nutrition, Rest, and Mobility
Sandra G. Funk, PhD, Elizabeth M. Tornquist, MA, Mary T. Champagne, PhD, RN, Ruth Wiese, MSN, RN, and Laurel Archer Copp, PhD, RN, FAAN
1990 Winner, AJN Book of the Year Award

Key Aspects of Comfort: Management of Pain, Fatigue, and Nausea
Sandra G. Funk, PhD, Elizabeth M. Tornquist, MA, Mary T. Champagne, PhD, RN, Ruth Wiese, MSN, RN, and Laurel Archer Copp, PhD, RN, FAAN
1990 Winner, AJN Book of the Year Award

Sandra G. Funk, PhD, is professor and associate dean for research in the School of Nursing at the University of North Carolina at Chapel Hill. In addition, she serves as director of the school's Research Support Center and associate director of the NIH-funded Center for Research on Chronic Illness. She has been a faculty member of the School of Nursing for over 20 years, having taught graduate research methods and statistics for many of those years. She has been principal and coinvestigator of numerous grants and has published widely on various aspects of research dissemination and utilization, preschool developmental screening, decision making, and data analysis techniques.

Elizabeth M. Tornquist, MA, has been a member of the faculty of the School of Nursing at the University of North Carolina at Chapel Hill for over 20 years, where she teaches scientific writing and serves as editor in residence. Ms. Tornquist is also on the faculty of the Public Health Leadership Program, School of Public Health, University of North Carolina at Chapel Hill. She is a former journalist and freelance writer and is the author of *From Proposal to Publication: An Informal Guide to Writing about Nursing Research* (1986), as well as numerous articles on writing, presenting, and reading research.

Jennifer Leeman, DrPH, MDiv, is project coordinator for the Center for Research on Chronic Illness, an NIH-funded research center at the School of Nursing at the University of North Carolina at Chapel Hill. She is a member of the School of Nursing faculty, where she teaches courses in health policy and public health. Prior to her doctoral education, Dr. Leeman was responsible for a large, multispecialty ambulatory care program in an academic medical center with a major emphasis on research and the education of health care providers.

Margaret S. Miles, PhD, RN, is professor of nursing at the School of Nursing at the University of North Carolina at Chapel Hill, where she teaches students at all levels. She has been a clinician, educator, and researcher in nursing for over 40 years. As principal investigator on numerous grants, she has published widely in the areas of parenting children with serious illness, parenting of prematurely born children, grief, and African-American women with HIV.

Joanne S. Harrell, PhD, RN, is Professor of Nursing and director of the Center for Research on Chronic Illness at the University of North Carolina at Chapel Hill, where she has been a faculty member for 16 years. Dr. Harrell's program of research involves preventing cardiovascular disease across the life span and caring for adults who have heart disease. Dr. Harrell's current research focuses on activity-based energy expenditure in children, school-based interventions to improve the cardiovascular health of children, and development of type 2 diabetes in childhood and adolescence.

KEY ASPECTS

OF

PREVENTING AND MANAGING

CHRONIC ILLNESS

Sandra G. Funk, PhD
Elizabeth M. Tornquist, MA
Jennifer Leeman, DrPH, MDiv
Margaret S. Miles, PhD, RN
Joanne S. Harrell, PhD, RN

Editors

Springer Publishing Company
New York

Springer Publishing Company, Inc.
536 Broadway
New York, NY 10012-3955

Acquisitions Editor: Ruth Chasek
Production Editor: Janice Stangel
Cover design by Susan Hauley

Library of Congress Cataloging-in-Publication Data

Key aspects of preventing and managing chronic illness / Sandra G.
   Funk . . . [et al.], editors.
      p. ; cm.
   Includes bibliographical references and index.
   ISBN 0-8261-1352-4
   1. Chronic diseases—Prevention. 2. Health promotion. I. Funk,
Sandra G.
   [DNLM: 1. Chronic Disease—nursing. 2. Health Education—
methods. 3. Health Promotion—methods. 4. Long-Term Care—
methods. WY 152 K447 2001]
   RC108 .K48 2001
   616.044—dc21
                                                              00-030056
                                                                    CIP

Printed in the United States of America

Contents

Part III.   The Illness Experience

Contributors

Alice S. Ammerman, DrPH, RD
Associate Professor, Department of
Nutrition, Schools of Public
Health and Medicine, University
of North Carolina at Chapel
Hill

Jan R. Atwood, PhD, RN
Professor, Colleges of Nursing and
Medicine, University of Ne-
braska Medical Center, and As-
sociate Director, Cancer
Prevention and Control Center,
University of Nebraska Medical
Center/Eppley Cancer Center,
Omaha

Brian Austin
Manager, The MacColl Institute
for Healthcare Innovation, Cen-
ter for Health Studies, Group
Health Cooperative of Puget
Sound, Seattle

Donald E. Bailey, Jr., MS, RN
Doctoral Student, School of Nursing, University of North Carolina at Chapel Hill

Shrikant I. Bangdiwala, PhD
Research Associate Professor, Department of Biostatistics, University of North Carolina at Chapel
Hill

Susan J. Barnes, PhD, RN
Assistant Professor, College of
Nursing at Lawton, University of
Oklahoma Health Sciences
Center

Julie Barroso, PhD, ANP, CS
Assistant Professor, Department of
Adult and Geriatric Health,
School of Nursing, University of
North Carolina at Chapel Hill

Michael Belyea, PhD
Research Associate Professor, So-
cial and Administration Systems,
School of Nursing, University of
North Carolina at Chapel Hill

Beth Black, MSN, RN
Research Assistant Professor, De-
partment of Children's Health,
School of Nursing, University of
North Carolina at Chapel Hill

Chyrise B. Bradley, MA
Research Assistant Professor, De-
partment of Adult and Geriatric
Health, School of Nursing, Uni-
versity of North Carolina at
Chapel Hill

Dale E. Brashers, PhD
Assistant Professor, Department of Speech Communication, University of Illinois, Urbana-Champaign

Kathleen C. Buckwalter, PhD, RN
Professor, Department of Adult and Gerontological Nursing, College of Nursing, and Associate Provost for the Health Sciences, University of Iowa, Iowa City

Sharon Ogden Burke, PhD, RN
Professor, School of Nursing, Queen's University, Kingston, Ontario, Canada

Perri E. Cagle, MS, PT
Assistant Professor, Physical Therapy, School of Allied Health, University of Kansas, Kansas City

Connie J. Canam, MSN, RN
Assistant Professor, School of Nursing, University of British Columbia, Vancouver

Linda W. Cardillo, MA
Doctoral Student, School of Journalism and Communication, Ohio State University, Columbus

Katherine Carlson, BS
Research Assistant, Fairway, KS

Mary T. Champagne, PhD, RN
Dean, School of Nursing, Duke University, Durham, NC

Wenyaw Chan, PhD
Associate Professor, School of Public Health, University of Texas, Houston

Brenda L. Cleary, PhD, RN
Executive Director, North Carolina Center for Nursing, Raleigh

Brenda Cobb, PhD, RN
Postdoctoral Fellow, School of Nursing, Emory University, Atlanta

Cynthia Fryhling Corbett, PhD, RN
Assistant Professor, Intercollegiate Center for Nursing Education, College of Nursing, Washington State University, Spokane

Dorothy Craig, MSc, RN
Professor, Faculty of Nursing, University of Toronto, Ontario, Canada

Linda R. Cronenwett, PhD, RN
Dean, School of Nursing, University of North Carolina at Chapel Hill

Judy Dahl, MSN, RN
Assistant Professor, William Jewell College of Nursing, Liberty, MO

Connie Davis, MN, ARNP
Clinical Research Specialist, The MacColl Institute for Healthcare Innovation, Center for Health Studies, Group Health Cooperative of Puget Sound, Seattle

Pamela Dawson, MN, RN
Director, Collaborative Research Program on Long Term Care, Faculty of Nursing, University of Toronto, Ontario, Canada

Linda K. Dobbs, PhD
Visiting Assistant Professor, Department of Communication, University of Tulsa, OK

Julie Fleury, PhD, RN
Associate Professor, Department of Adult and Geriatric Health, School of Nursing, University of North Carolina at Chapel Hill

Susan Folkman, PhD
Professor, School of Medicine, University of California, San Francisco

Stuart A. Gansky, DrPH
Research Assistant Professor, Department of Dental Public Health and Hygiene, University of California, San Francisco

Barbara B. Germino, PhD, RN
Associate Professor, Department of Adult and Geriatric Health, School of Nursing, University of North Carolina at Chapel Hill

Stephen M. Haas, PhD
Assistant Professor, Department of Communication, Rutgers University, New Brunswick, NJ

Lorna Harris, PhD, RN
Professor and Dean, North Carolina Agricultural and Technical University, Greensboro

Margaret B. Harrison, PhD, RN
Nurse Specialist, Nursing Research and Education, Ottawa Civic Hospital, Ontario, Canada

Martha N. Hill, PhD, RN
Professor, Center for Nursing Research, Johns Hopkins University, Baltimore

Ruthellyn Hinton, MS, MN, RNCS
Professor, Department of Nursing, Pittsburg State University, Pittsburg, KS

Diane Holditch-Davis, PhD, RN
Professor and Chair, Department of Children's Health, School of Nursing, University of North Carolina at Chapel Hill

James D. Hosking, PhD
Research Associate Professor, Department of Biostatistics, School of Public Health, University of North Carolina at Chapel Hill

Laurence Katz, MD
Assistant Professor, Department of Emergency Medicine, School of Medicine, University of North Carolina at Chapel Hill

Elizabeth Kauffmann, MEd, RN
Assistant Professor, School of Nursing, Queen's University, Kingston, Ontario, Canada

Lisa S. Kelley, MSN, RN
Doctoral Candidate, College of Nursing, University of Iowa, Iowa City

Thomas C. Keyserling, MD, MPH
Assistant Professor, Department of Medicine, School of Medicine, University of North Carolina at Chapel Hill

Diane Kjervik, JD, RN
Professor and Associate Dean for Community Outreach and Practice, School of Nursing, University of North Carolina at Chapel Hill

Beth Kramer, MSN, RN
Advanced Practice Nurse, Alvin, TX

Cristina Krasny, BA
Division of Community Health,
North Carolina Department of
Health and Human Services,
Raleigh

Michael J. Lichtenstein, MD, MPH
Professor, School of Medicine, University of Texas Health Science
Center, San Antonio

Patricia Liehr, PhD, RN
Associate Professor, School of Nursing, University of Texas,
Houston

Herbert B. Lindsley, MD
Professor, Department of Rheumatology, School of Medicine, University of Kansas, Kansas City

Adrianne D. Linton, PhD, RN
Associate Professor, Department of
Chronic Nursing Care, School
of Nursing, University of Texas
Health Science Center, San Antonio

Kate Lorig, DrPH, RN
Associate Professor, School of Medicine, Stanford University, Stanford, CA

Jennifer D. Lowe, MSN, RN
Research Assistant, School of Nursing, Queen's University, Kingston, Ontario, Canada

Meridean L. Maas, PhD, RN
Professor and Chair, Department
of Adult and Gerontological
Nursing, College of Nursing,
University of Iowa, Iowa City

Peter A. Margolis, MD, PhD
Associate Professor of Pediatrics
and Epidemiology and Codirector, Children's Primary Care Research Group, School of
Medicine, University of North
Carolina at Chapel Hill

Mary Ann Matteson, PhD, RN
Professor and Interim Chair, Family Nursing Care, School of
Nursing, University of Texas
Health Science Center, San Antonio

Robert G. McMurray, PhD
Professor, Department of Physical
Education, Exercise and Sport
Science, University of North Carolina at Chapel Hill

Janet C. Meininger, PhD, RN
Jamail Distinguished Professor,
Schools of Nursing and Public
Health, University of Texas,
Houston

Merle H. Mishel, PhD, RN
Professor, Department of Adult
and Geriatric Health, School of
Nursing, University of North
Carolina at Chapel Hill

James Mohler, MD
Associate Professor, Department of
Urology, School of Medicine,
University of North Carolina at
Chapel Hill

William H. Mueller, PhD
Professor, School of Public Health,
University of Texas, Houston

Judith L. Neidig, PhD, RN
Assistant Professor, Department of
Internal Medicine, Ohio State
University, Columbus

Geri B. Neuberger, EdD, MN, RN
Professor, School of Nursing, University of Kansas, Kansas City

Barbara D. Powe, PhD, RN
Associate Professor, College of
Nursing, Medical University of
South Carolina, Charleston

Allan N. Press, PhD
Associate Professor, Department of
Social Welfare, University of
Kansas, Lawrence

Dorothy Pringle, PhD, RN
Professor, Faculty of Nursing, Uni-
versity of Toronto, Ontario,
Canada

David Reed, PhD
Statistician, College of Nursing,
University of Iowa, Iowa City

Greg Roberts, PhD
Research Associate, College of Edu-
cation, University of Texas at
Austin

Cary Robertson, MD
Associate Professor, Department of
Urology, School of Medicine,
Duke University, Durham, NC

Jane A. Russell, BSN, RN
Research Nurse, AIDS Clinical Tri-
als Unit, Ohio State University,
Columbus

Judith Schaefer, MPH
Research Associate, The MacColl
Institute for Healthcare Innova-
tion, Center for Health Studies,
Group Health Cooperative of
Puget Sound, Seattle

Debra Schutte, MSN, RN
Doctoral Candidate, College of
Nursing, University of Iowa,
Iowa City

Stephen Scott, MSN, RN, CRN
Instructor, Neosho Community
College, Ottawa, KS

Anne Seraphine, PhD
Assistant Professor, Department of
Educational Psychology, Univer-
sity of Florida, Gainesville

Souraya Sidani, PhD, RN
Assistant Professor, Faculty of Nursing, University of Toronto, Ontario, Canada

Janet P. Specht, PhD, RN
Clinical Associate Professor, De-
partment of Adult and Geronto-
logical Nursing, College of
Nursing, University of Iowa,
Iowa City

Barbara J. Speck, PhD, RN
Assistant Professor, School of Nursing, University of Louisville, KY

Rachel Stevens, EdD, RN
Deputy Director, School of Public
Health, North Carolina Institute
for Public Health School, Uni-
versity of North Carolina at
Chapel Hill

Janet Stewart, MS, RN
Doctoral Student, School of Nursing, University of North Carolina at Chapel Hill

Alexa K. Stuifbergen, PhD, RN
Associate Dean for Research, School of Nursing, University of Texas at Austin

Elizabeth Swanson, PhD, RN
Associate Professor, Department of Adult and Gerontological Nursing, College of Nursing, University of Iowa, Iowa City

Debbie Travers, MSN, RN
Research Assistant Professor, Department of Emergency Medicine, School of Medicine, University of North Carolina at Chapel Hill

Toni Tripp-Reimer, PhD, RN
Professor, Department of Adult and Gerontological Nursing, College of Nursing, and associate dean, Office of Research, University of Iowa, Iowa City

Michael Von Korff, DSc
Investigator, The MacColl Institute for Healthcare Innovation, Center for Health Studies, Group Health Cooperative of Puget Sound, Seattle

Edward H. Wagner, MD, MPH, FACP
Director, The MacColl Institute for Healthcare Innovation, Center for Health Studies, Group Health Cooperative of Puget Sound, Seattle

Sally Weinrich, PhD, RN
Professor, College of Nursing, University of Louisville, KY

JoAnne Weiss, PhD, FNP-CS
Assistant Professor, School of Nursing, University of Central Florida, Orlando

Donna L. Wells, PhD, RN
Associate Professor, Faculty of Nursing, University of Toronto, Ontario, Canada

Charlene A. Winters, DNSc, RN, CS
Assistant Professor, Bozeman College of Nursing, Montana State University, Missoula

Carol Wong, MSN, RN
Professional Leader—Nursing, London Health Sciences Centre, London, Ontario, Canada

Betty H. Worthy, RN, MPH
Administrator of Personal Health Services, Gaston County Health Department, Gastonia, NC

Hany Zayed, MSc
Biostatistician, Family Health International, Research Triangle Park, NC

Acknowledgments

Support for this project was provided in part by a conference grant, "Key Aspects of Preventing and Managing Chronic Illness," from the Agency for Health Care Policy and Research (Grant # R13 HS09839; principal investigators: Sandra G. Funk and Elizabeth M. Tornquist) and by the Center for Research on Preventing and Managing Chronic Illness in Vulnerable People at the School of Nursing at the University of North Carolina at Chapel Hill, which is funded by a grant from the National Institute of Nursing Research at the National Institutes of Health (Grant # P30 NR03962; principal investigators: Joanne S. Harrell and Sandra G. Funk). We are most appreciative of the support provided by both agencies for this project.

We also gratefully acknowledge those who were instrumental in the success of the conference on which this volume is based: Dr. Margaret Miller, director of Continuing Education at the School of Nursing, UNC-CH, and Kathryn Lowe, administrative assistant for the Continuing Education Department; our advisory committee (Jacqueline Dunbar-Jacobs, Peter Margolis, Patricia Moritz, Thomas Sibert, Darlene Trandel-Korenchuk, and June Lunney); and our five cosponsoring nursing research centers at the Universities of California–San Francisco, Iowa, Pennsylvania, Pittsburgh, and Washington.

We are especially grateful to Julia Khanova and Dr. Leah Rutchik for their work in preparing the graphs, tables and text for this volume.

S.G.F.

Part I

PREVENTING AND MANAGING CHRONIC ILLNESS: AN OVERVIEW

[1]

Chronic Illness: Improving Nursing Practice through Research

Sandra G. Funk and Elizabeth M. Tornquist

Over 45% of the American population now have one or more chronic conditions (Hoffman, Rice, & Sung, 1996), and almost 30% of these individuals have sufficient disability to limit their normal daily activities (Aday, 1994; Lambert & Lambert, 1987). With the graying of the population, the prevalence of chronic conditions will continue to increase. Further, it is not only the elderly who suffer from chronic conditions: Thirty-one percent of children under the age of 18 years are estimated to be affected by chronic conditions such as respiratory allergies, repeated ear infections, and asthma; for over a third of these children, the severity of the condition results in limitation of activity (Newacheck & Taylor, 1992).

Patients with chronic illnesses use by far the greatest proportion of health care dollars. Currently, three fourths of health care expenditures are to provide direct care to those who are chronically ill (Hoffman et al., 1996). The rising costs of health care have made it crucial to prevent the development of chronic illnesses and, when prevention is not possible, manage chronic illness more effectively and efficiently. Scientists from nursing and other disciplines have studied the nature of chronic illnesses and successfully tested ways to prevent and more effectively manage them. However, few of these interventions reach the practice community. They often languish in

3

the scientific literature, unread and unused in practice. In part, that is because the research is scattered across disciplines and journals, and articles often lack the specificity needed to guide implementation. Further, there is little examination of issues of applicability and implementation. As one part of a multifaceted approach to moving research into practice, this book assembles the latest nursing research on preventing and managing chronic illness in one volume, presents the research in sufficient detail so clinicians can begin to evaluate its applicability to their settings, and provides a discussion of each study's implications for practice. To lay the foundation for the studies that follow, we present here a brief overview of the state of current knowledge of chronic illness.

The major causes of mortality and morbidity in the United States have shifted from infectious diseases to chronic illnesses, and in the next 25 years this shift will occur worldwide. Heart disease, cancer, arthritis, diabetes, stroke, respiratory illness, neuromuscular disorders, dementia, and AIDS are but a few of the major chronic illnesses facing us today. Virtually all are disproportionately represented among the most vulnerable populations—those who live in poverty, lack access to care, are of minority ethnic status, or are very young or very old (U.S. Department of Health and Human Services [USDHHS], 1991b).

Chronic illnesses are caused by pathological changes in the body that are nonreversible, permanent, or leave residual disability; they may be characterized by periods of recurrence and remission; and they generally require extended periods of supervision, observation, care, and rehabilitation (Kerson & Kerson, 1985). Chronic illnesses have a major impact on all aspects of a person's life—physical, psychological, familial, social, vocational, and economic (Falvo, 1991; Lubkin, 1990). They may result in impaired functioning, limitations in self-care and activities of daily living, loss of independence, pain and discomfort, emotional problems, and self-image changes (Lubkin, 1990; McBride, 1993). Further, because people are surviving longer with some chronic illnesses, they need more health care services (Haan et al., 1997).

Some chronic illnesses are genetic, but others can be shown to be related to personal health behaviors and therefore may be preventable. McGinnis and Foege (1993) present evidence that the most prominent contributors to mortality due to chronic diseases in the United States in 1990 were tobacco use (400,000 deaths), diet and activity patterns (300,000 deaths), and alcohol. Smoking, poor nutrition, and physical inactivity have all been shown to be related to heart disease, cancer, stroke, and pulmonary disease (Eddy, 1986; Fletcher et al., 1992; Leupker et al., 1996; McGinnis & Foege, 1993; National Center for Health Statistics [NCHS], 1993; USDHHS, 1991a, 1991b). Thus, the major causes of morbidity and mortality in society today have a strong behavioral component. Research has clearly demonstrated that lifestyle behaviors are amenable to change through community and individual health promotion and disease prevention interventions (Epstein, Saelens, Myers, & Vito, 1997; Harrell et al., 1996; Jette et al., 1999; Katzel et al., 1995; Miller, Balady, & Fletcher, 1997; Sorensen et al., 1996). For example, in recent decades, dramatic changes have occurred in smoking—the proportion of men who smoke dropped from 52% in 1965 to 26% in 1991 (NCHS, 1997). Patterns of food intake have also changed somewhat, with reductions in the consumption of fatty and high-cholesterol foods and increases in consumption of grains (Subar, Ziegler, Patterson, Ursin, & Graubard, 1994). Despite this improvement in eating habits, however, the prevalence of obesity has increased in both adults (Kuczmarski, Flegal, Campbell, & Johnson, 1994) and children (Troiano, Flegal, Kuczmarski, Campbell, & Johnson, 1995), perhaps because of the primarily sedentary lifestyles of Americans today (Anderson, Crespo, Bartlett, Cheskin, & Pratt, 1998).

Research also shows that many chronic illnesses may be curtailed or successfully managed if found early. Recently, studies of interventions to promote participation in early screening and detection programs have shown increased participation rates in screening for chronic illness and, in turn, increased detection rates (Champion & Huster, 1995; Powe, 1998).

However, even with managed care, which ideally focuses on prevention and early detection to avoid illness, plans vary widely in their use of preventive measures such as smoking cessation programs, beta blocker treatment, breast cancer screening, cervical cancer screening, childhood immunization, diabetic eye exams, and prenatal care in the first trimester. The 1998 report of the National Committee for Quality Assurance (NCQA), based on its Health Plan Employer Data and Information Set (HEDIS), notes that "if all health plans were performing at the level of the best plans, it would have a significant impact on the overall health of America" (NCQA, 1998, p. 12). Clearly, more needs to be done to ensure that health plans (and fee-for-service providers) are helping clients prevent chronic illness and implementing measures known to prevent chronic illness or enable early management.

When chronic illness cannot be prevented, the goal is to manage it successfully—to minimize its impact and progression and maximize normal functioning. Nurses in community settings, home health, long-term care facilities, and hospitals play key roles in caring for the chronically ill—from neonates to the elderly—and in helping these patients and their families maintain their quality of life. In managed care organizations, nurses often are the case managers and first-line providers for those with chronic illnesses. Nurses help patients and their families deal with acute episodes of the illness, ease transitions between hospital and community, and promote functional independence. They also assist patients and families to deal with high-tech home care, manage complex regimens, and live with persistent problems (Funk, Tornquist, Champagne, & Wiese, 1993). Even more importantly, they deal with patients and families over time, through the long and often complicated course of chronic illness.

There is a substantial body of descriptive literature to help nurses understand what it is like to live with a chronic illness (Sexton & Munro, 1988), what the adaptation process is like (Grey, Cameron, Lipman, & Thurber, 1994; Patterson, Thorne, & Dewis, 1998; Shaul, 1995), and how people manage the challenges of caring for themselves (DiIorio, Faherty, & Manteuffel, 1992). The demands of caring for the chronically ill (Bull, 1990), the impact that chronic illness has on the family (Knafl, Breitmayer, Gallo, & Zoeller, 1996; Quittner et al., 1998), and the importance of adequate support (Badger, 1996) have also been well described, as has the quality of life of the chronically ill and their families (Padilla, Ferrell, Grant, & Rhiner, 1990).

This rich descriptive base has guided efforts to develop interventions to improve the management of chronic illness. Research has found several interventions to be successful in enhancing functionality (de Jong, Grevink, Roorda, Kaptein, & van der Schans, 1994; Jensen et al., 1996; Neuberger et al., 1997) and promoting self-care, coping, and symptom management (Boland & Grey, 1997; Burke, Handley-Derry, Costello, Kauffmann, & Dillon, 1997; Mishel et al., 1998). Studies have also documented ways to improve the transition from hospital to home (Brooten et al., 1986) and to adapt the hospital environment for those who are chronically ill (Douglas et al., 1995; Swanson, Maas, & Buckwalter, 1994). Other interventions have successfully enhanced social support (Hansell et al.,1998) and the quality of home care (Archbold et al., 1995; McCorkle et al., 1994).

Studies such as these have provided the foundation for the new research on preventing and managing chronic illness presented in this volume. The studies here are organized into four broad areas that are critical in chronic illness: preventing chronic illness, the illness experience, illness and disease management, and caregiving. We have chosen research on different diseases so that those caring for individuals with one type of illness have ready access to the creative approaches tested with individuals who have other chronic illnesses. In the prevention section, significant attention is given to helping children, adults, and elders increase their levels of physical activity and maintain those levels over time in order to reduce obesity and risks for cardiovascular disease. Strategies to identify individuals at risk for illness and increase participation in screening programs are also highlighted, as are programs for risk reduction.

The studies presented on the illness experience add depth to our understanding of living with a chronic illness. They document what it is like to live with continual uncertainty about one's illness and one's ability to function, to live with secondary symptoms such as fatigue, and to struggle to take care of oneself on a daily basis. They also describe the challenges of enacting advance directives when emergent care is required and, most poignantly, the bewilderment and distress experienced by those for whom new drugs have significantly, and unexpectedly, extended their lives. A conceptual model captures the process of maximizing health in the context of chronic illness, and chronic disease management programs are reviewed. Studies focusing on illness and disease management examine the positive benefits of exercise for those who are chronically ill, strategies to manage symptoms such as dyspnea, cognitive approaches to reduce problem behavior, and ways to enhance self-care.

Since much of chronic illness care is now provided by the family, several studies presented here examine ways to help parents of children with chronic conditions and to help families become more involved in the care of an institutionalized, chronically ill relative. A new intervention also aids caregivers in long-term care to provide better care by focusing on the unique abilities of care recipients.

The book concludes with a discussion of the implications of the new research for practice and policy formation—the changes required at practitioner and organizational levels and the factors that influence the ability to change.

Care of the chronically ill is the task of today and tomorrow. It is nurses who will take the lead in making it a caring future, one in which the ill and disabled and those facing death are not simply "maintained" but are nurtured, supported, and encouraged to live life fully. Nurses must build on the research presented here and further develop and test cost-effective interventions to promote health and prevent illness, assist the chronically ill to maintain or recover function, and thus enhance quality of life. It is equally imperative that those who are responsible for promoting healthy lifestyles and caring for the chronically ill use the results presented here to enhance the effectiveness and efficiency of their care. We must make progress in both prevention and management of chronic illness if we are to meet the goals set forth in *Healthy People 2010* (USDHHS, 2000) and reduce the pervasive impact of chronic illness on our lives and on society.

ACKNOWLEDGMENTS

This work was supported in part by grants from the Agency for Health Care Policy and Research (R13 HS09839) and the National Institute of Nursing Research (P30 NR03962).

REFERENCES

Aday, L. A. (1994). Health status of vulnerable populations. *Annual Review of Public Health, 15,* 487–509.

Anderson, R. E., Crespo, C. J., Bartlett, S. J., Cheskin, L. J., & Pratt, M. (1998). Relationship of physical activity and television watching with body weight and level of fatness among children: Results from the Third National Health and Nutrition Examination Survey. *Journal of the American Medical Association, 279*(12), 938–942.

Archbold, P. G., Stewart, B. J., Miller, L. L., Harvath, T. A., Greenlick, M. R., Van Buren, L., Kirschling, J. M., Valanis, B. G., Brody, K. K., Schook, J. E., & Hagan, J. M. (1995). The PREP system of nursing interventions: A pilot test with families caring for older members . . . preparedness (PR), enrichment (E), and predictability (P). *Research in Nursing & Health, 18,* 3–16.

Badger, T. A. (1996). Family members' experiences living with members with depression. *Western Journal of Nursing Research, 18,* 149–171.

Boland, E. A., & Grey, M. (1996). Coping strategies of school-age children with diabetes mellitus. *Diabetes Educator, 22,* 592–597.

Brooten, D., Kumar, S., Brown, K., Finkler, S., Bakewell-Sachs, S., Gibbons, A., & Delivoria-Papadapoulos, M. (1986). A randomized clinical trial of early discharge and home follow-up of very low birthweight infants. *New England Journal of Medicine, 315,* 934–939.

Bull, M. J. (1990). Factors influencing family caregiver burden and health. *Western Journal of Nursing Research, 12,* 758–770.

Burke, S. O., Handley-Derry, M. H., Costello, E. A., Kauffmann, E., & Dillon, M. C. (1997). Stress-point intervention for parents of repeatedly hospitalized children with chronic conditions. *Research in Nursing & Health, 20,* 475–485.

Champion, V., & Huster, G. (1995). Effect of interventions on stage of mammography adoption. *Journal of Behavioral Medicine, 18,* 169–187.

de Jong, W., Grevink, R. G., Roorda, R. J., Kaptein, A. A., & van der Schans, C. P. (1994). Effect of a home exercise training program in patients with cystic fibrosis. *Chest: The Cardiopulmonary Journal, 104,* 463–468.

DiIorio, C., Faherty, B., & Manteuffel, B. (1992). Self-efficacy and social support in self-management of epilepsy. *Western Journal of Nursing Research, 14,* 292–307.

Douglas, S., Daly, B., Rudy, E., Song, R., Dyer, M. A., & Montenegro, H. (1995). The cost-effectiveness of a special care unit to care for the chronically critically ill. *Journal of Nursing Administration, 25,* 47–53.

Eddy, D. M. (1986). Setting priorities for cancer control programs. *Journal of the National Cancer Institute, 76,* 187–199.

Epstein, L. H., Saelens, B. E., Myers, M. D., & Vito, D. (1997). Effects of decreasing sedentary behaviors on activity choice in obese children. *Health Psychology, 16,* 107–113.

Falvo, D. R. (1991). *Medical and psychosocial aspects of chronic illness and disability.* Gaithersburg, MD: Aspen Publishers.

Fletcher, G. B., Blair, S. N., Blumenthal, J., Caspersen, C., Chaitman, B., Epstein, S., Falls, H., Froelicher, E. S. S., Froelicher, V. F., & Pina, I. L. (1992). Statement on exercise: Benefits and recommendations for physical activity programs for all Americans. *Circulation, 86*(1), 340–344.

Funk, S. G., Tornquist, E. M., Champagne, M. T., & Wiese, R. A. (Eds.). (1993). *Key aspects of chronic illness: Hospital and home.* New York: Springer.

Grey, M., Cameron, M. E., Lipman, T. H., & Thurber, F. W. (1994). Initial adaptations in children with newly diagnosed diabetes and healthy children. *Pediatric Nursing, 20,* 17–22.

Haan, M. N., Selby, J. V., Quesenberry, C. P., Schmittdiel, J. A., Fireman, B. H., & Rice, D. P. (1997). The impact of aging and chronic disease on use of hospital and outpatient services in a large HMO: 1971–1991. *Journal of the American Geriatrics Society, 45,* 667–674.

Hansell, P. S., Hughes, C. B., Caliandro, G., Russo, P., Budin, W. C., Hartman, B., & Hernandez, O. C. (1998). The effect of a social support boosting intervention on stress, coping, and social support in caregivers of children with HIV/AIDS. *Nursing Research, 47,* 79–86.

Harrell, J. S., McMurray, R. G., Bangdiwala, S. I., Frauman, A. C., Gansky, S. A., & Bradley, C. B. (1996). Effects of a school-based intervention to reduce cardiovascular disease risk factors in elementary-school children: The Cardiovascular Health in Children (CHIC) Study. *Journal of Pediatrics, 128,* 797–805.

Hoffmann, C., Rice, D., & Sung, H. (1996). Persons with chronic conditions: Their prevalence and costs. *Journal of the American Medical Association, 276,* 1473–1479.

Jensen, B. E., Fletcher, B. J., Rupp, J. C., Fletcher, G. F., Lee, J. Y., & Oberman, A. (1996). Training level comparison study: Effect of high and low intensity exercise on ventilatory threshold in men with coronary artery disease. *Journal of Cardiopulmonary Rehabilitation, 16,* 227–232.

Jette, A. M., Lachman, M., Giorgetti, M. M., Assmann, S. F., Harris, B. A., Levenson, C., Wernick, M., & Krebs, D. (1999). Exercise—It's never too late: The Strong-for-Life program. *American Journal of Public Health, 89,* 66–72.

Katzel, L. I., Bleecker, E. R., Colman, E. G., Rogus, E. M., Sorkin, J. D., & Goldberg, A. P. (1995). Effects of weight loss vs. aerobic exercise training on risk factors for coronary disease in healthy, obese, middle-aged and older men. *Journal of the American Medical Association, 274,* 1915–1921.

Kerson, T. S., & Kerson, L. A. (1985). *Understanding chronic illness: The medical and psychosocial dimensions of nine diseases.* New York: The Free Press.

Knafl, K. A., Breitmeyer, B., Gallo, A., & Zoeller, L. (1996). Family response to childhood chronic illness: Description of management styles. *Journal of Pediatric Nursing: Nursing Care of Children & Families, 11,* 315–326.

Kuczmarski, R. J., Flegal, K. M., Campbell, S. M., & Johnson, C. L. (1994). Increasing prevalence of overweight among U.S. adults. The National Health and Nutrition Examination Surveys, 1960 to 1991. *Journal of the American Medical Association, 272*(3), 205–211.

Lambert, V. A., & Lambert, C. E., Jr. (1987). Psychosocial impacts created by chronic illness. *Nursing Clinics of North America, 22,* 527–533.

Lubkin, I. M. (1990). *Chronic illness: Impact and interventions* (2nd ed.). Boston: Jones & Bartlett.

Luepker, R. V., Perry, C. L., McKinlay, S. M., Nader, P. R., Parcel, G. S., Stone, E. J., Webber, L. S., Elder, J. P., Feldman, H. A., Johnson, C. C., Kelder, S. H., Wu, M., for the CATCH Collaborative Group. (1996). Outcomes of a field trial to improve children's dietary patterns and physical activity: The Child and Adolescent Trial for Cardiovascular Health (CATCH). *Journal of the American Medical Association, 275,* 768–776.

McBride, A. B. (1993). Managing chronicity: The heart of nursing care. In S. G. Funk, E. M. Tornquist, M. T. Champagne, & R. A. Wiese (Eds.), *Key aspects of caring for the chronically ill* (pp. 8–20). New York: Springer.

McCorkle, R., Jepson, C., Malone, D., Lusk, E., Braitman, L., Buhler-Wilkerson, K., & Daly, J. (1994). The impact of posthospital home care on patients with cancer. *Research in Nursing & Health, 17,* 243–251.

McGinnis, J. M., & Foege, W. H. (1993). Actual causes of death in the United States. *Journal of the American Medical Association, 270*(18), 2207–2212.

Miller, T. D., Balady, G. J., & Fletcher, G. F. (1997). Exercise and its role in the prevention and rehabilitation of cardiovascular disease. *Annals of Behavioral Medicine, 19,* 220–229.

Mishel, M., Germino, B., Harris, L., Belyea, M., Mohler, J., & Robinson, C. (1998, April). *Effectiveness of the managing uncertainty intervention in stage B prostate cancer.* Paper presented at the Family Caregiver Education Program, School of Medicine, Pennsylvania State University, Hershey.

National Center for Health Statistics (NCHS). (1993). *Health United States 1992 and Healthy People 2000 Review.* Hyattsville, MD: Public Health Service.

National Committee for Quality Assurance (NCQA). (1998). *The state of managed care quality.* Available: http://www.ncqa.org/news/report.htm.

Neuberger, G. G., Press, A. N., Lindsley, H. B., Hinton, R., Cagle, P. E., Carlson, K., Scott, S., Dahl, J., & Kramer, B. (1997). Effects of exercise on fatigue, aerobic fitness, and disease activity measures in persons with rheumatoid arthritis. *Research in Nursing & Health, 20,* 195–204.

Newacheck, P. W., & Taylor, W. R. (1992). Childhood chronic illness: Prevalence, severity, and impact. *American Journal of Public Health, 82,* 364–371.

Padilla, G. V., Ferrell, B., Grant, M. M., & Rhiner, M. (1990). Defining the content domain of quality of life for cancer patients with pain. *Cancer Nursing, 13,* 108–115.

Patterson, B. L., Thorne, S., & Dewis, M. (1998). Adapting to and managing diabetes. *Image, 30,* 57–62.

Powe, B. (1998). An intervention to decrease cancer fatalism among African American elders. *Oncology Nursing Forum.*

Quittner, A. L., Espelage, D. L., Opipari, L. C., Carter, B., Eid, N., & Eigen, H. (1998). Role strain in couples with and without a child with a chronic illness: Associations with marital satisfaction, intimacy, and daily mood. *Health Psychology, 17,* 112–124.

Sexton, D. L., & Monro, B. H. (1988). Living with a chronic illness: The experience of women with chronic obstructive pulmonary disease (COPD). *Western Journal of Nursing Research, 10,* 26–44.

Shaul, M. P. (1995). From early twinges to mastery: The process of adjustment in living with rheumatoid arthritis. *Arthritis Care & Research, 8,* 290–297.

Sorensen, G., Thompson, G., Glanz, K., Feng, Z., Kinne, S., DiClemente, C., Emmons, K., Heimendinger, J., Probart, C., & Luchtenstein, E. (1996). Work site-based cancer prevention: Primary results from the Working Well Trial. *American Journal of Public Health, 86*, 939–947.

Subar, A. F., Ziegler, R. G., Patterson, B. H., Ursin, G., & Graubard, B. (1994). U.S. dietary patterns associated with fat intake: The 1987 National Health Interview Survey. *American Journal of Public Health, 84*(3), 359–366.

Swanson, E. A., Maas, M. L., & Buckwalter, K. C. (1994). Alzheimer's residents' cognitive and functional measures: Special and traditional care unit comparison. *Clinical Nursing Research, 3*, 27–41.

Tornquist, E. M., & Funk, S. G. (1993). How to report research with clarity, coherence and grace. *Journal of Emergency Nursing, 19*, 498–502.

Troiano, R. P., Flegal, K. M., Kuczmarski, R. J., Campbell, S. M., & Johnson, C. L. (1995). Overweight prevalence and trends for children and adolescents: The National Health and Nutrition Examination Surveys, 1963 to 1991. *Archives of Pediatrics and Adolescent Medicine, 149*(10), 1085–1091.

U.S. Department of Health and Human Services (USDHHS). (1991a). *Health status of minorities and low-income groups* (3rd ed.). Washington, DC: Government Printing Office.

U.S. Department of Health and Human Services (USDHHS). (2000). *Healthy people 2010*. Washington, DC: ODPHP.

[2]

Closing the Gap Between Information and Action

Martha N. Hill

Tremendous advances in biology are providing new knowledge about genetics, physiology, pathophysiology, and disease, creating exciting opportunities for clinical research. From the laboratory this research evolves into new applications for diagnosis, therapy, and prevention in humans. At the same time, important advances in behavioral science, clinical outcomes, and health care delivery have provided needed knowledge about prevention and treatment. However, there is a gap between the efficacy of interventions in studies and their effectiveness in practice, a gap between potential and reality, intention and action, and information and behavior. This chapter addresses the need to integrate the social and behavioral sciences with the biologic sciences to effectively prevent and manage chronic illness, and notes the importance of cross-disciplinary work. Both strategies will be essential if we are to close the gap between what we know works and what is actually happening in practice.

To prevent and manage chronic illness, the challenge now is to incorporate the sciences beyond biology in order to address the important role that environment and behavior play in illness. Let me illustrate, using heart disease as an example. Lifestyle constitutes about 54% of the estimated contribution of various factors to heart disease. The influence of the environment is 9%, health care services is about 12%, and biology is about 25% (Centers for Disease Control and Prevention, 1980). These statistics are a little deceptive because the factors are not mutually exclusive; rather, there are interactions among them. We need to understand those interactions and the complexity of the factors that influence the development of disease as well as the factors that influence prevention and treatment. If we are going to reduce death and disability due to heart disease and stroke, we need to understand the biologic mechanisms of disease, but we also need to understand the social and behavioral aspects of illness. We need to understand the behaviors of patients, providers, and systems. Only by studying behaviors will we be able to bridge the gap between what we know works, that is, which interventions are shown by research to be effective, and what actually happens in practice. Traditionally, medical research has been laboratory based. When medical researchers talk about translational research, they mean translating findings from bench to bedside, and the bedside they are talking about is in the clinical research center or the coronary care unit. When I speak of going from bench to bedside, I mean going not only from the basic science laboratory to the bedside in the hospital research unit, but also from the hospital bed to the ambulatory care setting, and to the beds in people's homes in the community. We need to recognize that when we do research, we are only establishing the potential to make things better. The real challenge is to translate the potential into reality, to move from intention to action. To do this, we need to move from information to behavior.

Let me offer some examples to illustrate the gap that currently exists between information and behavior. Over the past three decades the National Health and Nutrition Examination Surveys (NHANES) have found an impressive increase in the awareness, treatment, and control of hypertension (Burt et al., 1995). However, even with this increase, the control rate for hypertension is only 27.4%. A 27% control rate for hypertension in the United States is shockingly low. We had nurse-run clinics in Philadelphia in the 1970s with an 80% control rate, including justifiable exceptions (Hill & Reichgott, 1979; Reichgott, Pearson, & Hill, 1983). Something is very wrong when, despite all the research that has been done on the very clear benefit of controlling blood pressure to prevent strokes and heart failure, we have only a 27% control rate.

Another example is the baseline data from the Heart and Estrogen-Progestin Replacement Study (HERS) (Schroft, Bittner, Vittinghoff, Herrington, & Hully, 1997). Between 1993 and 1994, that study recruited elderly women with established coronary artery disease and evaluated their lipids and lipoproteins, their use of lipid-lowering medications, and the frequency with which they achieved national adult treatment panel (ATP) guideline goals for cholesterol levels. About 37% of the women met the ATP 1 goal of a low-density lipoprotein cholesterol (LDLC) less than 130, but only 9%

met the ATP 2 goal of LDLC less than 100. Further, 63% of the women whose cholesterol levels were at the ATP 1 goal were on medication. Only a third of those whose levels were over 220 were on medication. The point here is that we know from multiple studies that medication will lower lipid levels and that lowering lipid levels will reduce coronary artery disease and save lives. So why is it that so few women with established disease were being effectively treated?

Here is a third example. The most prevalent cause of stroke is hypertension. Atrial fibrillation is the second most prevalent cause, and it is the most common arrhythmia associated with adverse prognosis. About 2.2 million Americans have sustained or intermittent atrial fibrillation. In a recent study, a group of investigators did retrospective chart reviews of physician practices regarding anticoagulation before cardioversion (Schlict, Davis, Naqi, Cooper, & Rao, 1996). They found that doctors did not follow national consensus guidelines for about 35% of their cases. Another group of investigators reviewed hospital charts of Medicare patients age 65 or older with a history of atrial fibrillation before admission. Only 38% (117/304) had been prescribed warfarin. Of those not prescribed warfarin, 63% (117/187) were also not taking aspirin (Brass, Krumholz, Scinto, Mathur, & Radford, 1998). This underutilization rate was confirmed in a subsequent study of adherence to practice guidelines in a population-based cohort of elderly persons age 70 years or older with atrial fibrillation (White et al., 1999). These are but a few examples; anywhere you look in the literature, on almost any condition, you find evidence that providers are not implementing recommended guidelines and patients are not making recommended behavioral changes.

One reason for the gap between research and practice is that the bulk of the funding spent on biomedical research has been spent on basic research. Far less money has been spent on major treatment trials in populations that represent more of what we might call "free-range" people. Because they are testing whether or not a treatment will work, clinical trials have to have highly selected, very homogeneous populations in order to control for confounding factors. Once those studies are done, that is often the end of the research. The National Institutes of Health and other organizations spend very little money on application or demonstration research. This is the missing piece in the funding continuum that has kept us from having a greater understanding of what it will take to generalize the findings from those beautifully done controlled trials to real people in the real world.

A second reason for the gap between what we know and what happens in practice is our overproduction of guidelines. There are now over 3,000 sets of guidelines for the average American family practitioner. How could you possibly keep up and know what it is you are supposed to be doing?

In my view, the government and many other agencies believe they have done their job if they have gotten a task force together to write some guidelines. What is not attached to the writing of those guidelines is practical, real-world techniques and strategies for implementing them. Nor are funds put into health services research to study what it takes at system, provider, and patient levels to implement guidelines. We need to pay attention to closing this gap between what we know works and what is actually happening, because there is a global epidemic in cardiovascular diseases and stroke, as well as in other chronic illnesses.

To help close this gap, we need to recognize the broad continuum of science. We need to extend the science agenda beyond the laboratory and the clinical research center, taking advantage of the current interest in research done in ambulatory care settings and communities. The pressure to cut costs and improve outcomes is actually creating a gold mine of opportunities for the social and the behavioral sciences. Our colleagues in medicine now realize they will not be able to achieve the outcomes they are going to be held accountable for without collaborating with other disciplines. This calls for recognizing the broad continuum of influences that determine whether or not effective treatments are actually adopted by providers, by patients and families, and by the public. We need to be able to make changes at the level of an individual's trip to the grocery store, for example. Change at this level requires that we incorporate the sciences of cognitive processing, decision making, and reasoning—the sciences that go into having the vision and the ability to read food labels, make healthy food choices, and prepare a meal. Likewise, exercise physiology is one component of the exercise sciences, but exercise psychology is another. Measuring what happens when people are moving is quite interesting in terms of energy expenditure, but getting people up and moving is the real challenge.

We are not going to successfully prevent chronic illness if we do not look at the full continuum of sciences from the laboratory sciences to the clinical and community sciences. It is not enough to do research and publish statements about what people need to do; we also need to look at whether people are aware of those statements or those research findings and whether they lead to behavior change. It is critical to increase people's awareness, knowledge, motivation, and skills related to behavior change.

We must also reexamine the issue of compliance and stop blaming patients for the poor outcomes that occur. People cannot take prescription medications that are not prescribed. We need to look at compliance as a multilevel issue. We have known for over 35 years that preappointment reminders can double appointment keeping by patients with hypertension (Finnerty, Shaw, & Himmelsbach, 1973). My cat gets a preappointment reminder to come in for her feline leukemia shot. Even my Volvo gets a preappointment reminder. Yet I do not get one from any health care provider, except the dentist. Preappointment letters are an inexpensive intervention for health care organizations to implement. The return on that expenditure would be seen in patients' increased use of scheduled services and a reduction in the waste associated with no-shows. Another effective strategy involves developing individuals' health promotion skills. The demand for self-help materials can be seen in every bookstore, where one of the fastest growing sections is the health psychology, self-care section. The Internet is ablaze with people who are looking for and wanting to share information. People are looking for skills. They know they need to do things differently, to stop doing some things and to do other things better. We need to educate professionals about how to help patients, in a succinct and timely manner.

My own program of research illustrates the themes that I have been laying out. The research team is cross-disciplinary and includes colleagues from the school of nursing, the school of medicine, and the school of public health. The investigator team also includes various levels of seniority and experience, incorporating postdoctorates, new investigators, and established scientists. We also have graduate students, undergraduates, and high school students working with us on various aspects of the project. The study is a partnership between Johns Hopkins Medical Institutions, which include the hospital and the Schools of Hygiene and Public Health, Nursing, and Medicine, and the East Baltimore community. East Baltimore is a community in transition. The community is experiencing a decline in population and increases in crime, substance abuse, abandoned housing, and poverty. The community is also suffering a shocking and saddening decline in the quality of the public schools and a decline in social services.

We are conducting a clinical trial of a cross-disciplinary intervention with young, urban African-American men with hypertension. African Americans, particularly men, in low socioeconomic urban settings suffer earliest from severe complications of hypertension: they have disproportionately high rates of both end-stage renal disease and stroke. These men typically achieve poor control of their blood pressure, and they have very low rates of continuing care for their high blood pressure. Yet they are vastly understudied. Historically, the majority of participants in studies were recruited from clinic populations. They therefore were predominantly women, because women had higher rates of participating in continuing care than did men. As one of the young men in the study said to me, "I don't do doctors." You cannot sit in the clinic waiting for people to come to you. You have to go and find the people where they are. If we do not pair advanced practice clinic-based nursing with community outreach, we will only be taking care of the people who come to us; we will not be taking care of many of the people who need us.

The purpose of our study is to demonstrate sustained lowering of blood pressure over time and the effect of this lowered blood pressure on biologic outcomes. We also plan to conduct ancillary studies of the economic impact of the intervention. We know from the biomedical sciences and from the social sciences that numerous genetic, social, psychological, and behavioral factors are associated with uncontrolled blood pressure. Our conceptual framework is based on the model of health promotion and planning developed by Green and Kreuter (1991). This framework incorporates (1) predisposing factors, such as knowledge, attitudes, and beliefs; (2) enabling factors, such as whether one has a doctor, health insurance, and skills; and (3) reinforcing factors, such as social support. We are interested, first of all, in getting the men to take their antihypertensive medication. Then we look at modifying lifestyle, specifically the need to deal with substance abuse, which is a huge, prevalent confounder. Our primary hypothesis is that the more intensive intervention group will have significantly lower mean blood pressure and greater probability of blood pressure control than the less intensive intervention group, and they will have higher rates of continuing care, taking medication, and decreasing substance abuse. The secondary hypotheses are that compared to the less intensive group, the more intensive intervention group will have significantly less left ventricular mass and central vascular stiffness, and a lower albumin-creatinine ratio than the less intensive intervention group. We also hypothesize that they will have less left ventricular dysfunction, and they will have lower costs of care due to fewer major hypertensive complications involving emergency room visits and admissions, new starts on dialysis, and stroke.

Three hundred nine men have been enrolled in the study and their physical and psychosocial characteristics, including barriers to hypertension care and control, assessed (Hill et al., 1999). The subjects are young, with an average age of 41. They have an average of 11 years of education. About 40% are unemployed, and about 32% are disabled, mostly due to substance abuse; 64% have jail experience. More than 70% have incomes less than $10,000 a year, and half have no health insurance. Their alcoholism risk by CAGE score is about 62%. The percentage with a positive screen for illicit drugs on urine tests is 46%. Current cigarette smoking is extremely high, and half of the men report that they eat salty food all or most of the time. In terms of end organ damage, 20% of them have full-blown left ventricular hypertrophy (LVH), and 42% of them have microalbuminuria. This is a vulnerable high-risk group that already has target organ damage.

In an initial pilot study we randomized the men to a minimal intervention from a nurse-supervised community health worker who called them and went to their house. This study showed that we could find the men, we could recruit them, we could track them, and they would agree to be randomized. However, though the pilot was successful in demonstrating feasibility, the minimal intervention was not enough to cause significant improvement in subjects' control of their blood pressure (Hill et al., 1999). We then did a pilot study in which we randomly selected 18 men to be followed for 12 weeks by a nurse practitioner. The second pilot achieved 64% blood pressure control among men seen by the nurse practitioner and 0% among men referred to usual care in the community.

In the ongoing study we have randomized subjects to a less or a more intensive intervention. All the men come in annually for a visit, and trained observers who do not know group assignment obtain lab samples, measure blood pressure, and collect other information and measurements. The more intensive intervention is individualized nursing care from a nurse practitioner partnered with a community health worker and a cardiologist. The community health worker makes home visits, not to the study subjects but to the person to whom the men turn for help with health matters. The health workers all come from inner-city Baltimore. Our thinking here is based on literature that shows the value of helping the helper to be a helper. Helpers need help in navigating the fine line between being a helper and being a nag. We do telephone follow-up and also log in the calls the men make to us. We accept collect calls because the men call us if they are jailed or when they have no money. This rapport, this open dialogue and availability, has turned out to be very important. We provide transportation money to a maximum of $3 per visit if needed. Finally, we make referrals as necessary, primarily to social services.

Our unadjusted follow-up rates for the study are over 84% 2 years after enrollment. If we account for subjects whose whereabouts and reasons for not coming are known and who are not available to attend the annual evaluation visit by subtracting them from the denominator, our follow-up rates are about 95%. Subjects who are not available include those who are deceased, are incarcerated or in a nursing home, or have moved out of state.

The results of the study to date are very promising. On the first preliminary analysis at 12 months of follow-up, blood pressures had decreased by clinically important and statistically significant amounts from baseline levels in the more intensive group.

This is an innovative model of integrated cross-disciplinary research, which brings the behavioral and bio-behavioral sciences together and reaches out to bring in the community. A major aspect of preventing and managing chronic illness is recognizing the importance of partnerships. Today, as nurses, we are partnering not only with other health care providers, but also with patients and their families. More and more we are going to partner with community organizations and agencies. None of us can do this alone, and the burden and the scope of chronic illness are only going to increase. In our study we work with the American Heart Association, the Baltimore City Jail, the Broadway Center for Substance Abuse, and Clergy United for East Baltimore. We work with Bridges to Work because the greatest need the men have is jobs. We ask the men, "When you lie awake at night, what do you worry about?" Their number one answer is getting or keeping a job. Their number two answer is their children, and the number three answer is the rest of their family or themselves. In addition to partnering with community and nonprofit organizations, we have corporate partners. Merck & Co. has given us free medication, which I was pleased to accept because the medication is very well tolerated and has an extremely low rate of side effects. W. A. Baum and Co. gave us the sphygmomanometers and the blood pressure cuffs. Partnering with health workers from the community is also central to our success.

As we move forward in our efforts to prevent and manage chronic illness, we need to think about looking at the sciences within the context of the broader picture. Nurses are recognized as being very good collaborators and very collegial. We have opportunities to reach out and extend invitations to others to participate in our work, and to enrich our work by integrating in it people who represent other sciences. We also have our students, our staffs, and our clinical colleagues. For those nurses who work in clinical settings, it is helpful to think of researchers as an ancillary army, as people who have both knowledge and interest, with whom clinical problems and information can be shared so that the researchers address the questions that are clinically most relevant. Finally, partnerships with our patients, with their families, and with the community will be essential if we are to successfully prevent and manage chronic illness.

REFERENCES

Brass, L. M., Krumholz, H. M., Scinto, J. D., Mathur, D., & Radford, M. (1998). Warfarin use following ischemic stroke among Medicare patients with atrial fibrillation. *Archives of Internal Medicine, 158,* 2093–2100.

Burt, V. L., Cutler, J. A., Higgins, M., Horan, M., Labarthe, D., Whelton, P., Brown, C., & Roccella, E. (1995). Trends in the prevalence, awareness, treatment, and control of hypertension in the adult U.S. population: Data from the Health Examination Surveys, 1960–1991. *Hypertension, 26,* 60–69.

Centers for Disease Control and Prevention. (1980). Health analysis and planning for preventive services. In *Ten leading causes of death in the United States, 1977.* Atlanta: U.S. Department of Health and Human Services, Health Analysis and Planning for Preventive Services.

Finnerty, F. A., Jr., Shaw, L. W., & Himmelsbach, C. K. (1973). Hypertension in the inner city: II. Detection and follow-up. *Circulation, 47,* 76–78.

Green, L. W., & Kreuter, M. W. (1991). *Health promotion planning: An educational and environmental approach* (2nd ed.). Mountain View, CA: Mayfield.

Hill, M. N., Bone, L. R., Kim, M. K., Miller, D. J., Dennison, C. R., & Levine, D. M. (1999). Barriers to hypertension care and control in young urban black men. *American Journal of Hypertension, 12*(10 Pt. 1), 951–958.

Hill, M. N., Bone, L. R., Roary, M. C., Hilton, S. C., Kelen, G., & Levine, D. M. (1999). A clinical trial to improve HBP care in young urban African American men. *American Journal of Hypertension, 12,* 548–554.

Hill, M. N., & Reichgott, M. J. (1979). Achievement of standards for quality care of hypertension by physicians and nurses. *Clinical and Experimental Hypertension, 1,* 665–684.

Reichgott, M. J., Pearson, S., & Hill, M. N. (1983). The nurse practitioner's role in complex patient management: Hypertension. *Journal of the National Medical Association, 75,* 1197–1204.

Schlicht, J. R., Davis, R. C., Naqi, K., Cooper, W., & Rao, B. V. (1996). Physician practices regarding anticoagulation and cardioversion of atrial fibrillation. *Archives of Internal Medicine, 156,* 290–294.

Schroft, H. G., Bittner, V., Vittinghoff, E., Herrington, D. M., & Hully, S., for the HERS Research Group. (1997). Adherence to National Cholesterol Education Program treatment goals in postmenopausal women with heart disease. *Journal of the American Medical Association, 277,* 1281–1286.

White, R. H., McBurnie, M. A., Manolio, T., Furberg, C. D., Gardin, J. M., Kittner, S. J., Bovill, E., & Knepper, L. (1999). Oral anticoagulation in patients with atrial fibrillation: Adherence with guidelines in an elderly cohort. *American Journal of Medicine, 106,* 165–171.

[3]

Promoting Healthier Behaviors

Joanne S. Harrell and Jennifer Leeman

Healthy People 2000 distinguishes three categories of "prevention": disease prevention, health protection, and health promotion (U.S. Department of Health and Human Services, USDHHS, 1991). Disease prevention strategies include counseling, screening, and immunization. Health protection strategies address environmental or regulatory measures that protect health at the population level. Related issues include unintentional injury, occupational safety, environmental health, and food and drug safety. *Healthy People 2000's* third category, health promotion strategies, is the focus of this chapter. Health promotion strategies are "those related to individual lifestyle—personal choices made in a social context—that can have a powerful influence over one's health prospects" (USDHHS, 1991, p. 6). Clinicians encounter tremendous challenges in their efforts to promote healthy behaviors. Researchers and clinicians know what behaviors will lower the risk of chronic illness; what we need to learn is how to motivate people to engage in those healthier behaviors. In the words of Martha Hill, "What happens when people are moving is quite interesting in terms of energy expenditure, but getting people up and moving is the real challenge" (chapter 2, p. 15).

This chapter reviews the state of our knowledge on promoting healthier behaviors. The chapter focuses on *Healthy People 2000's* top three priority areas for health promotion: physical activity and fitness, nutrition, and tobacco use (USDHHS, 1991). For each priority area, the evidence establishing the prevalence of the problem behavior and its relationship to chronic illness is briefly reviewed. Then successes and challenges in the research on interventions to promote healthier behaviors are outlined. Finally, the chapter provides an overview of possible future directions for clinical practice.

PHYSICAL INACTIVITY, FOOD INTAKE, AND OBESITY

Recent national studies have found that a large percentage of Americans do not engage in any leisure-time physical activity. In the 1994 Behavioral Risk Factor Survey System (BRFSS), a third of Americans reported no leisure-time physical activity (Centers for Disease Control and Prevention, 1997), while in the third National Health and Nutrition Evaluation Survey (NHANES III), 22% reported no leisure-time physical activity (Crespo, Keteyian, Heath, & Sempos, 1996). In both of these studies the least active groups were women, older people, Hispanics, African Americans, those living in southern states, and those who were overweight. Although exercise or physical activity can help prevent cardiovascular disease (CVD), inactivity is still widespread. Several studies have shown that inactivity begins in childhood. Many children are not active, and their activity levels decrease as they pass through adolescence (Aarts, Paulssen, & Schaalma, 1997; Gavarry et al., 1998; Goran, Gower, Nagy, & Johnson, 1998; Miller, Balady, & Fletcher, 1997; Sallis, 1993). That is to say, physical inactivity tracks over time, so that inactive children are very likely to become inactive adults.

Both physical inactivity and diet contribute to obesity, a health problem that has reached epidemic proportions in the United States (Kuczmarski, Flegal, Campbell, & Johnson, 1994; Troiano, Flegal, Kuczmarski, Campbell, & Johnson, 1995). Increased total body fat, increased amount of visceral fat, and increased weight gain are all associated with increased risk of death (Solomon & Manson, 1997). In the United States more than 50% of all-cause mortality of adults ages 20 to 74 can be attributed to overweight (Bray, 1997). Americans have been following the public health recommendations to reduce fat intake, as shown by the results of the NHANES III study (Heini & Weinsier, 1997). Unfortunately, the study shows that while the percent of fat in the diet has decreased, the prevalence of obesity has increased.

The percentage of children, adolescents, and adults in the United States who are overweight or obese continues to increase. The proportion of overweight youth ages 12 to 17 increased from 15.2% at NHANES II in the 1970s to 22.3% at NHANES III in the 1990s (Troiano & Flegal, 1998; Troiano et al., 1995). In one longitudinal study of youth, the prevalence of overweight doubled between 1973 and 1994 (Freedman, Srinivasan, Valdez, Williamson, & Berenson, 1997). As with physical activity, obesity tends to track from childhood into adulthood. Adolescent obesity has been shown to be associated with being overweight as an adult and is associated with increased long-term morbidity and mortality (Harlan, 1993; Must, Jacques, Dallal, Bajema, & Dietz, 1992; Srinivasan, Bao, Wattigney, & Berenson, 1996).

Obesity can lead to premature death through many pathways. Obesity and weight gain have been shown to increase the risk of hypertension, hypercholesterolemia, coronary heart disease (CHD), and non-insulin-dependent diabetes (Colditz, Willett, Rotnitsky, & Manson, 1995; Manson, Colditz, & Stampfer, 1990; Van Itallie, 1985). In the U.S. Nurses' Health Study, the risk for CHD was 3.3 times greater in those with a body mass index (BMI) greater than 29 kg/m² than in those with a BMI less than 21 kg/m² (Manson et al., 1995). In addition, weight gain after the age of 18 increases the risk of CHD in middle-aged women (Willett et al., 1995). Van Itallie (1985) has estimated that 19% of the 406,923 deaths caused by coronary heart disease and 62% of the 55,110 deaths caused by diabetes may be attributable to obesity. Even more frightening, the increase in obesity in youth has increased the incidence of type 2 diabetes in children: More than a third of children ages 12 to 18 who developed diabetes in 1994 had type 2 diabetes (Glaser, 1997; Pinhas-Hamiel et al., 1996).

Obesity has also been shown to be associated with certain types of cancer. Obese men have an increased risk for neoplasms of the rectum, colon, and prostate, while obese women are at increased risk for cancer of the gallbladder and cancers of the reproductive system, including breast cancer (Huang et al., 1997). The musculoskeletal system is also markedly affected by obesity. Osteoarthritis, which is common in the obese, may be directly related to the trauma associated with excess body weight, especially when the knees and ankles are involved. However, the obese also have increased osteoarthritis in non-weight-bearing joints, particularly the fingers, which suggests that there may be other aspects of the obesity syndrome, independent of weight bearing, that alter cartilage and bone metabolism (Bollet, 1992; Bray, 1997).

In order to be beneficial, physical activity does not need to be vigorous aerobic exercise, as was once recommended (Anderson et al., 1999). Although this type of exercise is probably necessary to improve physical fitness (i.e., reduce weight and improve muscular endurance and aerobic power), a vigorous program is not necessary to produce considerable health benefits. The current public health recommendation for physical activity is that all adults and children accumulate at least 30 minutes of moderately vigorous physical activity at least 5 days a week, preferably every day. Numerous studies have pointed to the value of moderate-intensity physical activity for improving health (Dunn et al., 1998; Pate et al., 1995). Dunn and colleagues (1999) conducted a randomized trial in which subjects were assigned to two interventions: a traditional, structured exercise program or a lifestyle activity intervention designed to increase moderate physical activity. After 24 months, the lifestyle and structured exercise interventions produced comparable improvements in physical activity, cardiorespiratory fitness, blood pressure, and percent body fat. A Mayo clinic study (Levine, Eberhardt, & Jensen, 1999) found that total activity was more important than the length of exercise sessions. For example, "fidgeters" (those who squirm in chairs, swing legs, tap fingers, pace the floor, etc.) lost more weight than nonfidgeters.

We have tended to focus our attention on encouraging physical fitness among the younger and healthier segments of the population. However, there is increasing evidence that regular exercise and physical activity can improve functional capacity and quality of life at all stages of life (Mazzeo et al., 1998). In the Strong-for-Life Program, Jette and colleagues (1999) randomly assigned 215 older persons to either a home-based resistance exercise training group or a wait list control group. Intervention subjects were taught movement patterns associated with functional activities. They were expected to do the program three times a week in their homes. Subjects receiving the intervention improved in lower extremity strength and movement, in shoulder abduction and elbow extension, and in tandem gait. In addition, they had a significantly greater reduction in overall disability than the controls.

Diet habits have been implicated in the etiology of cancer of the colon, stomach, pancreas, and breast (Giovannucci, Stampfer, Colditz, Rimm, & Willett, 1992; Steinmetz, Kushi, Bostick, Folsom, & Potter, 1994). There is controversy over the specific role of diet in these cancers, but certainly a healthy diet may help reduce the risk of cancer. Cancer prevalence is lower in countries where fat is low in the usual diet and complex carbohydrates provide most of the calories. In addition, the fiber from vegetables, especially green vegetables, and from fruits and grains has been shown to protect against heart disease and cancer (Stefanick et al., 1998; Willet, 1994; Zhang et al., 1999). The DASH (Dietary Approaches to Stop Hypertension) study showed that a diet low in saturated fat and rich in fruits, vegetables, and low-fat dairy food can lower blood pressure substantially (Appel et al., 1997). Although there is acceptance of the importance of diet, interventions to permanently change the diet have not been very successful (Fitzgibbon, Stolley, Avellone, Sugerman, & Chavez, 1996).

TOBACCO USE

Over the past several years we have seen increases in tobacco use, which had been steadily decreasing since the 1960s. In 1997, 24.7% of U.S. adults, about 48 million people, were current smokers. Slightly more men (27.4%) than women (23.3%) were smokers. Smoking prevalence was highest among people with 9 to 11 years of education (35.4%) and lowest in those with at least 16 years of education (11.6%). Further, smoking was most common (33.3%) in those living below the poverty level (Office on Smoking and Health, 1999). Smoking among U.S. high school students has increased markedly, from 27.5% in 1991 to 36.4% in 1997 (USDHHS, 1998). Also, the age of initiation of smoking is younger than many realize. In a study following children from third through eighth grade, we found a mean age of initiation of 12.3 years (Harrell, Bangdiwala, Deng, Webb, & Bradley, 1998). According to the U.S. Surgeon General, among adults who have ever tried smoking a cigarette, 88% did so by the age of 18 and 71% of daily smokers were daily smokers before they were 18 years old (Centers for Disease Control and Prevention, 1994).

In 1990 tobacco use accounted for 400,000 deaths in the United States (McGinnis & Foege, 1993), including deaths from cancer (9 types), cardiovascular disease (coronary artery disease [CAD], stroke, peripheral arterial disease, hypertension), lung diseases (chronic obstructive pulmonary disease [COPD], chronic bronchitis, pneumonia), low birth weight and other problems of infancy, and burns. In addition, smoking alters the effects of some medications (USDHHS, 1989). Because of these profound health effects, it is critically important to prevent initiation of smoking and encourage smoking cessation. Unfortunately, many of the interventions tried to date have had little or no impact on smoking cessation.

THE RESEARCH ON INTERVENTIONS TO PROMOTE HEALTHIER BEHAVIORS

While the research clearly supports the importance of physical activity, a healthy diet, and avoidance of tobacco, interventions to promote behavior change have had mixed results. While some have had success over the short term, few have demonstrated enduring changes in behavior. Further, few have been effective in achieving changes at the physiologic level.

For example, one large study found that a low-intensity nutrition intervention delivered by physicians increased fiber and reduced fat consumption somewhat; however, there was no change in BMI (Beresford et al., 1997). In a trial of dietary advice for patients with hypertension or a family history of premature CVD, nurses provided intervention group subjects with health education every 2 months (Bakx, Stafleu, van Staveren, van den Hoogen, & van Weel, 1997). Although there was a significant decrease in blood pressure and serum cholesterol after 1 year, long-term follow-up showed that these benefits were not sustained. In a study of overweight subjects who had parents who were diabetic, subjects ($n = 154$) were randomly assigned to diet (decreasing calories and percent of calories from fat), exercise, diet plus exercise, or a control group (Wing, Venditti, Jakicic, Polley, & Lang, 1998). All treatment groups met weekly for the first 6 months, then biweekly for 6 months, with two 6-week refresher courses during year 2. After 6 months, subjects in the combined group showed greater weight loss than those in the other two groups, and these losses were associated with beneficial changes in lipids, serum insulin, and systolic blood pressure (SBP). However, all of these benefits were lost at 12 months and 24 months.

Several large school-based studies have provided activity and knowledge/attitude interventions to promote health and reduce cardiovascular disease risk factors in children. The Child and Adolescent Trial for Cardiovascular Health (CATCH) study, conducted in four sites around the United States, involved parents and changed schools' physical education and lunch programs (Luepker et al., 1996); but the CATCH interventions produced no demonstrable effect on physiologic outcomes. A similar lack of effect was found in a large community-based project in England that included school-based interventions (Baxter et al., 1997). However, the Cardiovascular Health in Children (CHIC) study found that school-based interventions decreased total cholesterol and body fat in third and fourth graders (Harrell, McMurray, Gansky, Bangdiwala, & Bradley, 1999). The CHIC study was conducted in 18 schools in North Carolina and only changed the schools' PE program and classroom teaching but still had significant effects.

The Community Intervention Trial for Smoking Cessation (COMMIT) was funded by the National Cancer Institute to test the effectiveness of a multifaceted, 4-year community-based intervention to promote smoking cessation in adults ages 25 to 64 (Ross & Taylor, 1998). The study was conducted in 11 intervention communities, with 11 communities serving as controls. Unfortunately, the intervention had no effect on the prevalence of heavy smoking or on overall smoking (Cummings, Hyland, Ockene, Hymowitz, & Manley, 1997).

Through the Alliance of Black Churches Health Project, a smoking cessation program was implemented in churches in a rural county in Virginia (Schorling et al., 1997). The intervention incorporated feedback from community members and included one-on-one counseling by church members, provision of self-help materials, and community-wide activities. However, the intervention did not result in a significant decrease in smoking.

Enforcing laws to ban tobacco sales to minors is widely advocated as a way to reduce the access of youth to tobacco. However, a study comparing the access of youth to tobacco in three communities that strictly enforced the laws with three that did not found no difference in adolescents' perceived access to tobacco or in their smoking (Rigotti et al., 1997). Another study that evaluated the effects of a law requiring a locking device on cigarette vending machines found that it did not limit minors' access to cigarettes (Forster, Hourigan, & Kelder, 1992).

While many interventions have failed to change behaviors, some approaches have been successful. A meta-analysis of 17 randomized controlled trials of interventions with a nutrition component found that individual dietary intervention achieved modest improvements in diet and CVD risk factors that were maintained from 9 to 18 months (Brunner et al., 1997). Interventions may be more successful when they are tailored to individuals' cultural contexts and to their stage of readiness to change. In one large office practice, a physician-nurse team set up a smoking cessation program that included systematic assessment of current smoking and stage of change in smoking behavior at each patient visit using "Smoke Cards" placed on the outside of the patient's chart (Pine, Sullivan, Sauser, & David, 1997). The physician or nurse gave a brief smoking cessation message based on assessment of the patient's stage of readiness to change. Self-help materials were available, there were posters about smoking cessation in the examining rooms, and no smoking was allowed in the office. Follow-up was provided to support those who quit; 17.6% of the 142 smokers quit smoking for at least 6 months.

Low-income, pregnant, Hispanic, and African-American women attending WIC clinic sites were the target of a smoking cessation study designed by nurses (Lillington, Royce, Novak, Ruvalcaba, & Chlebowski, 1995). The program included a 15-minute one-on-one counseling session and an incentive contest, was culturally appropriate, and required few reading skills. Almost twice as many smokers in the intervention group (43%) as in the controls (25%) reported quitting smoking at 9 months. At 6 weeks after giving birth, 25% of women in the intervention group were still abstinent, as compared with 12% in the control group.

This brief review of the research can give us an appreciation of how difficult it is to change behaviors and provide guidance on potential strategies to promote behavior change. We know that we need to start working for behavior change early in life; behaviors developed in childhood tend to continue into adulthood. We also know that we need to continue to promote healthful behaviors throughout the life span and throughout the trajectory of chronic illness. Finally, the research suggests that interventions may need to be tailored to individuals' cultural context and to their stage of readiness to change.

DIRECTIONS FOR CLINICAL PRACTICE

The health promotion chapters in this book move us closer to understanding what will be required if we are to promote healthy lifestyles. Several chapters suggest that bringing about behavior change will require a fundamental change in the relationship between patients and clinicians. Both players must recognize that control over behavior rests with the patient. The clinician's role is not to make the rules for patients, but to facilitate and inform patients' decision making as they plan self-care. Patient decisions about their behaviors are influenced by a wide range of factors that are beyond the scope of the clinician-patient encounter. In order to influence patient decision making, clinicians must pay attention to the many and complex factors influencing those decisions. Clinicians must also become more cognizant of the broader contexts of patients' lives—their families, their communities, and their religious and social organizations.

Chapter 15, "Self-Care Decision Making in Clients with Diabetes and Hypertension," presents a model for understanding the factors that influence behavior change in patients. Weiss shows how we can move beyond the "provider view of adherence (following the rules) to the broader client view of responsibility for self-care (determining the rules)." She encourages clinicians to approach behavior change from patients' perspectives by viewing self-care decision making within the context of patients' social networks, their past experience, their perceptions of risk, and their perceptions of the cost of change. Weiss's model highlights the need to recognize the uniqueness of each patient's approach to behavior change and to tailor intervention strategies accordingly.

Several other chapters advance our understanding of differences across social groups. Chapter 8, "Regular Physical Activity in Older African Americans," describes contextual and other factors important to behavior change in rural, elderly African Americans. For this group, perceived social support and the presence and perception of chronic illness are significant predictors of regular physical activity. In Chapter 9, "Maintenance of Regular Physical Activity in Working Women," Speck explores factors that support behavior change among working women. In her study, support from friends was the strongest predictor of maintenance of physical activity. Both of these studies suggest that clinicians can better facilitate patients' self-care decision making if they attend to patients' social networks, family, friends, and community.

In their communications with patients, clinicians tend to focus on the benefits of change to the individual patient. To promote healthier self-care decision making, providers also need to attend to patients' concerns about costs, whether financial, physical, emotional, or social. Barriers such as financial burdens, transportation, and conflicting demands of family members need to be considered and addressed. In Chapter 12, "Development of a Public Health Nurse–Delivered Cholesterol Intervention Program," Keyserling and colleagues discuss the value of addressing patients' concerns about costs. This program facilitated public health nurses' use of nutrition interventions by providing them with a structured assessment and intervention tool, strategies for overcoming obstacles to change, and a southern-style recipe book.

If we are to address patients within the context of their lives, it also makes sense to move efforts to change behavior beyond the one-on-one encounter in the clinician's office. Chapter 11, "Early Interventions: A Systems Approach," reports on an intervention that employed nurses as agents for change at the level of the family, primary care practices, and the community. Chapter 7, "School-based Interventions to Improve the Health of Children with Multiple Cardiovascular Risk Factors," describes an intervention delivered in public school classrooms. The intervention produced large reductions in cholesterol, slight reductions in body fat, and an increase in health knowledge.

We know that physical inactivity and obesity have reached epidemic proportions in the United States. We also know that there are strong associations between these behaviors and increased risk for premature morbidity and mortality. What we still do not know is how to get people to make the behavior changes necessary to reduce their risks and improve their health. Getting individuals and populations to make long-lasting behavior change remains a major challenge for both clinicians and researchers. It is a challenge that we need to continue struggling with if we are to turn the tide on the increasing prevalence of inactivity and poor diet. Improving health behaviors will play a critical role in the long-term health of the population. Increasing physical activity and improving diets will improve health by reducing the rates of obesity, osteoarthritis, cancer, cardiovascular disease, and diabetes. Convincing people to stop smoking will reduce many of the same illnesses and also reduce the prevalence of chronic obstructive pulmonary disease and emphysema.

While we have a beginning understanding of how to assist individuals with behavior change, we still have not opened the black box; that is, we still do not know what interventions will be most effective in promoting health and preventing disease. We do not know enough about how to motivate people to make enduring changes in their behaviors. The chapters in this book move us a little closer to the understanding that will be required if we are to improve health by promoting healthy lifestyles.

ACKNOWLEDGMENT

This work was partially funded by NIH, NINR grant # P30 NR03962 to the Center for Research on Chronic Illness, University of North Carolina at Chapel Hill, School of Nursing.

REFERENCES

Aarts, H., Paulssen, T., & Schaalma, H. (1997). Physical exercise habit: On the conceptualization and formation of habitual health behaviors. *Health Education Research, 12*(3), 363–374.

Anderson, R. E., Wadden, T. A., Bartlett, S. J., Zemel, B., Verde, T. J., & Franckowiak, S. C. (1999). Effects of lifestyle activity vs. structured aerobic exercise in obese women. *Journal of the American Medical Association, 281*, 335–340.

Appel, L. J., Moore, T. J., Obarzanek, E., Vollmer, W. M., Svetkey, L. P., Sacks, F. M., Bray, G. A., Vogt, T. M., Cutler, J. A., Windhauser, M. M., Lin, P. H., & Karanja, N. (1997). A clinical trial of the effects of dietary patterns on blood pressure. *New England Journal of Medicine, 336*(16), 1117–1124.

Bakx, J. C., Stafleu, A., van Staveren, W. A., van den Hoogen, H. J., & van Weel, C. (1997). Long-term effect of nutritional counseling: A study in family medicine. *American Journal of Clinical Nutrition, 65*(Suppl. 6), 1946S–1950S.

Baxter, A. P., Milner, P. C., Hawkins, S., Leaf, M., Simpson, C., Wilson, K. V., Owen, T., Higginbotton, G., Nicholl, J., & Cooper, N. (1997). The impact of heart health promotion on coronary heart disease lifestyle risk factors in school children: Lessons learnt from a community-based project. *Public Health, 111*, 231–237.

Beresford, S. A. A., Curry, S. J., Kristal, A. R., Lazovich, D., Feng, Z., & Wagner, E. H. (1997). A dietary intervention in primary care practice: The Eating Patterns Study. *American Journal of Public Health, 87*(4), 610–616.

Bollet, A. J. (1992). Obesity and musculoskeletal disease. In P. Bjorntorp & B. N. Brodoff (Eds.), *Obesity* (pp. 563–567). Philadelphia: Lippincott.

Bray, G. A. (1997). Health hazards of obesity. *Endocrinology and Metabolism Clinics of North America, 25*, 907–919.

Brunner, E., White, J., Thorogood, M., Bristow, A., Curle, D., & Marmot, M. (1997). Can dietary interventions change diet and cardiovascular risk factors? A meta-analysis of randomized controlled trials. *American Journal of Public Health, 87*(9), 1415–1422.

Centers for Disease Control and Prevention. (1994). Preventing tobacco use among young people: A report of the Surgeon General (Executive Summary). *Morbidity and Mortality Weekly Review, 43*(RR-4).

Centers for Disease Control and Prevention. (1997). Monthly estimates of leisure-time physical inactivity—United States, 1994. *Morbidity and Mortality Weekly Report, 46*(18), 393–397.

Colditz, G. A., Willett, W. C., Rotnitsky, A., & Manson, J. E. (1995). Weight-gain as a risk factor for clinical diabetes-mellitus in women. *Annals of Internal Medicine, 122*, 481–486.

Crespo, C. J., Keteyian, S. J., Heath, G. W., & Sempos, C. T. (1996). Leisure-time physical activity among U.S. adults: Results from the Third National Health and Nutrition Examination Survey. *Archives of Internal Medicine, 156,* 93–98.

Cummings, K. M., Hyland, A., Ockene, J. K., Hymowitz, N., & Manley, M. (1997). Use of the nicotine skin patch by smokers in 20 communities in the United States, 1992–1993. *Tobacco Control, 6*(Suppl. 2), S63–70.

Dunn, A. L., Garcia, M. E., Marcus, B. H., Kampert, J. B., Kohl, H. W., & Blair, S. N. (1998). Six-month physical activity and fitness changes in Project Active: A randomized trial. *Medicine, Science, Sports and Exercise, 30,* 1076–1083.

Dunn, A. L., Marcus, B. H., Kampert, J. B., Garcia, M. E., Kohl, H. W., & Blair, S. N. (1999). Comparison of lifestyle and structured interventions to increase physical activity and cardiorespiratory fitness: A randomized trial. *Journal of the American Medical Association, 281,* 327–334.

Fitzgibbon, M. L., Stolley, M. R., Avellone, M. E., Sugerman, S., & Chavez, N. (1996). Involving parents in cancer risk reduction: A program for Hispanic American families. *Health Psychology, 5*(6), 413–422.

Forster, J. L., Hourigan, M. E., & Kelder, S. (1992). Locking devices on cigarette vending machines: Evaluation of a city ordinance. *American Journal of Public Health, 82*(9), 1217–1219.

Freedman, D. S., Srinivasan, S. R., Valdez, R. A., Williamson, D. F., & Berenson, G. S. (1997). Secular increases in relative weight and adiposity among children over two decades: The Bogalusa Heart Study. *Pediatrics, 99*(3), 420–426.

Gavarry, O., Bernard, T., Giacomoni, M., Seymat, M., Euzet, J. P., & Falgairette, G. (1998). Continuous heart rate monitoring over 1 week in teenagers aged 11–16 years. *European Journal of Applied Physiology and Occupational Physiology, 77*(1–2), 125–132.

Giovannucci, E., Stampfer, M. J., Colditz, G., Rimm, E. B., & Willett, W. C. (1992). Relationship of diet to risk of colorectal adenoma in men. *Journal of the National Cancer Institute, 84*(2), 1991–1992.

Glaser, N. S. (1997). Non-insulin-dependant diabetes mellitus in childhood and adolescence. *Pediatric Clinics of North America, 44,* 307–331.

Goran, M. I., Gower, B. A., Nagy, T. R., & Johnson, R. K. (1998). Developmental changes in energy expenditure and physical activity in children: Evidence for a decline in physical activity in girls before puberty. *Pediatrics, 101*(5), 887–891.

Harlan, W. R. (1993). Epidemiology of childhood obesity: A national perspective. *Annals of the New York Academy of Sciences, 699,* 1–5.

Harrell, J. S., Bangdiwala, S. I., Deng, S., Webb, J. P., & Bradley, C. (1998). Smoking initiation in youth. *Journal of Adolescent Medicine, 23,* 271–279.

Harrell, J. S., McMurray, R. G., Gansky, S. A, Bangdiwala, S. I., & Bradley, C. B. (1999). A public health vs. a risk-based intervention to improve cardiovascular health in elementary school children: The Cardiovascular Health in Children Study. *American Journal of Public Health, 89,* 1529–1535.

Heini, A. F., & Weinsier, R. L. (1997). Divergent trends in obesity and fat intake patterns: The American paradox. *American Journal of Medicine, 102,* 259–264.

Huang, Z., Hankinson, S. E., Colditz, G. A., Stampfer, M. J., Hunter, D. J., Manson, J. E., Hennekens, C. H., Rosner, B., Speizer, F. E., & Willett, W. C. (1997). Dual effects of weight and weight gain on breast cancer risk. *Journal of the American Medical Association, 278,* 1407–1411.

Jette, A. M., Lachman, M., Giorgette, M. M., Assmann, S. F., Harris, B. S. A., Levenson, C., Wernick, M., & Krebs, D. (1999). Exercise—It's never too late: The Strong-for-Life Program. *American Journal of Public Health, 98,* 66–72.

Kuczmarski, R. J., Flegal, K. M., Campbell, S. M., & Johnson, C. L. (1994). Increasing prevalence of overweight among U.S. adults. *Journal of the American Medical Association, 272,* 205–211.

Levine, J. A., Eberhardt, N. L., & Jensen, M. D. (1999). Role of nonexercise activity thermogenesis in resistance to fat gain in humans. *Science, 283*(5399), 212–214.

Lillington, L., Royce, J., Novak, D., Ruvalcaba, M., & Chlebowski, R. (1995). Evaluation of a smoking cessation program for pregnant minority women. *Cancer Practice, 3,* 157–163.

Luepker, R. V., Perry, C. L., McKinlay, S. M., Nader, P. R., Parcel, G. S., Stone, E. J., Webber, L. S., Elder, J. P., Feldman, H. A., Johnson, C. C., Kelder, S. H., & Wu, M. (1996). Outcomes of a field trial to improve children's dietary patterns and physical activity: The Child and Adolescent Trial for Cardiovascular Health. *Journal of the American Medical Association, 275*(10), 768–776.

Manson, J. E., Colditz, G. A., & Stampfer, M. J. (1990). A prospective study of obesity and risk of coronary heart disease in women. *New England Journal of Medicine, 322,* 882–889.

Manson, J. E., Willett, W. C., Stampfer, M. J., Colditz, G. A., Hunter, D. J., Hankinson, S. E., Hennekens, C. H., & Speizer, F. E. (1995). Body weight and mortality among women. *New England Journal of Medicine, 333,* 677–685.

Mazzeo, R. S., Cavanagh, P., Evans, W. J., Flatarone, M., Hagberg, J., McAuley, E., & Startzell, J. (1998). Exercise and physical activity in older adults. *Medicine and Science in Sports and Exercise, 30*(6), 992–1008.

McGinnis, J. M., & Foege, W. H. (1993). Actual causes of death in the United States. *Journal of the American Medical Association, 270,* 2207–2212.

Miller, T. D., Balady, G. J., & Fletcher, G. F. (1997). Exercise and its role in the prevention and rehabilitation of cardiovascular disease. *Annals of Behavioral Medicine, 19*(3), 220–229.

Must, A., Jacques, P. F., Dallal, G. E., Bajema, C. J., & Dietz, W. H. (1992). Long-term morbidity and mortality of overweight adolescents: A follow-up of the Harvard Growth Study of 1922 to 1935. *New England Journal of Medicine, 327*(19), 1350–1355.

Office on Smoking and Health. (1999). Tobacco use—United States, 1900–1999. *Morbidity and Mortality Weekly Report, 48,* 986–996.

Pate, R. R., Pratt, M., Blair, S. N., Haskell, W. L., Macera, C. A., Bouchard, C., Buchner, D., Ettinger, W., Heath, G. W., King, A. C., Kriska, A., Leon, A. S., Marcus, B. H., Morris, J., Paffenbarger, R. S., Patrick, K., Pollock, M. L., Rippe, J. M., Sallis, J., & Wilmore, J. H. (1995). Physical activity and public health: A recommendation from the Centers for Disease Control and Prevention and the American College of Sports Medicine. *Journal of the American Medical Association, 273*(5), 402–407.

Pine, D., Sullivan, S., Sauser, M., & David, C. (1997). Effects of a systematic approach to tobacco cessation in a community-based practice. *Archives of Family Medicine, 6*, 363–367.

Pinhas-Hamiel, O., Dolan, L. M., Daniels, S. R., Standiford, D., Khoury, R. P., & Zietler, P. (1996). Increased incidence of non-insulin-dependant diabetes mellitus among adolescents. *Journal of Pediatrics, 128*, 608–615.

Rigotti, N. A., DiFranza, J. R., Chang, Y., Trisdale, T., Kemp, B., & Singer, D. E. (1997). The effect of enforcing tobacco-sales laws on adolescents' access to tobacco and smoking behavior. *New England Journal of Medicine, 337*, 1044–1051.

Ross, N. A., & Taylor, S. M. (1998). Geographical variation in attitudes towards smoking: Findings from the COMMIT communities. *Social Science and Medicine, 46*, 703–717.

Sallis, J. F. (1993). Epidemiology of physical activity and fitness in children and adolescents. *Critical Reviews in Food and Science, 33*(4/5), 403–408.

Schorling, J. B., Roach, J., Siegel, M., Baturka, N., Hunt, D. E., Guterbock, T. M., & Stewart, H. L. (1997). A trial of church-based smoking cessation interventions for rural African Americans. *Preventive Medicine, 26*(1), 92–101.

Solomon, C. G., & Manson, J. E. (1997). Obesity and mortality: A review of the epidemiologic data. *American Journal of Clinical Nutrition, 66*(Suppl.), 10445–10505.

Srinivasan, S. R., Bao, W., Wattigney, W. A., & Berenson, G. S. (1996). Adolescent overweight is associated with adult overweight and related multiple cardiovascular risk factors: The Bogalusa Heart Study. *Metabolism, 45*(2), 235–240.

Stefanick, M. L., Mackey, S., Sheehan, M., Ellsworth, N., Haskell, W. L., & Wood, P. D. (1998). Effects of diet and exercise in men and postmenopausal women with low levels of HDL cholesterol and high levels of LDL cholesterol. *New England Journal of Medicine, 339*, 12–20.

Steinmetz, K. A., Kushi, L. H., Bostick, R. M., Folsom, A. R., & Potter, J. D. (1994). Vegetables, fruit, and colon cancer in the Iowa Women's Health Study. *American Journal of Epidemiology, 139*(1), 1–15.

Troiano, R. P., & Flegal, K. M. (1998). Overweight children and adolescents: Description, epidemiology, and demographics. *Pediatrics, 101*(3), 497–504.

Troiano, R. P., Flegal, K. M., Kuczmarski, R. J., Campbell, S. M., & Johnson, C. L. (1995). Overweight prevalence and trends for children and adolescents: The National Health and Nutrition Examination Surveys, 1963–1991. *Archives of Pediatric and Adolescent Medicine, 149*, 1085–1091.

U.S. Department of Health and Human Services (USDHHS). (1989). *Reducing the health consequences of smoking—25 years of progress: A Report of the Surgeon General.* Washington, DC: U.S. Government Printing Office.

U.S. Department of Health and Human Services (USDHHS). (1990). *Healthy people 2000: National health promotion and disease prevention objectives* (DHHS Publication No. (PHS) 91-50212). Washington, DC: Public Health Service.

U.S. Department of Health and Human Services (USDHHS). (1998). Tobacco use among high school students—United States, 1997. *Morbidity and Mortality Weekly Report, 47*, 229–234.

Van Itallie, T. B. (1985). Health implications of overweight and obesity in the United States. *Annals of Internal Medicine, 103,* 983–988.

Willett, W. C. (1994). Diet and health: What should we eat? *Science, 264,* 532–537.

Willett, W. C., Manson, J. E., Stampfer, M. J., Colditz, G. A., Rosner, B., Speizer, F. J., & Hennekens, C. H. (1995). Weight, weight change and coronary heart disease in women. *Journal of the American Medical Association, 274,* 461–465.

Wing, R. R., Venditti, E., Jakicic, J. M., Polley, B. A., & Lang, W. (1998). Lifestyle intervention in overweight individuals with a family history of diabetes. *Diabetes Care, 21*(3), 350–359.

Zhang, S., Hunter, D. J., Forman, M. R., Rosner, B. A., Speizer, F. E., Colditz, G. A., Manson, J. E., Hankinson, S. E., & Willett, W. C. (1999). Dietary carotenoids and vitamins A, C, and E and risk of breast cancer. *Journal of the National Cancer Institute, 91*(6), 547–556.

[4]

Self-Management in Chronic Illness

Kate Lorig

This chapter focuses on self-management and its fit with the health care system. We have a few basic models for nursing and medical care, which can be illustrated by the metaphor of a person falling into a river. The medical model works very well for acute diseases. When somebody falls into the river of illness—for example, when a person has appendicitis or a broken leg—the medical model saves the person by pulling him out. This was the predominant model of health care until the mid-twentieth century, and it is still the model that is most commonly taught. Those of us in public health, however, think it is possible to go upstream and build barriers to keep people from falling into the river. We do this by giving inoculations, by having clean water supplies, by providing sanitation, and, most recently, by sponsoring health promotion programs to help people stop smoking and prevent heart attacks. Many of these programs have been highly successful. For example, in the United States there has not been a large cholera outbreak for many years as a result of public health measures.

However, neither the public health nor the medical model can deal with chronic disease, the number one cost of health care today and the number one demand on the system. Neither the medical model nor the public health model can solve this problem. It is too late. On average, people over the age of 60 have two chronic illnesses. We might prevent some chronic illnesses, but no matter what we do, the fact is that, as people live longer, the prevalence of chronic illness will continue to increase. Therefore, I would like to suggest a new model—a self-management model. In this model the patients themselves, the individuals with the chronic illness, manage their disease on a day-to-day basis. In chronic illness, when people fall into the river we need to be able to help them learn how to swim—quickly.

Gregory Bateson, noted anthropologist, philosopher, and author, once said, "You cannot not communicate." I'd like to change that to say "You cannot not manage." A person with a chronic illness has to manage the disease. He or she can manage the disease by staying home and becoming totally unfunctional, a burden on society and the family. Or the person can be proactive and manage the disease, and continue to lead a full and happy life. The difference between those two has very little to do with the disease process. It has to do with self-management. What I have been doing for the last 20 years is helping people learn how to manage disease.

To put this into a public policy context, in the traditional view, the health care system in the United States provides primary, secondary, and tertiary care. But in fact, these represent only 20% of health care. About 80% of health care today is self-care, care that individuals do for themselves (Kemper, 1984). Did you brush your teeth this morning? If yes, then you have done at least one self-care activity. If you took vitamins, or walked, or did a number of other different things, then you participated in self-care. If we were able to increase the amount of self-care by just 5%, we might be able to reduce the amount of health care by a full 25% (Kemper, 1984). That is why the whole area of self-care, or self-management, has become a very important health policy issue.

Self-care used to be perceived as a nice "extra." When I was attending Boston University, I used *Textbook of the Principles and Practice of Nursing* (1955), by Harmer and Henderson. Mary Ann Garrigan, one of my professors, said that health care professionals should keep their books because they are very important, and I did. I recently skimmed my copy of the textbook to see what it said about patient education and health education. There is one line in the book: "Whether the nurse likes it or not, teaching is inherent in her profession, and her position makes health guidance one of her obligations" (Harmer & Henderson, 1955, pp. 534–535). (The line is sexist, but so was the profession at that time.) As far as I can remember, in my 4 years of nursing education, that was the extent of what I was taught about patient education. We can no longer afford to do this.

To introduce self-management, let me begin by pointing to the ways in which the views of patients and nurses differ. Patients want to know why they feel so bad; nurses are interested in anatomy and physiology. Patients are interested in behaviors that will solve the problems they have; nurses are interested in behaviors to maintain health. Patients have beliefs about disease, whereas nurses want them to know the facts about disease. Patients want skills to maintain their normal lives, but nurses want to teach them skills to perform health behaviors. Patients are frustrated about living with disease, and nurses are frustrated because patients do not comply with what they tell the patients to do. Finally, patients fear the future, whereas clinicians fear malpractice suits.

Clearly health professionals and patients have different worldviews. As a result, professionals often target health education at the wrong place. Self-management begins with the patient's perceived problems, not with what health professionals think the patient needs to learn.

What problems do patients need help dealing with? Corbin and Strauss (1988), in their study of the tasks and work of chronic illness, discovered three sets of tasks. First, people with chronic illness need to deal with the medical management of the disease. Medical management covers taking medications, doing prescribed exercises, eating a prescribed diet, and so on. Medical management thus includes the tasks that are part of traditional patient education and self-help programs. The second set of tasks Corbin and Strauss outlined are those that people with chronic disease have to do to maintain their roles in life. These roles might include grandmother, fixer of Thanksgiving turkey, reader at the Seder service during Passover, and basketball player. Helping people with the tasks they need to do to maintain meaningful roles is something most traditional patient education programs do not do very well. The third task for people with chronic illness is dealing with the emotional sequelae of the disease, especially those that come from having an indefinite future. Folkman (see chapter 25) has spoken eloquently about these tasks, about dealing with fear, frustration, depression, and anger. Again, health professionals do not do a very good job of helping people deal with these powerful emotions, but they are always there, in one form or another. In my work I have learned that people use a range of language to express these emotions. People will tell me that they do not get angry or frustrated. They will say, "I'm not angry, I'm depressed," or "I'm not depressed, I'm angry." The language is not important. What is important is that we find ways to help people deal with the negative emotions involved with living with chronic illness.

These are the tasks, then, that need to be considered when we speak of self-management. And where does self-management fit into the labyrinth of health and patient education? First, there is what patients "must know," the education that happens in the examining room (e.g., "You must take these pills three times a day"). Then there is the "need to know" (e.g., "This is the way you count carbohydrates when you are a diabetic"; "This is the way you use your inhaler"). "Need to know" information is usually covered in traditional patient education programs and materials. Finally, there is the third level of information that is important for patients but unfortunately is not often provided. Patients want to know, given the circumstances of their chronic illness, how to get on with the rest of their lives, what new life skills they need to carry on with their lives, and how to acquire these skills. This third level is where I see self-management fitting into patient education.

At the center I have headed at Stanford University, we offer arthritis self-management programs in both English and Spanish. The Spanish and English programs are different programs, not translations. We also offer programs on low back pain in two forms. We offer the programs in a small group format and also through an e-mail discussion group on the Internet (Von Korff et al., 1998). There is also a pain self-management program, and we are piloting a diabetes self-management program in Spanish. The chronic disease self-management program combines people with various illnesses in the same intervention group. This program is offered only in English at present, but we are currently evaluating a Spanish version. Table 4.1 outlines the topics covered in the chronic disease self-management program.

All of the programs, except for the one on the Internet, are community-based. The programs are offered in senior centers, in church basements, at regional shopping centers, and in community health centers. We try to go where people are and not require them to come to us. Since they are community-based, the courses are also given at various times. Many of the courses are given on Saturday mornings. Recently we began to offer courses for Seventh-Day Adventists on Sunday afternoons because that seems to be preferable. We will give courses whenever and wherever they are needed. The groups are small, and all of the courses are taught by chronically ill

TABLE 4.1   Topics Covered in Chronic Disease Self-Management Program

Developing Patient/Physician Partnerships
Use of Community Resources
Healthful Eating
Managing Medications
Advance Directives for Health Care
Disease-related Problem Solving
Managing Emotions
Exercise
Cognitive Symptom Management
Communication Skills

people we have trained. We invite participants to bring anybody they want to the program with them. They can bring a family member or significant other, and about 20% to 30% of the people do bring someone with them. The programs are structured in such a way that family members are full participants, so they also make action plans, do problem solving, and take part in all the activities.

The programs are from 4 to 7 weeks in length, depending on the topic. Sessions range from 2 to 2 1/2 hours each week. All are built on an assessment of patient needs and taught according to a very detailed protocol. Our courses use a "Sesame Street" approach. If you have ever watched the children's TV show "Sesame Street," you know that young viewers do not work on the color red one day, the word *yes* on the second day, and the number 1 on the third day. Instead, they work on all three topics during one show, then build on them over a week's time. Unfortunately, patient education typically focuses on one topic per session: one week covers medication, the next week exercise, and the next emotions. We have traditionally done education that way because it is convenient for health professionals. However, it is not very effective, nor does it make a lot of sense educationally. In our classes, any one session will deal with three or four topics. We then build on those topics and revisit them over a period of 4, 5, or 6 weeks. The leaders act as facilitators rather than instructors. The longest lecture in any of our courses is 5 minutes.

We depend fairly heavily on ritual. By ritual I do not mean candles and incense; what I mean is that every session looks pretty much like every other session. Participants begin by giving feedback, they learn something, they have a break, they learn something else, they learn something else, they make action plans, and they go home. What ritual does for participants is give them a sense of security. While there are some ritualistic aspects to our programs, if you asked the participants, they would probably not tell you they were ritualistic. In fact, that is not a word I have ever heard from a participant. We also do a lot of mutual support. When we ask participants what they get out of the courses, they tell us "sharing," and what they mean by sharing is that they are helping others (Campbell, Sengupta, Santo, & Lorig, 1995). Another process we use is problem solving (D'Zurilla, 1986).

We provide our leaders with very detailed manuals, and we standardize our patient materials. Participants are given one of the books that we have written for each of our courses (Gifford, Lorig, Laurent, & González, 1997; Lorig & Fries, 1995; Lorig et al., 1993; Moore, Lorig, Von Korff, González, & Laurent, 1999). While we provide all participants with books, nothing in the program depends on literacy. Our Spanish speakers have an average literacy level of grade 4. Therefore, in the Spanish courses we originally planned to use pictures and simplified text, but our Spanish-speaking participants told us they wanted a book like everyone else. They told us that if they could not read it, they would find someone in their household who could. We now give our Spanish speakers a 250-page book, and participants with only 2 years of education are ordering and paying for two and three extra copies to give to their friends.

The courses rely heavily on self-efficacy theory. Early in our research we asked people why they got better when they went to the arthritis course, and they said that they felt more in control. We then tested a number of different theories: learned helplessness, congruence, locus of control, stress and coping, and self-efficacy, and we found that self-efficacy gave us the best explanation for our effects. As a result, over the years we have continued to work with self-efficacy theory. To increase self-efficacy, our courses incorporate skills mastery, modeling, work on changing beliefs about the symptoms or problems, and social persuasion.

In every class we teach skills mastery by asking participants to make specific action plans for the coming week. For example, my action plan for this week is that I will not eat any candy between lunch and dinner 4 days this week. On a scale from 0 (totally uncertain) to 10 (totally certain), my confidence or my sureness that I can do this is 7 or 8. We ask participants to do this at every class, every week.

We use modeling by having people with chronic disease teach others with chronic disease. It is harder for someone to say "You don't know what it's like," when in fact you do. In addition, all of our materials model people of different sizes and races, both male and female, because we want participants to look at the photographs in the book and see themselves. We work on changing beliefs about symptoms by making sure that every time we talk about symptoms, we talk about them as having multiple causes, and therefore multiple solutions. Finally, we incorporate social persuasion by doing many things in the class to encourage participants to help each other and to report back on what they are doing.

We have completed a study of the Stanford chronic disease self-management program with funding from the Agency for Health Care Policy and Research and have replicated the study in Spanish with funding from the National Institute of Nursing Research. Our initial study was a randomized trial of just over a thousand people. To be included in the study, subjects had to have heart disease, lung disease, stroke, or arthritis. They could have other problems, but they had to have at least one of these four diseases in order to be enrolled. Over half had arthritis (54%), almost half had lung disease (45%), and about one third had heart disease (35%). The mean number of diseases per participant was 2.2. Enrollees were randomized to either a control group or a treatment group who participated in the chronic disease self-management program.

At the end of 6 months, the treatment group did more minutes per week of exercise, spent more time per week practicing cognitive symptom management, and reported better communication with their physicians than the control group. The treatment group had less disability than the control group, reported less fatigue and more energy, and showed an improvement in self-rated health, measured by the question, "How healthy are you?" Interestingly, that one question has been shown to be a better predictor of future hospitalization, future death, and future health than any other measure (Lorig et al., 1999). The treatment group also reported having better social and role function than the control group, as well as less distress about their health. Finally, we looked at health care utilization; the treatment group had fewer hospitalizations and eight-tenths fewer days of hospitalization over 6 months. When we costed this out, we found that the treatment group was spending about $800 less on medical care costs over 6 months than the control group. The cost of the intervention was about $100, so this was a very large payback for a very low cost intervention. We also saw trends toward fewer emergency room visits and fewer outpatient visits, but they did not reach the level of significance (Lorig et al., 1999).

Stanford's disease self-management program has become very popular, and it is being used by many voluntary agencies. One agency that is disseminating it is the Liver Trust in Great Britain. A number of managed care plans are also using the program. Kaiser Permanente is disseminating it nationwide. Group Health Cooperative of Puget Sound is using the program, as well as Henry Ford Health System in Detroit. Blue Cross and Blue Shield is using it in New Hampshire and other states. The Department of Veterans' Affairs is using it in the southern region and in Puerto Rico. The state health department of California is using it. If an organization wants to use the program, we have licensing agreements and a system to help train people.

In summary, the care of chronic disease depends on a partnership between health care providers and patients. Although nurses and other providers can advise and counsel patients, it is up to each patient to manage the disease on a day-to-day basis. We now have strong evidence that it is possible to teach self-management skills and to improve self-management. Such improvements lead to improved health and lower health care utilization. Harmer and Henderson were right: Facilitating patients' learning of self-management skills is a nursing obligation.

REFERENCES

Campbell, B., Sengupta, S., Santo, C., & Lorig, K. (1995). Balanced incomplete block design: Description, case study, and implications for practice. *Health Education Quarterly, 22,* 201–210.

Corbin, J., & Strauss A. (1988). *Unending work and care: Managing chronic illness at home.* San Francisco: Jossey-Bass.

D'Zurilla, T. J. (1986). *Problem solving therapy.* New York: Springer.

Gifford, A. L., Lorig, K., Laurent, D., & González, V. (1997). *Living well with HIV & AIDS.* Palo Alto, CA: Bull.

Harmer, B., & Henderson, V. (1955). *Textbook of the principles and practice of nursing* (5th ed.). New York: Macmillan.

Kemper, D. (1984, June). The art of healing thyself. *Business and Health,* 32–34.

Lorig, K., & Fries, J. (1995). *The arthritis helpbook* (4th ed.). Reading, MA: Addison-Wesley.

Lorig, K., Holman, H., Sobel, D., Laurent, D., González, V., & Minor, M. (1993). *Living a healthy life with chronic conditions.* Palo Alto, CA: Bull.

Lorig, K. R., Sobel, D. S., Stewart, A. L., Brown, B. W., Jr., Bandura, A., & Ritter, P. (1999). Evidence suggesting that a chronic disease self-management program can improve health status while reducing hospitalization: A randomized trial. *Medical Care, 37*(1), 5–14.

Moore, J. E., Lorig, K., Von Korff, M., González, V. M., & Laurent, D. D. (1999). *The back pain helpbook.* Reading, MA: Perseus Books.

Von Korff, M., Moore, J., Lorig, K., Cherkin, D. C., Saunders, J. D., & González, V. M. (1998). A randomized trial of a lay person–led self-management group intervention for back pain patients in primary care. *Spine, 23,* 2608–2615.

[5]

The Interplay of Biology, Environment, and Behavior in the Prevention and Management of Chronic Illness

Mary T. Champagne

The term *chronic illness* comes from the Latin word *chronicus*, meaning "for the time." For those of us who do not have a chronic illness, I suspect it is only "for the time." For those who are chronically ill, however, it is for the time remaining—ever present. The challenge is to create a functional, fulfilling life with chronic illness. From an etiologic point of view and thus also from the point of view of prevention and management, chronic illness interfaces with three sciences: the biomedical, the environmental, and the behavioral. While the specifics may differ in particular diseases, there is good reason to believe that most chronic illnesses represent the interplay of these three sciences, and therefore prevention and management must incorporate them as well.

In 1994 we were riveted by the discovery of the BRCA 1 and 2 breast cancer susceptibility genes (Claus, Schildkraut, Iversen, Berry, & Parmigiani, 1999). Shortly after that, we learned of the apolipoprotein E gene–e4 allele and its relationship to Alzheimer's Disease (Roses, 1998). It is likely that there is a genetic susceptibility to almost all chronic illnesses, and thus all of us are carrying in our genes the susceptibility to the chronic illnesses that we will develop (Pyeritz, 1997). At present, people recognize that a familial history of a disease and a mother or a sister with breast cancer or a father who dies in his 30s are markers of risk for individuals. Aggressive mapping of the human genome will lead in the near future to the ability to identify personal risks of chronic illness at birth. Thus, in the not too distant future, it is likely that newborns will be screened and personal individualized health promotion/disease prevention prescriptions given. While this may create ethical concerns, the very early identification of susceptibility to chronic illnesses will help us to better target interventions. Geno-mapping will not, however, lead to successful interventions. It will only help us predict a patient's risk for given problems and advise how those problems might be avoided (Eisenberg, 1998).

Environmental causes can alter genes or turn on a programmed genetic or physiologic response that can lead to illness. The environment includes social mores and stresses and how we live. Environmental threats are broad and range from asbestos in ceilings, to dust mites and cockroaches in homes, to the Big Macs on the corner (every corner if you have children), to cigarette smoking in public places. Because the environment can be critical in the development of chronic illness, it should come as no surprise that it also looms large in the management of chronic illness. Social, economic, family, caregiver, and household circumstances all play a role in a person's ability to adapt to chronic illness. We know more about the environment than we have ever known, but it is not at all clear that a healthy choice is easy in this country. We need interventions and policy changes at the societal level to make it easier for people to make healthy choices. Individual changes—changes by the patient and the family—will never be sufficient in and of themselves. We need both personal and population-based approaches. Community partnerships or coalitions that address the health of the community can help move policy in the right direction (Flynn, Rider, & Ray, 1991).

We know a great deal about the lifestyle changes needed to promote health and reduce the risk of chronic illness. They are the same behavior changes that we advocate for people with chronic illness in order to ensure maximal health and function. However, as Chapter 2 has so clearly pointed out, people are not making the necessary changes to their lifestyles. We are nowhere near mastery of the science of behavior change. Genetic progress and molecular medicine will never realize their potentials until we find ways to empower patients to change their lifestyles. Chapter 3 speaks of the "black box" of mechanisms to connect what we know people should do with their actual behaviors. Our greatest challenge in preventing and managing chronic illness may be opening that black box.

Why do people choose to do what they do? How can clinicians and researchers provide people with the information, care, environmental support, and self-care strategies that will promote healthy lifestyles? One particularly useful behavioral model from the psychiatric and health promotion literature is the transtheoretical model (Prochaska & DiClemente, 1982, 1986, 1992). The transtheoretical model (TTM) has been used to develop interventions for adopting exercise, using mammography, changing diet, and reducing HIV risk, to name a few areas (Lipkus, Rimer, & Strigo, 1996; Prochaska et al., 1994; Rakowski et al., 1998). TTM proposes that people move through a series of progressively more committed stages of change as they advance toward modifying behaviors or adopting new health behaviors. The stages range from precontemplation of the behavior to maintenance. People move through these stages based on their perceptions of the benefits of the behavior change and the impact on themselves and others of trying to change their behavior. The TTM model can be used by clinicians to assess the individual's current stage, then to provide information and advice to facilitate movement to the next stage. For example, someone who is in the precontemplation stage in relation to exercise needs information about why exercise is beneficial. If the person is at the contemplation stage, it is helpful to develop an action plan for how to begin an exercise program.

Models such as TTM are useful both in discussing and planning interventions. Models like TTM are also helpful in delineating some of the commonalities of managing different chronic illnesses. First, people require information to move beyond the precontemplation stage and begin to make the behavior changes necessary to reduce the risk of illness or manage an existing illness—whatever the illness. People need information about the risks and benefits of behaviors, the incentives for making healthy decisions, and living with chronic illness. Second, behavior change occurs over time and relapse is not uncommon, no matter what the risk of illness is. Chapter 3 describes how diet interventions may be successful initially, but the real challenge comes in trying to sustain the behavioral change. I am reminded of the story of a man who has written a book on diet and rushes it to his publisher. When he hears that the book is titled *The 100-Year Diet*, the publisher says, "Nobody will buy this book. People don't want this. They want to know how to lose 20 pounds in 6 weeks." And the man says, "Yes, but my book is the only one that will tell them how to keep the weight off."

Finally, the whole question of self-management and who is in charge has to be very, very clear. The notion of personal responsibility for health has become fashionable—which can also trivialize it. Nevertheless, for health promotion to be successful, or for a person with chronic illness to live well, a passive-aggressive approach, with the provider aggressive and the patient passive, simply does not work. Individuals and their families must take responsibility for managing their risk factors or their chronic illness. To do so, patients and families need information and help with management skills and behavioral change. Those with chronic illness need information about their illness, explanations of treatment options, descriptions of medications, and clinical studies that might offer hope. They may need help in building or accessing needed support systems or resources. Their caregivers may need support and relief. Studies of the chronically ill demonstrate that teaching patients self-management skills decreases symptoms, improves function, and improves self-advocacy (Gifford, Laurent, Gonzales, Chesney, & Lorig, 1998; Von Korff et al., 1998). Our challenge is to find ways to provide what is needed, when it is needed, using the appropriate dose and the appropriate delivery system. Our challenge is to serve as healers, educators, and advisors. This book includes a number of studies that can help us with that.

Because there is an essential link between patient responsibility for self-management and the quality of the outcome for the patient, a key component in the prevention and management of all forms of chronic illness is education. However, the effectiveness of education in increasing healthful behaviors and in managing chronic illness varies. There is no question that appropriately delivered education is effective, but some educational programs are more effective than others (Mullen et al., 1997). Several factors influence the effectiveness of patient education. First, clinicians need to stage information, that is, provide information that matches the individual's state of readiness to adopt or continue a behavior. Further—and this may be most important—clinicians need to provide information that is culturally relevant and specific to a person's concerns and questions. Some very nice work in the literature and in this book has shown that tailored information, whether computer-generated or done over the telephone, is effective both in increasing preventive measures such as use of mammography and in reducing uncertainty in chronic illness (Longman, Braden, & Mishel, 1997; Morgan et al., 1996; Rakowski et al., 1998; Rimer & Glassman, 1998). Clinicians may also need to provide the information more than once, since behavior change is best fostered in steps, some regimes are complex, and relapse is not uncommon.

We also need to pay greater attention to how education is delivered. There is good evidence that electronic modalities can be timely and effective. A 1997 meta-analysis in the *Journal of the American Medical Association* reports on telephone calls for counseling. Interactive phone systems and even telephone systems that delivered prerecorded messages resulted in better preventive care and management of diseases ranging from osteoar-thritis to diabetes (Balas et al., 1997). The Internet is an increasingly im-portant modality for the delivery of health information and support to patients. A recent issue of *Computers in Nursing* included the article, "Cyber Solace," which reported a study of Internet support groups for cancer patients (Klemm, Hurst, Dearholt, & Trone, 1999). The findings were similar to those found in other studies that looked at Internet support groups. Patients provide each other with information and support, and they share personal experiences, hope, and humor. There are numerous chat groups for people with chronic illness on the Internet; they deliver support and information to the chronically ill, though we do not know what effect they have on outcomes. Another dimension of education that warrants mention is the use of patients as teachers. This model has been used in diseases related to addiction, such as alcohol or drug use, but now we are also seeing highly effective self-management programs for chronic illness that use patients as teachers (Agency for Health Care Policy and Research [AHCPR], 1999). Finally, there is evidence that education and counseling programs that involve patients' self-monitoring activities are more successful than those that do not (Mullen et al., 1997).

The amount of information available is rapidly becoming the greatest challenge to effective education. At times we seem to have daily reports of what is and what is not beneficial to our health. We are plagued daily by newspapers that tell us red wine is good, or maybe not so good; that beta-carotene works but maybe not in pill form; that our mother maybe really did know best when she gave us our childhood dose of cod liver oil. On TV it is possible to switch between commercials for garlic capsules, ginko, and prescription medications. Unfortunately, when people are besieged by information, they begin to consider the issues trivial. One important element in the prevention and management of chronic illness, therefore, may be to help patients sift through the latest news about the right thing to do and help them understand how the news is related to their illness. As health professionals, our job is to help people distinguish between behavior changes that are reasonable to adopt and those that are trivial and meaningless.

Consider exercise, for example. In recent years, there has been a para-digm shift in the way we think about physical activity for people with chronic illnesses. For patients with intermittent claudication, we now know that walking three times a week for 30 minutes improves the claudication and relieves pain (Gardner & Poehlman, 1995; Leng, Fowler, & Ernst, 1998), upper and lower extremity and inspiratory muscle training reduce dyspnea in patients with chronic obstructive pulmonary disease (Lacasse et al., 1996), and aerobic and resistance exercise improve pain and performance in patients with osteoarthritis (Ettinger, Burns, & Messier, 1997). From a clinical perspective, we need to know the specific dose and type of exercise beneficial for each disease; we need to recognize that these will vary for someone who has multiple sclerosis and someone who has asthma.

Behavior change for the chronically ill poses additional challenges beyond disease prevention and health promotion. With chronic illness, a patient has to manage a complex regime and has to do so under the burden of suffering, often with threats to physical and interpersonal function. Commonalities across chronic illnesses can be found in the research in this book. These common themes can also be found in patients' own stories. Here are a few:

Aaron's story: I am 12 years old now. I have had asthma since I was 6, but I play a lot of sports anyway. I play soccer, baseball, basketball, and I swim on a summer swim team. As I get older, I'm getting better about how I control my asthma. And I am always looking for ideas that will help.

Mary's story: In 1982 I was delivering telephone books and fell, causing a herniated disc, which resulted in a total of 11 back surgeries. I am never without pain. I am constantly taking pain pills just to make it through the day. The nights are always bad, waking several times a night and having a hard time getting back to sleep. I do try to keep busy, taking care of my family, husband, and cleaning my home. I take pride in having a clean home. Sometimes I wonder why I must endure so much pain. I am always wishing I could be the person I used to be, but that is just a dream. I have had to take notice of every single thing I do or want to try and do, always considering the effect. A lot of trial and error comes into play for me. I have always been active, but now I have had to adjust and learn to cope with a different set of rules to play by. Today I just have to go on, do what I can when I can, and try not to be depressed about this situation. This story is just to let anyone out there know you are not alone. Many people are in the same boat as you, rowing, rowing, and going on with life as best we can.

Frank's story: I believe that the progression of multiple sclerosis (MS) and the continued lost of functionality is most challenging. The slow loss of coordination and mobility allows time to adjust, but the need to make continued adjustments is difficult. With MS, one must continually admit to changes related to a new stage. As my family (three boys ages 7, 9, and 11) begins to age and I lose functionality, acceptance becomes even more difficult. And acknowledgment within the family unit, even though my disabilities are obvious, is more difficult still. I am lucky to have a wife who has been part of my life since the early stages of my life with MS.

These stories speak of how patients deal with symptoms, with treatments, with getting through the day, and with uncertainty. For the most part, chronic illness is an ongoing process. Depending on the particular illness and its trajectory, patient and family needs and concerns will change over time. Yet chronic illnesses include several broad commonalities, and for the most part these are our concern as nurses. They have to do with care, not cure, with comfort and function, and with sensible being. They have to do with a connectedness to others, in particular family, and a sense of meaning and purpose in one's life. While as nurses we should lay claim to work in these areas, we must do so with full appreciation for the role of other health care professions.

With managed care, we have seen increasing concern for cost-effective interventions. In this new health care environment, health plans are asking that we reduce the cost of care while demonstrating improvements in patient outcomes from new programs. Although many clinicians are justifiably concerned about the focus on cost, the new environment also brings opportunities. For example, managed care has encouraged systems approaches to managing chronic illness, which have the potential to greatly improve the coordination of care. A variety of disease-specific management programs are now being tested, most commonly by managed care companies. In general, the focus of these programs is on the use of interdisciplinary or multidisciplinary teams and organizational structures to manage patients with specific diseases such as congestive heart failure, diabetes, and asthma (Brunner & Hickey, 1997; Simons, Haim, Rizzo, & Zannad, 1996; Urden, 1998; Venner & Seelbinder, 1996). These are high-cost, highly prevalent diseases. The disease-specific management programs usually cut across settings, from hospital to home and everywhere in between. They use evidence-based guidelines for management; they focus on outpatient treatment; they are aggressive in their use of primary and secondary interventions; and they use advanced practice nurses, particularly nurse practitioners, to manage care for both the individual patient and for the disease-specific population enrolled in the plan. Most of the systems of disease management that are successful have very good information systems so that data are logged in and feedback is readily available to help with management of the patient. The most common outcomes monitored by these programs are related to disease control, that is, how well the disease is being managed. Measures include disease control or limitation of disease progression, hospital readmission rates, emergency department encounters, control of symptoms, and functional capacity. Satisfaction with care and cost-to-outcome ratios are also examined (Armstrong, 1996; Langley, 1996; Summers, 1996). We need to follow what happens with these management programs since we may find them very helpful.

When we think about prevention and management of chronic illness, one area where we see less attention than warranted is the area of the most vulnerable. Do health promotion or disease-specific management programs reach those in greatest need? What is our responsibility for seeking out those who do not come to us, at least in the traditional fashion? How do we know which people are at high risk or have chronic illnesses if they are outside the traditional mainstream insurance loop? What about those with chronic illnesses who are part of the 44 million uninsured or the underinsured, and what about that large proportion of Medicaid patients who do not use the health system in the "right way"? How do we reach these people?

Durham, North Carolina, can provide an example of how we might approach this problem. Durham is a relatively small county of only 200,000 people, though the population is diverse. Over the last few years, through the Division of Community Health at Duke University, we have formed a community coalition to look at the health of people in Durham and reach the most vulnerable people in the county who might have chronic illnesses. One of the first things we did was to look at state mortality data and compare them to the data in Durham. We found much higher rates of morbidity and mortality among minority populations. We then collected data on ambulatory care–sensitive conditions, that is, diseases that the Institute of Medicine has identified as conditions where appropriate management in the primary care setting should avoid admissions to the emergency department or the hospital (Millman, 1993). Such conditions include asthma, congestive heart failure, and diabetes. Sometimes people need to be admitted for these conditions, but in general they should be able to be treated in the community. We used small area analysis and compared different geographic areas in Durham to examine admission rates for ambulatory care–sensitive conditions. We plotted the records of all emergency department and hospital admissions for ambulatory care–sensitive conditions by zip code, and identified four zip codes that had significantly higher rates for ambulatory care–sensitive conditions than the rest of Durham. For example, zip code 27701 had a rate of 26.4 per 1,000 residents, whereas 27703 had a rate of 8.7.

We then collected data on the health care encounters of individuals living in the four zip codes with high rates of ambulatory care–sensitive conditions. We collected data on the specific diseases that resulted in admissions or emergency department visits, whether patients were self-pay or covered by Medicaid, and the cost of the care provided. We focused on three diseases that were high cost, important to health and function, highly prevalent, and amenable to community-based interventions—diabetes, asthma, and hypertension. Next, we worked with the health department to geomap encounters (emergency and hospital admissions) in Durham for these diseases for self-pay and Medicaid patients. Geomapping involves taking each encounter and pinpointing its location on a map. We found that 75% of the patient encounters for the targeted diseases were in the four zip codes we had identified using small area analysis. The geomapping further identified four "morbidity clusters," very small geographic areas that could be characterized as neighborhoods. When we mapped this out, we also found that these were poor neighborhoods with many of the socio-economic challenges you might expect. We are now doing a community-based intervention program in those four neighborhoods to work on risk reduction and management of the three targeted chronic illnesses.

As we address the management and prevention of chronic illness, we need to consider the commonalities of different illnesses, and examine the interfaces between the biological, environmental, and behavioral sciences. Interventions must target both individuals and populations. Effective delivery of information and reduction of barriers to care make a difference in patient outcomes. Self-management is crucial to positive outcomes, as is self-efficacy. As shifts occur in our management paradigms, we need to learn them well so we can share them with our patients. And we must not forget to care for the most vulnerable. Nursing is at the center of the interdisciplinary team for managing chronic illness. We need to lead.

REFERENCES

Agency for Health Care Policy and Research. (1999). Self-management program helps people with chronic diseases improve their health status and avoid hospitalization. *Research Activities, 225,* 1–2.

Armstrong, E. P. (1996). Monitoring and evaluating disease management: Information requirements. *Clinical Therapeutics, 18*(6), 1327–1233.

Balas, E. A., Jaffrey, F., Kuperman, G. J., Boren, S. A., Brown, G. D., Pinciroli, F. L., & Mitchell, J. A. (1997). Electronic communication with patients: Evaluation of distance medicine technology. *Journal of the American Medical Association, 278*(2), 152–159.

Brunner, L., & Hickey, M. E. (1997). Lovelace health systems episodes of care—a case study. *Best Practices and Benchmarking in Healthcare, 2*(6), 254–257.

Claus, E. B., Schildkraut, J., Iversen, E. S., Berry, D., & Parmigiani, G. (1998). Effect of BRCA1 and BRCA2 on the association between breast cancer risks and family history. *Journal of the National Cancer Institute, 90*(23), 1824–1829.

Eisenberg, L. (1998). The implications of the new genetics for health professional education. *The Chairman's Summary of the Conference,* Josiah Macy Jr. Foundation, 1–5.

Ettinger, W. H., Burns, R., & Messier, S. P. (1997). A randomized trial comparing aerobic exercise and resistance exercise with a health education program in older adults with knee osteoarthritis: The Fitness Arthritis and Seniors Trial. *Journal of the American Medical Association, 277*, 25–31.

Flynn, B. C., Rider, M., & Ray, D. W. (1991). Healthy cities: The Indiana model of community development in public health. *Health Education Quarterly, 18*(3), 331–347.

Gardner, A. W., & Poehlman, E. T. (1995). Exercise rehabilitation programs for the treatment of claudication pain: A meta-analysis. *Journal of the American Medical Association, 274*, 975–980.

Gifford, A. L., Laurent, D. D., Gonzales, V. M., Chesney, M. A., & Lorig, K. R. (1998). Pilot randomized trial of education to improve self-management skills of men with symptomatic HIV/AIDS. *Journal of Acquired Immune Deficiency Syndromes and Human Retrovirology, 18*(2), 136–144.

Klemm, P., Hurst, M., Dearholt, S. L., & Trone, S. R. (1999). Cyber solace: Gender differences on Internet cancer support groups. *Computers in Nursing, 17*(2), 65–72.

Lacasse, Y., Wong, E., Guyatt, G. H., King, D., Cook, D. J., & Goldstein, R. S. (1996). Meta-analysis of respiratory rehabilitation in chronic obstructive pulmonary disease. *Lancet, 348*(9035), 1115–1119.

Langley, P. C. (1996). Assessing the input costs of disease management programs. *Clinical Therapeutics, 18*(6), 1334–1340.

Leng, G. C., Fowler, B., & Ernst, E. (1998). Exercise for intermittent claudication. *Cochrane Database of Systematic Reviews, 4.*

Lipkus, I. M., Rimer, B. K., & Strigo, T. S. (1996). Relationships among objective and subjective risk for breast cancer and mammography stages of change. *Cancer Epidemiology, Biomarkers and Prevention, 5*, 1005–1011.

Longman, A. J., Braden, C. J., & Mishel, M. H. (1997). Pattern of association over time of side-effects burden, self-help, and self-care in women with breast cancer. *Oncology Nursing Forum, 24*(9), 1555–1560.

Millman, M. (Ed.). (1993). *Access to health care in America.* Washington, DC: National Academy Press.

Morgan, G. D., Noll, E. L., Orleans, C. T., Rimer, B. K., Amfoh, K., & Bonney, G. (1996). Reaching midlife and older smokers: Tailored interventions for routine medical care. *Preventive Medicine, 5*(3), 346–354.

Mullen, P. D., Simons-Morton, D. B., Ramirez, G., Frankowski, R. F., Green, L. W., & Mains, D. A. (1997). A meta-analysis of trials evaluating patient education and counseling for three groups of preventive health behaviors. *Patient Education Counseling, 32*, 157–173.

Pyeritz, R. E. (1997). Family history and genetic risk factors: Forward to the future. *Journal of the American Medical Association, 278*(15), 1284–1285.

Prochaska, J. O., & DiClemente, C. C. (1982). Transtheoretical therapy: Toward a more integrative model of change. *Psychotherapy: Theory, Research, and Practice, 19*, 276–288.

Prochaska, J. O., & DiClemente, C. C. (1986). Toward a comprehensive model of change. In W. R. Miller & N. Heather (Eds.), *Treating addictive behaviors: Processes of change* (pp. 3–27). New York: Plenum.

Prochaska, J. O., & DiClemente, C. C. (1992). Stages of change in the modification of problem behaviors. In M. Hersen, R. M. Eisler, & P. E. Miller (Eds.), *Progress in behavior modification* (vol. 28, pp. 184–218). Newbury Park, CA: Sage.

Prochaska, J. O., Velicer, W. F., Rossi, J. S., Goldstein, M. G., Marcus, B. H., Rakowski, W., Fiore, C., Harlow, L. L., Redding, C. A., Rosenbloom, D., & Rossi, S. R. (1994). Stages of change and decisional balance for 12 problem behaviors. *Health Psychology, 13,* 39–46.

Rakowski, W., Ehrich, B., Goldstein, J. G., Rimer, B. K., Pearlman, D. N., Clark, M. A., Velicer, W. F., & Woolverton, H. (1998). Increasing mammography among women aged 40–74 by use of a stage-matched, tailored intervention. *Preventive Medicine, 27,* 748–756.

Rimer, B. K., & Glassman, B. (1998). Tailoring communications for primary care settings. *Methods of Information in Medicine, 37*(2), 171–177.

Roses, A. D. (1998). Apolipoprotein E and Alzheimer's disease: The tip of the susceptibility iceberg. *Annals of the New York Academy of Sciences, 855,* 738–743.

Simons, W. R., Haim, M., Rizzo, J., & Zannad, F. (1996). Effect of improved disease management strategies on hospital length of stay in the treatment of congestive heart failure. *Clinical Therapeutics, 18*(4), 726–746.

Summers, K. H. (1996). Measuring and monitoring outcomes of disease management programs. *Clinical Therapeutics, 18*(6), 1341–1348.

Urden, L. D. (1998). Heart failure collaborative care: An integrated partnership to manage quality and outcomes. *Outcomes Management for Nursing Practice, 2*(2), 64–70.

Venner, G. H., & Seelbinder, J. S. (1996). Team management of congestive heart failure across the continuum. *Journal of Cardiovascular Nursing, 10*(2), 71–84.

Von Korff, M., Moore, J. E., Lorig, K., Cherkin, D. C., Saunders, K., Gonzales, V. M., Laurent, D., Rutter, C., & Comite, F. (1998). A randomized trial of a lay person–led self-management group intervention for back pain patients in primary care. *Spine, 23*(23), 2608–2615.

Part II

PREVENTING CHRONIC ILLNESS

[6]

Identification of High-Risk Adolescents for Interventions to Lower Blood Pressure

Janet C. Meininger, Patricia Liehr, William H. Mueller, and Wenyaw Chan

Hypertension affects 50 million Americans ages 6 and older, but it is not equally distributed among subgroups of the population. The death rate from high blood pressure is approximately four times higher among black Americans than among white Americans (American Heart Association, 1998). Less is known about blood pressure levels among Hispanic Americans, but in general, the data point toward slightly lower blood pressure levels among Hispanic-American adults than among non-Hispanic black and white adults in the United States (Sorel, Ragland, Syme, & Davis, 1992).

The framework used for this study (see Figure 6.1) (Meininger, Liehr, Mueller, Chan, & Chandler, 1998) views prevention from a life span perspective, encompassing primary, secondary, and tertiary prevention (Leavell & Clark, 1965). Primary prevention includes health promotion and protection against environmental factors. Secondary prevention is important once it is determined that an individual is at risk or in the early phases of clinically apparent disease, such as stage 1 hypertension. Tertiary

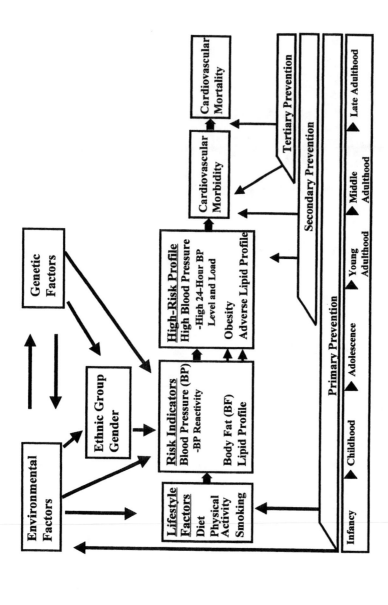

FIGURE 6.1 Emergence of risk for cardiovascular disease: A life span perspective on prevention.

Reprinted with permission from Meininger, J. C, Leihr, P., Mueller, W. H., Chan, W., & Chandler, P. S. (1998). Predictors of ambulatory blood pressure: Identification of high-risk adolescents. *Advances in Nursing Science, 20*(3), 50–64. © 1998, Aspen Publishers, Inc.

prevention is directed toward individuals with clinically diagnosed disease and is aimed toward restoration of functional capabilities, prevention of disability, and prevention of death from cardiovascular disease.

Because the precursors of cardiovascular disease are evident even during childhood and adolescence (Berenson et al., 1998; Sternby, Fernandez-Britlo, & Nordet, 1999; Williams & Wynder, 1993), primary prevention should begin very early in life to prevent the onset of pathological athero-sclerotic or hypertensive processes. Blood pressure increases with age in both boys and girls, but the pattern differs by gender. In boys, a modest increase with growth occurs during middle childhood, and this is followed by a rapid acceleration after age 10. In girls, a steady increase in systolic blood pressure is observed during childhood, but it levels off between 15 and 17 years of age. In general, boys have higher systolic blood pressure than girls throughout adolescence, but there is not a large, clear-cut gender difference in diastolic blood pressure (Rosner, Prineas, Loggie, & Daniels, 1993).

Blood pressure reactivity may be an earlier precursor of hypertension than elevated resting blood pressure levels. Reactivity refers to the magnitude, patterns, and mechanisms of cardiovascular response associated with exposure to stress (Sherwood & Turner, 1992). Several types of psychological stressors have been employed in laboratory protocols to measure reactivity, including video games and serial subtraction. Talking has also been established as a stressor accompanied by blood pressure reactivity in subjects of varying age and health status (Krantz et al., 1991; Matthews & Stoney, 1988; Thomas, Liehr, DeKeyser, & Friedmann, 1993). In several studies, blood pressure increased regardless of speech content, but talking about anger and other personally relevant content was associated with the greatest increases (Ewart & Kolodner, 1991; Siegman, 1993; Thomas et al., 1984).

There is a growing consensus that ambulatory blood pressure monitoring is more representative of the individual's true pressure than individual readings or averages of measurements taken in resting subjects (Monsoor & White, 1994; Perloff, Sokolow, Cowan, & Juster, 1989). There has been limited research on the extent to which blood pressure responses to standardized laboratory protocols predict levels of blood pressure during the course of daily activities, particularly in adolescent samples. However, two studies suggest the utility of examining the ability of blood pressure responses to a laboratory mental stress test to predict ambulatory blood pressure in adolescents. Ewart and Kolodner (1993), who studied 14- and 15-year-old adolescents with blood pressures at the upper end of the distribution (above the 66th percentile), found that their blood pressure responses to a self-disclosure speaking task in the laboratory predicted ambulatory blood pressure. Also, in a study of undergraduate students by

Linden and Con (1994), blood pressure responses to a discussion of recent interpersonal conflict predicted ambulatory blood pressure.

This study focused on blood pressure reactivity in adolescence, a transitional phase during which adult patterns of health behavior are established (Langer & Warheit, 1992), and a pivotal period in the evolution of risk for hypertension and other cardiovascular morbidity. To date, studies of adolescent blood pressure as a predictor of risk for adult hypertension have used resting blood pressure levels as predictors (Lauer & Clarke, 1989). This study investigated the potential of blood pressure reactivity of adolescents as a screening tool. Specifically, the study examined the extent to which blood pressure responses to standardized laboratory protocols predicted blood pressure over 24 hours among male and female adolescents from three ethnic groups: African, European, and Hispanic Americans. We hypothesized that blood pressure levels during laboratory reactivity testing would be better predictors of ambulatory blood pressure levels among adolescents than levels of blood pressure measured at rest using a standard protocol.

METHODS

Setting and Sampling Plan

The target population for the study was African-, European-, and Hispanic-American adolescents, 11 to 16 years old, residing in a large metropolitan city in southeast Texas with an ethnically diverse population. The sample of adolescents was accessed through middle and high schools in a public school district. Stratified sampling was used, taking into consideration chronological age, ethnic group, and gender. Because maturation affects blood pressure and females begin puberty about 2 years earlier than boys, younger girls and older boys were oversampled to ensure that males and females would overlap in terms of biological, rather than chronological, age.

Instruments

Blood Pressure

Three instruments were used to measure blood pressure: a mercury sphygmomanometer (Baumanometer) and stethoscope, and two automatic devices that use an oscillometric technique (Dinamap and Spacelabs monitors). With all three of these instruments, the bladder width of the cuff was 40% to 50% of the upper arm circumference. For auscultatory measurement of blood pressure with the Baumanometer and stethoscope, procedures outlined by the American Heart Association (1987) for measuring resting blood pressure were used after the adolescent had been resting for 5 minutes. The Dinamap (Model 825XT, Critikon, Tampa, FL) was used to record blood pressure during the laboratory protocol. For 24-hour ambulatory blood pressures, a Spacelabs monitor (Model 90207, Spacelabs, Inc., Redlands, WA) was selected because of its reported reliability (James et al., 1988), predictive validity (Parati, Pomidossi, Albini, Malaspina, & Mancia, 1987), and size (12.2 oz with batteries). Although all three instruments are considered valid if appropriate procedures are followed, there are some differences in the measurements. In a previous study that included adolescents, oscillometric systolic blood pressure readings were slightly higher than auscultatory systolic readings, but oscillometric diastolic blood pressure readings were slightly lower than auscultatory diastolic readings (Abcejo, Cardenas, & Leal, 1993).

Physical Activity and Diary Recordings During Ambulatory Monitoring

Because the conditions of blood pressure measurement during ambulatory monitoring are not under control and/or observation, and because blood pressure may be affected by the activity level of the subject at the time of measurement, activity of subjects was measured with a Motionlogger actigraph (Ambulatory Monitoring, Inc., Ardsley, NY). This instrument, which is the size of a large wristwatch, collects and stores data on subject activity as a continuous time series (Mason & Redeker, 1993). It was selected because of strong evidence of reliability and validity (Tryon, 1991). Five readings at 1-minute intervals immediately before each blood pressure reading were averaged and used to control for activity level.

Height and Maturation

Measurement of blood pressure during adolescence is complicated because this is a period of rapid growth and there is considerable variation in the stage of development of adolescents of the same chronological age. Sexual maturation and anthropometric characteristics such as height were measured, therefore, because they are closely linked with the increases in blood pressure that emerge during adolescence. Height was measured with an Accustat (Ross Laboratories) wall-mounted anthropometer. Subjects removed their shoes before this measurement. Tanner (1962) stages were used to rank physical maturation. Each adolescent was assessed by one of three pediatric nurse practitioners who had been trained and tested for interrater reliability with pediatric endocrinologists.

Procedures for Data Collection

Recruitment

Adolescents were recruited in general assemblies or required classes so that groups would not be systematically excluded on the basis of enrollment in particular courses. Those who volunteered to participate were required to have written parent/guardian consent. A Spanish translation of the consent form was available for parents who did not speak or understand English. To encourage completion of the study by those who agreed to participate, students who completed all components of the protocol including 24-hour blood pressure monitoring were reimbursed $30.

After signed parental consent was received, each adolescent was scheduled to complete the protocol within a 1- to 2-week period. Students were not removed from more than one class period per day to participate in the study. Laboratory testing and the physical exam were conducted on different days and were usually completed prior to the ambulatory monitoring; however, the order of data collection was not completely standardized because of student absences, holidays, exams, and other scheduling complications.

Laboratory Testing

The "laboratory" was a private, quiet room in the school where interruptions were unlikely to occur. The reactivity testing (also referred to as the laboratory protocol) was conducted in this room by a trained data collector. The participant was seated in a comfortable chair and was fitted with a Dinamap cuff of the appropriate size. The 26-minute protocol consisted of 6 minutes of resting followed by two counterbalanced series of 4 minutes of quiet, 2 minutes of talking, and 4 minutes of quiet. During one series the adolescent talked about a usual day (neutral talking); in the other series the subject talked about an anger-provoking situation (angry talking). Blood pressure was taken every 2 minutes throughout the 26-minute protocol except during talking, when it was taken every minute. Talking segments were conducted in English and audiotaped. The angry and neutral talking segments were randomly ordered and crossed over for each subject.

Participants were grouped in three categories of blood pressure reactor status on the basis of blood pressure recordings during the talking segments of the laboratory session. Separate classifications were made for systolic and diastolic blood pressures and for male and female subjects. Subjects were classified as consistently high reactors if they were in the highest quartile of the distribution of blood pressure for their same-sex counterparts during angry and neutral talking. Consistently low reactors were those in the lowest quartile of the distribution of blood pressure during angry and neutral talking. All other subjects were classified as mixed reactors.

Ambulatory Monitoring

Blood pressure was monitored for 24 hours using the Spacelabs ambulatory equipment with simultaneous monitoring by the actigraph. The participant was fitted with the appropriately sized cuff and Motionlogger on the non-dominant arm and wrist. The ambulatory blood pressure monitor was calibrated against a mercury sphygmomanometer, and blood pressure and activity monitors were synchronized. Participants were instructed to wear the monitor throughout the 24-hour period except during bathing and to keep their arms still when the blood pressure cuff automatically inflated every 30 minutes.

Reactor status variables were examined in relation to daytime ambulatory blood pressure load. Blood pressure load was defined as the percent of ambulatory blood pressure readings over a level considered hypertensive. Because there are no normative data for ambulatory blood pressure readings, the 95th percentile of resting blood pressure for age, gender, and percentile of height (National High Blood Pressure Education Program Working Group on Hypertension Control in Children and Adolescents, 1996) was used as the cut point for calculating blood pressure load.

Physical Exam

Nurse practitioners trained in this protocol conducted physical exams in the school setting to collect data on maturation, height, and resting blood pressure. Resting blood pressures were taken after the subject had been sitting quietly for 5 minutes. Two readings were averaged for the analysis.

RESULTS

The sample consisted of 383 adolescents from 11 to 16 years old. Data on 10 adolescents who classified their ethnic group as "other" were excluded, resulting in a sample size of 373. There was a slight preponderance of females (53.5%). There were proportionately more African-American respondents (37.5%) than European Americans (31.1%) or Hispanic Americans (31.4%).

Means for blood pressure measured during the physical exam, during the ambulatory monitoring, and during laboratory testing are shown by gender in Table 6.1. Blood pressures taken during the physical exam were compared with normative values. Seven adolescents, six boys and one girl, had systolic blood pressure over the 95th percentile for age and height. Four were Hispanic Americans, and three were European Americans. Five adolescents, two boys and three girls, were above the 95th percentile for diastolic blood pressure. Four of these were African Americans, and one was Hispanic American. As expected, ambulatory blood pressures were higher than blood pressures taken during the physical exam.

Laboratory baseline blood pressures were slightly lower than blood pressures taken during the physical exam. This may have been due to differences in the method of measuring blood pressure (auscultatory in the physical exam and oscillometric measurement during the laboratory protocol), the longer period of sitting during the laboratory protocol, or a "white coat" effect on blood pressures taken as part of the physical exam. Talking is associated with an increase in blood pressure, and talking about an anger-provoking situation elicited higher blood pressures than talking about a usual day.

High reactors comprised 17% of the sample for both systolic blood pressure (SBP) and diastolic blood pressure (DBP). Those who responded as low reactors during the laboratory protocol comprised 14.6% of the sample for SBP and 18.5% for DBP.

TABLE 6.1 Descriptive Statistics for Systolic and Diastolic Blood Pressure (mm Hg)

				Laboratory		
	(n)	Physical Exam	Ambulatory	Baseline	Talking Neutral	Talking Anger
Systolic BP						
Males	(171)	108.97	119.40	107.73	112.53	115.58
Females	(202)	104.75	115.91	103.02	107.65	111.27
Diastolic BP						
Males	(171)	61.97	68.68	59.42	65.78	68.38
Females	(202)	61.96	68.71	58.79	64.99	67.73

Mixed-effects analysis for repeated measures data (Laird & Ware, 1982) was applied with ambulatory SBP and DBP analyzed separately as the dependent variables. Complete data were available on 371 subjects for this analysis. The use of a two-stage model with each participant as the unit of analysis ($n = 371$) and each measurement of ambulatory SBP or DBP as the subunit ($n = 16,171$) provided a means to effectively deal with the lack of statistical independence of multiple measurements on the same individual. The independent variables were gender, ethnic group, blood pressure measured during the physical exam, and blood pressure reactor status during laboratory testing (high, low, mixed). To control for anthropometric differences related to blood pressure, the subject's height was included in each analysis. Five groups of Tanner stages were included in the analysis as four dummy variables. To control for level of subject activity, activity measurements recorded every minute for 5 minutes before each measurement of ambulatory blood pressure were averaged and used for this analysis.

The SBP reactor status variables were significant predictors ($p < .0001$) of 24-hour ambulatory blood pressure controlling for height, Tanner stage, activity, gender, and blood pressure measured during the physical exam. High SBP reactors had 24-hour ambulatory SBP 3.48 mm Hg higher than low reactors. Mixed SBP reactors had 24-hour SBP 2.48 mm Hg higher than low SPB reactors. Height, Tanner stage, and activity were significantly related to 24-hour ambulatory SBP. Boys had SBP 1.82 mm Hg higher than females ($p = .0001$); African Americans had significantly higher SBP than European Americans (1.39 mm Hg higher, $p = .001$). Hispanic Americans had lower 24-hour SBP than European Americans, but the difference was not significant.

For 24-hour DBP, the DBP reactor status variables were statistically significant. High DBP reactors had higher 24-hour ambulatory DBP (2.65 mm Hg, $p < .001$) than low reactors. Mixed DBP reactors had 24-hour ambulatory blood pressure 1.37 mm Hg higher than low reactors ($p = .002$). Height, Tanner stage, and gender were not significantly related to 24-hour DBP. The African-American group had higher 24-hour DBP than the European-American group (1.36 mm Hg, $p = .0004$), but the Hispanic-American group did not differ significantly from the European-American group.

To evaluate the validity of the laboratory protocol as an indicator of ambulatory blood pressure, the reactor status variables were examined in relation to daytime ambulatory blood pressure load. The percentage of SBP readings during the daytime that were above the 95th percentile of resting blood pressure for age, height, and gender are presented in Figure 6.2. Blood pressure load was defined as the percent of ambulatory blood pressure readings over the 95th percentile of the norms. Low reactors clustered at low levels of blood pressure load. High and mixed reactors

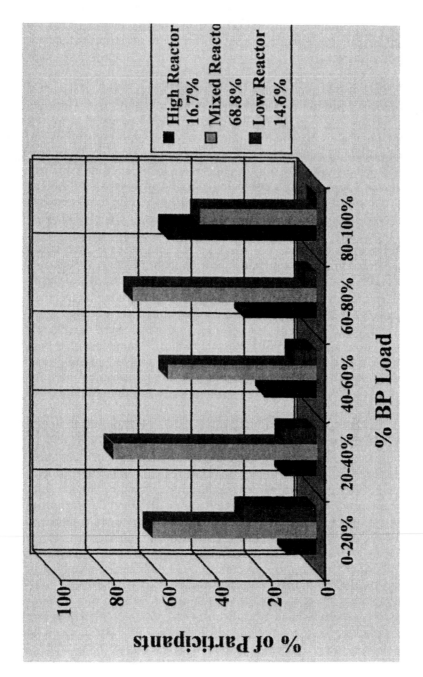

FIGURE 6.2 Distribution of systolic blood pressure (SBP) reactor status by levels of SBP load.

were more prevalent than low reactors at the highest levels of blood pressure load.

DISCUSSION

In multivariable analysis, African-American adolescents had higher levels of ambulatory blood pressure than European- and Hispanic-American adolescents, and males had significantly higher ambulatory systolic blood pressure than females. However, because height, maturation, and activity are closely linked with blood pressure in adolescents, it is extremely important to control for these effects in making inferences about gender and ethnic group differences in blood pressure.

As hypothesized, there was a significant relationship between blood pressures measured while talking during a laboratory session and blood pressures observed by 24-hour ambulatory monitoring as adolescents went about their usual activities. The effect was greater for systolic than diastolic blood pressure. High and mixed reactors in the laboratory had higher levels of 24-hour blood pressure and higher blood pressure load during the daytime. The fact that this association was evident in multivariate analyses that controlled for resting blood pressure, as well as activity, height, maturation, gender, and ethnic group, underlines its importance. A limitation of the study was that blood pressures taken during the laboratory protocol may have been better predictors of ambulatory blood pressure than resting blood pressures because of differences in instrumentation. Blood pressures during the physical exam were auscultatory measurements, whereas those taken during the laboratory protocol and ambulatory monitoring used oscillometric devices.

These results confirm the results of an earlier pilot study (Meininger et al., 1998) and are consistent with those of Ewart and Kolodner (1993), who studied African- and European-American adolescents in the same age group who had high blood pressure. They are also similar to the findings of Linden and Con (1994), who studied European- and Asian-American male and female undergraduates. When considered in conjunction with previous studies, the findings of the present study provide further evidence that blood pressure measured during laboratory tasks that require talking may be useful as a screening device to identify adolescents with high blood pressure. High and mixed SBP reactors were more prevalent than low reactors at the highest levels of SBP load. Low SBP reactors in the laboratory had ambulatory blood pressure readings that were clustered at very low levels of SBP load. Further study will be necessary to quantify the sensitivity and specificity of the laboratory protocol as an indicator of high blood pressure.

The study confirms the central importance of height as a predictor of blood pressure. When interpreting the blood pressure of a child or adolescent, it is essential to relate the individual's blood pressure to norms for that individual's percentile of height for age and gender (National High Blood Pressure Education Program Working Group on Hypertension Control in Children and Adolescents, 1996); guidelines are accessible through the National Heart, Lung and Blood Institute Web site (http://www.nhlbi.nih.gov/nhlbi/cardio/hbp/prof/hbp_ped.htm). Because blood pressure increases with height, tall children are likely to be misclassified as hypertensive, and hypertension in short children is likely to be missed unless blood pressure norms for percentile of height are used. A child's or adolescent's height percentile is determined from a standard growth chart. The measured blood pressure is compared with the 90th and 95th percentile of blood pressure in the gender-specific table for that individual's age and height. If blood pressure is below the 90th percentile, the child or adolescent is considered normotensive; between the 90th and 95th percentile the blood pressure is considered high-normal; if blood pressure (systolic or diastolic) is at or above the 95th percentile, the individual may be hypertensive.

Elevated blood pressure must be confirmed on repeated visits before characterizing an adolescent as hypertensive. Blood pressure is a dynamic rather than a static indicator, fluctuating from moment to moment and day to day in response to environmental stimuli, physical exertion, and mental stress (Thomas et al., 1993). For this reason, children and adolescents are not classified as hypertensive unless their systolic and/or diastolic blood pressure readings are at or above the 95th percentile on three separate occasions.

While ambulatory blood pressure monitoring is useful for understanding the dynamic nature of blood pressure, it is an impractical method in terms of time and expense (Liehr, Meininger, Mueller, Chandler, & Chan, 1997). The laboratory protocol using a Dinamap to measure blood pressure while adolescents talk may be a more feasible screening procedure. That is, blood pressure changes during talking may serve as a marker for those who have high blood pressure load during 24-hour ambulatory monitoring. Further work is needed to test the reliability and validity of this approach for screening large samples of adolescents.

ACKNOWLEDGMENTS

This research was funded by the National Institute of Nursing Research, NIH grant #'s R55 NR03052 and R01 NR03052.

REFERENCES

Abcejo, S. N., Cardenas, M. F., & Leal, M. A. (1993). *The relationship between physical activity and blood pressure measured by two indirect methods in adolescents and their parents.* Unpublished master's research project, The University of Texas-Houston Health Science Center, Houston.

American Heart Association. (1987). *Recommendations for human blood pressure determination by sphygmomanometers.* Dallas: Author.

American Heart Association. (1998). *1999 heart and stroke statistical update.* Dallas, TX.

Berenson, G. S., Srinivasan, S. R., Bao, W., Newman, W. P. I., Tracy, R. E., & Wattigney, W. A. (1998). Association between multiple cardiovascular risk factors and atherosclerosis in children and young adults. *New England Journal of Medicine, 338,* 1650–1656.

Ewart, C. K., & Kolodner, K. B. (1991). Social competence interview for assessing physiological reactivity in adolescents. *Psychosomatic Medicine, 53,* 289–304.

Ewart, C. K., & Kolodner, K. B. (1993). Predicting ambulatory blood pressure during school: Effectiveness of social and non-social reactivity tasks in black and white adolescents. *Psychophysiology, 30,* 30–38.

James, G. D., Pickering, T. G., Yee, L. S., Harshfield, G. A., Riva, S., & Laragh, J. H. (1988). The reproducibility of average ambulatory, home, and clinic pressures. *Hypertension, 11,* 545–549.

Krantz, D. S., Helmers, K. F., Bairey, C. N., Nebel, L. E., Hedges, S. M., & Rozanski, A. (1991). Cardiovascular reactivity and mental stress–induced myocardial ischemia in patients with coronary artery disease. *Psychosomatic Medicine, 53,* 1–12.

Laird, N. M., & Ware, J. H. (1982). Random effects models for longitudinal data. *Biometrics, 34,* 963–974.

Langer, L. M., & Warheit, G. J. (1992). The Pre-Adult Health Decision-Making Model: Linking decision-making directedness/orientation to adolescent health-related attitudes and behaviors. *Adolescence, 27,* 919–994.

Lauer, R. M., & Clarke, W. R. (1989). Childhood risk factors for high adult blood pressure: The Muscatine Study. *Pediatrics, 84,* 633–641.

Leavell, H. R., & Clark, E. G. (1965). *Preventive medicine for the doctor in his community, an epidemiologic approach.* New York: McGraw-Hill.

Liehr, P., Meininger, J. C., Mueller, W., Chandler, P. S., & Chan, W. (1997). Blood pressure reactivity in urban youth during angry and normal talking. *Journal of Cardiovascular Nursing, 11*(4), 84–94.

Linden, W., & Con, A. (1994). Laboratory reactivity models as predictors of ambulatory blood pressure and heart rate. *Journal of Psychosomatic Research, 38,* 217–228.

Mason, D. J., & Redeker, N. (1993). Measurement of activity. *Nursing Research, 42,* 87–92.

Matthews, K. A., & Stoney, C. M. (1988). Influence of sex and age on cardiovascular responses during stress. *Psychosomatic Medicine, 50,* 46–56.

Meininger, J. C., Liehr, P., Mueller, W. H., Chan, W., & Chandler, P. S. (1998). Predictors of ambulatory blood pressure: Identification of high-risk adolescents. *Advances in Nursing Science, 20*(3), 50–64.

Monsoor, G. A., & White, W. B. (1994). Ambulatory blood pressure and cardiovascular risk stratification. *Journal of Vascular Medicine and Biology, 5,* 61–68.

National High Blood Pressure Education Program Working Group on Hypertension Control in Children and Adolescents. (1996). Update on the 1987 task force report on high blood pressure in children and adolescents: A working group report from the National High Blood Pressure Education Program. *Pediatrics, 98,* 649–658.

Parati, G., Pomidossi, G., Albini, F., Malaspina, D., & Mancia, G. (1987). Relationship of 24-hour blood pressure mean and variability to severity of target-organ damage in hypertension. *Journal of Hypertension, 5,* 93–98.

Perloff, D., Sokolow, M., Cowan, R. M., & Juster, R. P. (1989). The prognostic value of ambulatory blood pressure measurements: Further analysis. *Journal of Hypertension, 7*(Suppl. 3), S3–10.

Rosner, B., Prineas, R. J., Loggie, J. M. H., & Daniels, S. R. (1993). Blood pressure nomograms for children and adolescents, by height, sex, and age, in the United States. *Journal of Pediatrics, 123,* 871–886.

Sherwood, A., & Turner, J. R. (1992). Individual differences in cardiovascular response to stress. In J. R. Turner, A. Sherwood, & K. C. Light (Eds.), *A conceptual and methodological overview of cardiovascular reactivity research.* New York: Plenum, 3–32.

Siegman, A. W. (1993). Cardiovascular consequences of expressing, experiencing, and repressing anger. *Journal of Behavioral Medicine, 16,* 539–569.

Sorel, J. E., Ragland, D. R., Syme, S. L., & Davis, W. B. (1992). Educational status and blood pressure: The Second National Health and Nutrition Examination Survey 1976–1980 and the Hispanic Health and Nutrition Examination Survey 1982–1984. *American Journal of Epidemiology, 135,* 1339–1348.

Sternby, N. H., Fernandez-Britlo, J. E., & Nordet, P. (1999). Pathobiological determinants of atherosclerosis in youth (PBDAY Study) 1986–96. *Bulletin of the World Health Organization, 77*(3), 250–257.

Tanner, J. M. (1962). *Growth at adolescence.* London: Blackwell.

Thomas, S. A., Liehr, P., DeKeyser, F., & Friedmann, G. (1993). Nursing blood pressure research. 1980–1990: A bio-psychosocial perspective. *Image: Journal of Nursing Scholarship, 25,* 157–164.

Thomas, S. A., Lynch, J. J., Friedmann, E., Suginohara, M., Hall, P. S., & Peterson, C. (1984). Blood pressure and heart rate changes in children when they read aloud in school. *Public Health Report, 99,* 77–84.

Tryon, W. (1991). *Activity measurement in psychology and medicine.* New York: Plenum.

Williams, C., & Wynder, E. (1993). A child health report card 1992. *Preventive Medicine, 22*(4), 604–628.

[7]

School-Based Interventions to Improve the Health of Children with Multiple Cardiovascular Risk Factors

Joanne S. Harrell, Stuart A. Gansky, Robert G. McMurray, Shrikant I. Bangdiwala, Annette C. Frauman, and Chyrise B. Bradley

Many studies have shown that risk factors for cardiovascular disease (CVD), particularly high cholesterol, hypertension, physical inactivity, and obesity, are present in children and adolescents, and these tend to remain risk factors through adulthood (Dennison, Straus, Mellits, & Charney, 1988; Enos & Beyer, 1955; McNamara, Molot, Stremple, & Cutting, 1971; Raitakari, Porkka, Rasanen, Ronnemaa, & Viikari, 1994; Tracy, Newman, Wattigney, & Berenson, 1995; Wissler & PDAY Research Group, 1995). Although there is general agreement on the need to reduce these risk factors and increase physical activity in children, we do not know the best way to deliver such health-promoting interventions to this population. Should interventions be given only to children who are at greatest risk for future heart disease, or should they be given to all children, given the wide prevalence of CVD?

To date, no studies have systematically compared the effects of a population-based intervention to the effects of a risk-based intervention on children with multiple CVD risk factors. The study reported here compared a risk-based, individualized program given only to children with at least two identified risk factors and a classroom-based intervention received by all children. We examine here the effects on a subset of children in the classroom intervention who had the same risk factors as those receiving the risk-based intervention. A control group was composed of children with similar risk factor profiles who received their usual health and physical education curriculum.

METHODS

Setting and Sample

This study was part of a larger study, the Cardiovascular Health In Children (CHIC) study, which was conducted in 18 schools or school clusters in North Carolina. Study schools were randomly selected from 33 rural and urban schools that agreed to participate. Three school clusters were randomly selected within each of six strata or blocks (defined by the three state geographic regions and rural or urban setting) and randomized to one of the two intervention groups or to the control group.

Subject inclusion criteria for the CHIC study included assignment to the third or fourth grade regardless of age; ability to read and write English; no mental, emotional, or physical handicap identified by parents or teachers; no chronic illness such as diabetes or moderate to severe asthma reported by parents, teachers, or child; and ability to participate in an exercise program. Most (60.4%) of the third and fourth graders in the 18 study schools participated in the study.

An additional inclusion criterion for the study reported here was the presence of low aerobic power (an analog for physical inactivity) and at least one of the following CVD risk factors: high cholesterol or obesity. Children were classified as physically inactive based on standards by gender and age for predicted aerobic power (pVO_2max) results (Shvartz & Reibold, 1990). Children were deemed hypercholesterolemic if they had a total cholesterol over the 75th percentile for age and sex using Lipid Research Clinic (LRC) standards (National Institutes of Health, 1980). Children were classified as obese if they had both a body mass index (BMI) and a sum of triceps and subscapular skinfolds over the 90th percentile for age and gender (National Institutes of Health, 1980; Johnston, Hamill, & Lemeshow, 1972). The study included only those children who had the combination of obesity and low fitness, or high cholesterol and low fitness, or all three.

Interventions

The classroom-based intervention was taught to all third and fourth graders in the schools randomly assigned to that intervention. Regular classroom teachers used the American Heart Association (AHA) Lower and Upper Elementary School Site Program Kits (American Heart Association, 1989) to provide instruction twice a week for 8 weeks. Content included information about selecting "heart healthy" foods, the importance of getting regular physical exercise, the dangers of smoking, and ways to combat pressure to smoke. In addition, children received a modified physical education (PE) program three times a week, taught by physical educators using lesson plans compiled by the exercise physiologist coinvestigator and derived from standard PE curriculum texts. Aerobic activities included jumping rope to music, endless relay, parachute games, and aerobic dance.

The children in schools assigned to the risk-based intervention received an intervention only if they were found at baseline to have at least two of the three CVD risk factors described. Two risk-based interventions were used: (1) physical activity classes, given to those at risk due to low aerobic capacity (all children reported herein); and (2) nutrition classes, given to those at risk due to elevated cholesterol levels and/or obesity. All interventions for the risk-based groups were conducted in groups of five to eight children, over 8 weeks, during regular school hours. The physical activity intervention was taught three times a week by physical educators, using the same activities as those in the classroom-based intervention, but involving only five to eight at-risk children at a time. The nutrition classes were taught by registered nurses twice a week. Children in the control group schools did not receive any intervention but had their regular health and PE classes.

Variables and Their Measurement

The primary outcome variables were health status, health behaviors, and health knowledge. In addition, selected family influences (parental education and smoking) and child developmental/personal characteristics (age, grade, race, and sex) from the Bruhn and Parcel (1982) Development of Positive Health Behavior model were measured as potential explanatory variables.

Health Status Outcomes

Health status measurements were taken by a team of trained research assistants (RAs) following standardized training and interrater reliability testing. Blood pressure (BP) was measured on the right arm using a Bauma-nometer mercury sphygmomanometer and appropriately sized cuffs according to AHA recommendations for children (Frohlich et al., 1988). Total serum cholesterol was measured nonfasting with the Reflotron (Boehringer Mannheim Diagnostics), using rigorous internal and external quality control procedures. Predicted aerobic power (pVO_2max) was determined using a Bodyguard Professional Cycle Ergometer (ÆGLÆND DBS A.S.) and a 6-minute, three-stage cycle test (the Eurofit protocol) for children (Klissouras & Tokmakidis, 1982). Polar Pacer heart rate monitors (Computer Corp.) were used to obtain heart rates continuously during the cycle test. Triceps and subscapular skinfolds were measured in mm on the right side of the body using Lange skinfold calipers (Cambridge Scientific). The skinfold sites were measured according to NHANES procedures (Najjar & Rowland, 1987). Weight was measured to the nearest 0.1 kg using a calibrated balance beam scale (Detecto Scales, Inc.), and height was measured to the nearest 0.1 cm using a stadiometer (Perspective Enterprises). Both measurements were taken with children clothed but shoeless. Body mass index (BMI) was calculated as weight divided by squared height (kg/m^2).

Health Behaviors

Health behaviors were physical activity (PA) and eating habits. To obtain a PA score, the children filled out a revised form of the Know Your Body Health Habits Survey (Williams, Carter, & Eng, 1980). To assess eating habits, children were given a short list of high- and low-fat foods and asked to circle how often they ate each one (not much, some, or a lot).

Health Knowledge

Health knowledge was assessed only at posttest, using an adaptation of the Heart Smart knowledge questionnaire (Oaks, Warren, & Harsha, 1987). We added five questions about the dangers of smoking and eliminated some of the original general questions about the cardiovascular system. Thus, the Healthy Heart Knowledge test was a 25-item, multiple-choice questionnaire covering nutrition, exercise, smoking, and general heart health.

Parental education, used as an indication of family socioeconomic status, was determined from parents' questionnaires. The highest grade the father had completed in school was used unless it was unavailable; then the mother's was used. Parental smoking items were included on parents' questionnaires.

Data Collection Procedures

After we obtained written parental consent and child assent, we collected baseline data from the children at their respective schools. Parental data were collected via mailed questionnaires. The intervention began after baseline testing; posttest data were collected in the same school order within 2 weeks of completion of the 8-week intervention.

A team of trained RAs administered the questionnaires to children in groups of 10 to 25. One to three days after administration of the question-naires, physiologic data were collected in empty classrooms, gyms, or media rooms; each measure was done at a separate "station." All variables were measured in the same sequence for each child. After completing the assess-ments, each child received a small prize. Baseline and posttest procedures were identical, and all measures were taken by the same team of RAs. Parents of children in the two intervention groups and in the control group received a written report of their child's physical testing results about 4 weeks after each test.

Statistical Methods

Two separate multivariate analyses assessed the short-range intervention effects. One analysis examined changes in health status variables, and the other looked at changes in health behaviors and postintervention health knowledge. Since significant overall effects were found for both of these, intervention effects were then examined for each outcome variable. To control for initial differences between groups that could either mask or inflate the actual intervention effects, each of these analyses was statistically adjusted for the study design (region and locale within region), for poten-tially significant demographic factors (gender, race, parental education, and age at pretest) and for the pretest value of the outcome variable.

RESULTS

Subjects in this study were 422 children (20% of the total group of 2,109 CHIC subjects) who, at baseline, had low aerobic power and either high total cholesterol or obesity. There were 164 children in the risk-based group, 108 in the classroom-based group, and 150 in the control group. The ages of the children ranged from 8 to 11, with a mean age of 9.0 years at pretest and 9.3 at posttest. Age, gender, grade, and level of parental education did not vary significantly by intervention group. However, there were significantly fewer white subjects in the control group than in the two intervention groups ($p = .047$).

At baseline, cholesterol ranged from 103 to 264 mg/dl; means for the three groups were between 178.4 and 181.6 mg/dl. Mean BMI values for the three groups ranged from 22.9 to 23.5 kg/m², and mean blood pressure was approximately 110/70 mmHg, with mean weight ranging from 45.0 to 46.4 kg and height from 139.6 to 140.3 cm. As expected given the inclusion criteria, aerobic power was low in all groups, with group means ranging from 29.6 to 30.6 ml/kg/min.

Changes after the Interventions

Figure 7.1 shows the unadjusted changes for each of the three groups, with a brief summary of the results of the adjusted statistical analyses. Each intervention group was first compared to the control group (using Dunnett's test $\alpha = .05$), then the two intervention groups were compared.

Health Status Outcomes

Cholesterol

The raw, unadjusted changes in cholesterol were marked: Cholesterol decreased 10.1 mg/dl in the risk-based intervention group, 11.7 in the classroom based intervention group, and 2.4 in the control group. Following the intervention, cholesterol was 7.7 mg/dl lower in the risk-based intervention group than in the control group, and it was 9.3 mg/dl lower in the classroom-based group than in the control group (see Figure 7.1). When adjusted for demographic variables and baseline values, the values for both intervention groups differed significantly from the controls, although there was no significant difference between the two intervention groups. Thus, the two interventions worked about equally well.

Systolic Blood Pressure (SBP)

The expected growth-related increase in systolic blood pressure differed among the three groups. Unadjusted changes were 2.9 mmHg (classroom-based), 3.3 mmHg (risk-based group), and 5.3 mmHg (control group). The adjusted change in the classroom-based intervention group was 1.95 mmHg less than in the control group, but this was not significant. However, the adjusted change in the risk-based intervention group was 2.41 mmHg

Changes in Total Cholesterol

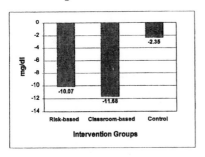

Note: Both intervention groups were significantly different from control ($p < .05$), but not different from each other ($p = .913$)

Changes in Systolic BP

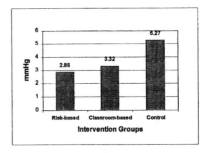

Note: Only the risk-based group was significantly different from control ($p < .05$), the two intervention groups were not significantly different from each other ($p = .371$)

Changes in Aerobic Power

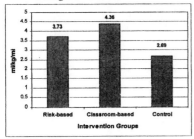

Note: Only the classroom-based group was significantly different from control ($p < .05$), the two intervention groups were not significantly different from each other ($p = .654$)

Changes in Skinfolds

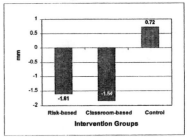

Note: Both intervention groups were significantly different from control ($p < .05$), but not different from each other ($p = .775$)

FIGURE 7.1 Changes in health status outcomes after the interventions.

less than in the controls, which was statistically significant. The adjusted difference between the two intervention groups (classroom-based and risk-based) was not significant (see Figure 7.1).

Diastolic Blood Pressure (DBP)

Unadjusted differences in DBP were 5.0 mmHg (risk-based group), 4.8 mmHg (classroom-based group), and 7.2 mmHg (control group). Mean

DBP rose more in the control group than in either intervention group, but these differences were not significant.

Other Physiologic Variables

Aerobic power (pVO$_2$max) increased in all three groups (3.7 mg/kg/min for risk-based group, 4.4 for classroom-based group, and 2.7 for control group). Adjusted pVO$_2$max was significantly higher for those in the classroom-based group (1.67 ml/kg/min higher) than for the controls. There were also small changes in skinfolds; adjusted skinfolds were significantly lower in both intervention groups than in the control group.

Health Behaviors and Knowledge

Physical Activity

Raw changes in physical activity (PA) showed an increase for each intervention group (0.4 units for classroom-based and 6.4 units for risk-based) and a decrease for the control group (−1.0). However, adjusted PA scores did not differ significantly between intervention and control groups. Differences among the three groups in eating a high-fat diet were also nonsignificant.

Knowledge

Unadjusted total knowledge scores at posttest were 64% correct for the risk-based group, 68% for the classroom-based group, and 60% for the control group. The adjusted mean percent correct was significantly higher in both the risk-based group and the classroom-based group than in the control group.

DISCUSSION

Significant improvements were observed in some risk factors in this school-based study of interventions for children with multiple risk factors for CVD. Both the risk-based and the classroom-based interventions produced large decreases in total serum cholesterol (−10.1 mg/dl and −11.7 mg/dl, respectively), whereas the control group had only a −2.5 mg/dl change. Also, SBP increased less in the risk-based intervention group than in the control group. Further, there was a significantly greater increase in aerobic power (pVO$_2$ max) in the classroom-based intervention group than in the controls, and there were significant decreases in skinfolds in both intervention groups.

Posttest health knowledge was significantly higher in both intervention groups than in the control group. Of course, because health knowledge was measured only at posttest, it could be argued that the difference between the groups existed at baseline. However, because the children were such young readers, we elected not to overburden them with questionnaires at the pretest.

The large drop in total cholesterol in both intervention groups after the brief, 8-week intervention is very encouraging. The effects of the intervention were stronger than the Dietary Intervention Study in Children (DISC), which used an intense nutrition intervention with children with high cholesterol (DISC, 1995); this suggests that physical activity should be part of interventions to reduce cholesterol.

Our intervention produced only small reductions in body fat and no change in BMI, perhaps because of the short duration of the intervention. Our team of examiners received standardized training on height, weight, skinfolds, and blood pressure measurements prior to data collection, and the same team conducted both baseline and posttesting. In addition, they were subjected to repeated interrater reliability testing and differences between raters were minimal, so examiner technique is not likely to have been a confounding factor.

Epstein, Coleman, and Myers (1996) say that their studies indicate that efforts to reduce obesity in children are more successful if there is direct involvement of at least one parent, if physical activity is part of the program, and if there is family and friend support. Our interventions included physical activity, but they did not involve parents. In addition, we did nothing to manipulate diet other than provide information to the child about wise food choices. Because children usually do not have much control over what food is purchased or prepared in the household, this may have been a factor in the rather small change observed in body fat. Also, as noted above, the intervention may not have been long enough to produce a large decrease in obesity. Because we wanted to be sure we targeted truly overfat children, we incorporated skinfold measurements with BMI measurements and used a strict definition of obesity. Although our definition was stringent, we still found approximately 26% of our overall sample to be obese (Harrell et al., 1996). The fact that the interventions did not strongly affect these obese subjects is most likely a result of several factors in combination, but particularly the lack of parental involvement.

SBP rose more in the control subjects than in the other two groups, with the greatest differences between the risk-based intervention children and the control children. Diastolic pressure rose more than SBP. There were no significant differences in DBP. It is possible that we might have seen greater effects on BP, especially DBP, had the interventions been longer.

Very few other studies have compared a population approach to a high-risk approach to promote cardiovascular health in either adults or children. Interventions for high-risk groups of children and adolescents are familiar to nurses and physicians, are relatively easy for them to incorporate into their practice (Lawrence, Arbeit, Johnson, & Berenson, 1991), and can be useful in working with high-risk families (Johnson et al., 1991). They have been shown to be effective in dealing with small groups of children with obesity (Epstein et al., 1996; Haddock, Shadish, Klesges, & Stein, 1994), high blood pressure (Hansen, Froberg, Hyldebrandt, & Nielsen, 1991), and hyperlipidemia (DISC, 1995). However, studies have shown that pediatricians and family practice physicians do not routinely assess family history for CVD and seldom emphasize CVD risk factors in their routine practice with children and adolescents (Arneson, Luepker, Pirie, & Sinaiko, 1992; Jennings & Leon, 1992).

We have shown that both a risk-based intervention and a population-based intervention can produce improvements in the CVD risk profile of children with multiple risk factors. Although both approaches appeared to work, they were not equally feasible. In practical terms, the risk-based intervention was much more difficult to incorporate into the school day, required hiring additional nurses to teach the children, and thus used more resources.

The relatively inexpensive population or classroom-based intervention was as effective in improving the CVD risk profiles of children with multiple CVD risk factors as the more intensive, risk-based intervention. The classroom-based approach was easier to implement and it fit logically into the school curriculum. Also, it avoided stigmatization of at-risk children, used positive peer pressure, and avoided the potential problem of misclassifying children at risk. It had the added advantage of providing benefits to children from all risk groups, even those at low risk (Harrell et al., 1996).

The findings of this study are consistent with the recent study of Tosteson and colleagues (1997), who concluded that population-based programs can lengthen life and save resources, and who recommend that "population-wide programs should be a part of any national health strategy to reduce coronary heart disease" (p. 24). The classroom-based (population) strategy presented here should be used more widely, and its potential for primary prevention of CVD in adulthood tested further.

This school-based approach can be strongly advocated by nurses in a variety of settings. School nurses can present the intervention to school authorities and strongly suggest adoption of the program. Pediatric nurses can recommend such a program both to parents and to schools. Finally, nurses who work in critical care or coronary care units or in cardiac rehabilitation settings can talk with patients about the need to initiate heart-healthy habits in their children and grandchildren. All of these nurses can suggest that parents contact their local school boards and principals to request a program that incorporates regular, fun aerobic activities at least three times a week, and a related knowledge/attitude program. If a program similar to ours were adopted in many settings, we could expect to see a significant reduction in CVD risk factors in children.

ACKNOWLEDGMENTS

This work was supported by federal grant R01 NR01837 from the National Institute of Nursing Research, National Institutes of Health. Adapted from Harrell, J. S., Gansky, S. A., McMurray, R. G., Bangdiwala, S. I., Frauman, A. C., and Bradley, C. B. (1998). School-based interventions improve heart health in children with multiple cardiovascular disease risk factors. *Pediatrics* vol. 102, 371–380. Printed with permission.

REFERENCES

American Heart Association. (1989). *The AHA Schoolsite Program: Heart decisions elementary school package technical report.* Dallas: Author.

Arneson, T., Luepker, R., Pirie, P., & Sinaiko, A. (1992). Cholesterol screening by primary care pediatricians: A study of attitudes and practices in Minneapolis–St. Paul metropolitan area. *Pediatrics, 89,* 502–505.

Bruhn, J., & Parcel, G. (1982). Current knowledge about the health behavior of young children: A conference summary. *Health Education Quarterly, 9*(2, 3), 142–166.

Dennison, B. A., Straus, J. H., Mellits, E. D., & Charney, E. (1988). Childhood physical fitness tests: Predictor of adult physical activity levels. *Pediatrics, 82*(3), 324–330.

Dietary Intervention Study in Children (DISC). (1995). Efficacy and safety of lowering dietary intake of fat and cholesterol in children with elevated low-density lipoprotein cholesterol. *Journal of the American Medical Association, 273*(18), 1429–1435.

Enos, W. F., & Beyer, C. J. C. (1955). Pathogenesis of coronary disease in American soldiers killed in Korea. *Journal of the American Medical Association, 158,* 912–914.

Epstein, L. H., Coleman, K. J., & Myers, M. D. (1996). Exercise in treating obesity in children and adolescents. *Medicine and Science in Sports and Exercise, 28*(4), 428–435.

Frohlich, E. D., Grim, C., Labarthe, D. R., Maxwell, M. H., Perloff, D., & Weidman, W. H. (1988). Recommendations for human blood pressure determination by sphygmomanometers: Report of a special task force appointed by the Steering Committee, American Heart Association. *Hypertension, 11,* 209A–222A.

Haddock, C. K., Shadish, W. R., Klesges, R. C., & Stein, R. J. (1994). Treatments for childhood and adolescent obesity. *Annals of Behavioral Medicine, 16*(3), 235–244.

Hansen, H. S., Froberg, K., Hyldebrandt, N., & Nielsen, J. R. (1991). A controlled study of eight months of physical training and reduction of blood pressure in children: The Odense Schoolchild Study. *British Medical Journal, 303*(6804), 682–685.

Harrell, J. S., McMurray, R. G., Bangdiwala, S. I., Frauman, A. C., Gansky, S. A., & Bradley, C. B. (1996). Effects of a school-based intervention to reduce cardiovascular disease risk factors in elementary-school children: The Cardiovascular Health in Children (CHIC) study. *Journal of Pediatrics, 128,* 797–805.

Jennings, R. B., & Leon, S. P. (1992). Pediatric preventive cardiology: Experience in the Tidewater, Virginia, area. *Pediatrics, 31,* 89–93.

Johnson, C. C., Nicklas, T. A., Arbeit, M. L., Harsha, D. W., Mott, D. S., Hunter, S. M., Wattigney, W., & Berenson, G. S. (1991). Cardiovascular intervention for high-risk families: The Heart Smart Program. *Southern Medical Journal, 84*(11), 1305–1312.

Johnston, F. E., Hamill, P. V., & Lemeshow, S. (1972). Skinfold thickness of children 6–11 years, United States. *Vital and Health Statistics—Series 1: Programs and Collection Procedures, 11,* 1–60.

Klissouras, V., & Tokmakidis, S. (1982). Evaluation of physical fitness of school children: The Eurofit test. *Proceedings of the 15th Meeting of the International Council for Physical Fitness Research: Olympia Seminar, Switzerland,* 198–212.

Lawrence, M., Arbeit, M., Johnson, C. C., & Berenson, G. S. (1991). Prevention of adult heart disease beginning in childhood: Intervention programs. *Cardiovascular Clinics, 21*(3), 249–262.

McNamara, J. J., Molot, M. A., Stremple, J. F., & Cutting, R. T. (1971). Coronary artery disease in combat casualties in Vietnam. *Journal of the American Medical Association, 216*(7), 1185–1187.

Najjar, M. F., & Rowland, M. (1987). Anthropometric reference data and prevalence of overweight. *Vital and Health Statistics: Series 11, 238,* 1–73.

National Institutes of Health. (1980). *The Lipid research clinics population studies data book: Vol. 1. The Prevalence Study I* (NIH Publication No. 80-1527). Washington, DC: U.S. Government Printing Office.

Oaks, J., Warren, B., & Harsha, D. (1987). Cardiovascular health knowledge of children and school personnel in Louisiana public schools. *Journal of School Health, 57*(1), 23–27.

Raitakari, O. T., Porkka, K. V. K., Rasanen, L., Ronnemaa, T., & Viikari, J. S. (1994). Clustering and six-year cluster-tracking of serum total cholesterol, HDL-cholesterol and diastolic blood pressure in children and young adults: The Cardiovascular Risk in Young Finns Study. *Journal of Clinical Epidemiology, 47*(10), 1085–1093.

Shvartz, E., & Reibold, R. C. (1990). Aerobic fitness norms for males and females aged 6 to 75 years: A review. *Aviation, Space, and Environmental Medicine, 61,* 3–11.

Tosteson, A. N. A., Weinstein, M. C., Hunink, M. G. M., Mittleman, M. A., Williams, L. W., Goldman, P. A., & Goldman, L. (1997). Cost-effectiveness of population wide educational approaches to reduce serum cholesterol levels. *Circulation, 95*, 24–30.

Tracy, R. E., Newman, W. P., Wattigney, W. A., & Berenson, G. S. (1995). Risk factors and atherosclerosis in youth autopsy findings of the Bogalusa Heart Study. *American Journal of the Medical Sciences, 310*(Suppl. 1), S37–S41.

Williams, C. L., Carter, B. J., & Eng, A. (1980). The "Know Your Body" Program: A developmental approach to health education and disease prevention. *Preventive Medicine, 9*, 371–383.

Wissler, R. W., & PDAY Research Group. (1995). An overview of the quantitative influence of several risk factors on progression of atherosclerosis in young people in the United States. *American Journal of Medical Sciences, 310*(Suppl. 1), S29–S36.

[8]

Regular Physical Activity in Older African Americans

Julie Fleury, Joanne S. Harrell, and Brenda Cobb

Although coronary heart disease (CHD) and stroke mortality have declined in recent decades both in the total population and among African Americans, the age-adjusted death rates for CHD and stroke remain higher for African Americans than for the total population (National Center for Health Statistics, 1996). According to the *Healthy People 2000* progress report, these disparities between African Americans and the total population are due to a higher prevalence of risk factors among African Americans, including hypertension, obesity, cigarette smoking, higher cholesterol levels, and physical inactivity (U.S. Department of Health and Human Services [USDHHS], 1995).

Among the major modifiable risk factors for cardiovascular disease, physical inactivity affects the largest proportion of the population (King, 1995). Moderate physical activity has been positively linked to a number of cardiovascular health benefits, and it reduces the risk of chronic illness (Pate et al., 1995; USDHHS, 1996). Yet population-based surveys indicate that 40% of adults in the United States are sedentary and fewer than 10% engage in levels of physical activity consistent with positive health outcomes (Lewis, Raczynski, Heath, Hilyer, & Cutter, 1993).

In studies that included African Americans, regular physical activity has been found to positively affect blood lipid levels, diabetes, and obesity, and improve the management of hypertension (Arroll & Beaglehole, 1992;

Macera et al., 1993; Miller, Balady, & Fletcher, 1997). Yet comparative studies have shown that African Americans participate in regular physical activity less often than Caucasians (Broman, 1995). However, little is known about the social and cultural processes influencing the initiation and maintenance of regular physical activity by minority populations. Few studies have targeted African-American communities for primary and secondary prevention programs, and even fewer have addressed cultural and socioeconomic factors in the process of health behavior change. The research reported here was a pilot study designed to identify motivational predictors of regular physical activity in elderly, rural African Americans. The long-term goal is to develop effective, feasible, and acceptable intervention strategies to promote regular physical activity among rural African Americans and thus maintain or improve cardiovascular health.

THEORETICAL FRAMEWORK

Wellness motivation theory provides a framework for understanding the process through which regular physical activity is initiated and maintained over time (Fleury, 1991, 1994). Wellness motivation theory conceptualizes individual motivation for health behavior change as a dynamic process of intention formation and goal-directed behavior leading to new and positive health patterns. The theory consists of three major concepts: contextual influences, behavioral change processes, and action (see Figure 8.1).

Contextual Influences

Contextual influences refer to factors that originate either within the individual or as a part of the individual's sociocultural and physical environ-

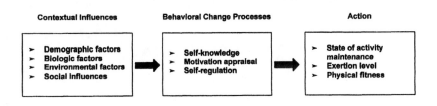

FIGURE 8.1 Wellness motivation theory.

ment. Contextual influences are thought to have a significant impact on behavioral change processes and physical activity maintenance (USDHHS, 1996).

Behavioral Change Processes

Behavioral change processes reflect the ways in which individuals create and evaluate goals, establish standards for behavioral change, determine behavioral strategies, and regulate and strengthen patterns of behavioral change (Bandura, 1989; Carver & Scheier, 1982; Ewart, 1991; Fleury, 1991, 1996). Behavioral change processes, which involve self-knowledge, motivation appraisal, and self-regulation, reflect the human propensity to strive toward new goals and move beyond goals that have been achieved (Fleury, 1991, 1996).

Self-Knowledge

Self-knowledge frames and guides the generation of individual goals and behavioral intentions as well as perceived capability to achieve goals (Bandura, 1989; Fleury, 1991, 1996; Hooker & Kaus, 1992). Individuals select goals that represent not just desired outcomes, but outcomes related to valued representations of the self, or enduring self-definitions (Fleury, 1991; Markus & Nurius, 1986). Culturally and socially formed self-schemas have motivational force because they determine our interpretation of the world, direct our actions in it, organize our experiences, set goals for action, and include personal desires and values for specific self-definitions (D'Andrade, 1990).

Motivation Appraisal

Motivation appraisal involves intention formation as a basis for goal-directed behavior. In the appraisal of readiness to initiate and sustain health behavior change, individuals examine their present behavior in relation to personal beliefs and values, evaluate the relevance and severity of symptom patterns, identify information and resources available for changing their health behavior, establish goals and standards for behavior, and evaluate their ability to successfully initiate valued change (Fleury, 1991).

Self-Regulation

Self-regulation in change reflects the cognitive, affective, and behavioral strategies used to achieve valued goals. Strategies for health behavior change are guided by individual determination of personal, environmental, and economic resources as well as responses to personal and contextual cues such as the family environment, stressful situations, and economic concerns. Self-regulation includes the use of monitoring behaviors focused on symptom patterns and the use of structured activities aimed at managing risk modification efforts and environmental cues.

Action

Action, in this case physical activity, incorporates the individual's response to contextual influences and behavioral change processes. Physical activity may be evaluated on a number of levels, including subjective response, objective evaluation, and physiologic or biologic response. The ability to relate physical activity to health outcomes depends on accurate, precise, and reproducible measures (USDHHS, 1996).

METHODS

Data collection for the study reported here proceeded in two phases designed first, to obtain contextual and culturally relevant information specific to motivational predictors of physical activity among older African Americans, and second, to examine motivational predictors of regular physical activity in elderly, rural African Americans. The study was implemented in collaboration with Joint Orange-Chatham Community Action (JOCCA), located in rural North Carolina. JOCCA includes 10 rural community sites that provide human services programs and assist families and individuals to achieve self-sufficiency and improve the quality of their lives. JOCCA leaders worked with the investigators to facilitate the conduct of the community-based focus groups and data collection efforts at community sites and through community health fairs.

In phase 1, community-based focus groups were convened to explore cultural differences in the meaning, measurement, and interpretation of motivational predictors of physical activity. Focus group interviews were conducted with elderly African Americans using a semi-structured interview format, at rural community sites over a period of 2 months. Focus groups consisted of 6 to 10 men and women. Based on the recommendations of the focus groups, items on the study instruments (see below) were revised to enhance item clarity, relevance, and meaning for this population. Questionnaire response formats were also revised to facilitate face-to-face administration and reduce respondent burden among elderly African Americans.

For example, cards color-coded in decreasing shades of blue were used to enhance understanding of the gradations in the Likert format scales. During face-to-face interviews, respondents were asked to point to the color, ranging from dark blue (strongly agree) to light blue (strongly disagree) that best corresponded to their thoughts about a given questionnaire item.

In phase 2, a convenience sample of English-speaking African-American elders were recruited from within JOCCA community sites in rural North Carolina. Data collection visits to the community sites were arranged with community leaders to fit with existing activities, including lunch, crafts, and Bible study. Participant recruitment and data collection were also conducted during two community health fairs organized by investigators in collaboration with JOCCA leaders. The study was introduced by the investigators as one designed to understand the health and health behaviors of community members. After participants gave informed consent, they were administered a standardized interview, which consisted of measures of contextual influences, self-knowledge, motivation appraisal, self-regulation, and indices of regular physical activity. In addition, participants were evaluated on the physiologic measures of weight, height, and blood pressure.

Measurement

Contextual Influence

Contextual influence was operationalized as including participant health status, perceived well-being, health values, and social support. Health status included biologic factors, risk assessment, and physiologic parameters. Biologic factors included cardiac diagnosis and personal and family history of cardiovascular disease. Associated comorbidities were evaluated through self-report of chronic illnesses. Cardiovascular risk assessment included assessment of tobacco use, blood pressure, and body mass index (BMI). Tobacco use was assessed through self-report questions indexing smoking patterns and the use of smokeless tobacco, including snuff. Items asked about individual smoking history and, for ex-smokers, the number of years since quitting. Blood pressure was measured with a random zero mercury sphygmomanometer using the protocol outlined by the American Heart Association (1993). Participants were also asked if they were currently taking antihypertensive medication, and if they had ever been told by a health care provider that they were hypertensive. BMI was computed as weight in kilograms divided by a squared term of height in meters. Height was measured to the nearest 0.1 cm with a stadiometer, with the individual standing erect with heels against the base of the stadiometer. Weight was measured to the nearest 0.1 kg using a balance beam metric scale, with the participant clothed.

Perceived well-being was measured using a modification of the Perceived Well-Being Scale (PWB) (Reker, Peacock, & Wong, 1987), which measures both psychological and physical well-being. Internal consistency reliability estimates for the modified PWB scales range from .70 to .82. Construct validity has been established through confirmatory principal components factor analysis.

Health value orientation was measured using a modification of the Value Orientation Scale (VOS) (Murdaugh, 1982). The modified VOS provides a measure of individual health value orientation within the dimensions of time, relationships, and spirituality. Internal consistency reliability estimates have ranged from .70 to .86. Construct validity has been established by confirmatory principal components factor analysis.

Perceived social support was measured using the Tilden Interpersonal Relationship Inventory (IPRI) (Tilden, Nelson, & May, 1990). The IPRI measures social support, including indices of network function and conflict. Internal consistency reliability estimates range from .83 to .92. Construct validity has been established by confirmatory principal components factor analysis.

Behavioral Change Processes

Behavioral change processes were evaluated as motivation appraisal and self-regulation. Motivation appraisal was measured using the Index of Readiness (IR) (Fleury, 1992). The IR includes three subscales measuring individual reevaluation of lifestyle, identification of barriers to health behavior change, and goal commitment. The IR consists of nine items rated on a scale ranging from 1 to 5 (strongly disagree to strongly agree). Internal consistency estimates range from .72 to .86. Construct validity has been established through scale convergence with measures of health locus of control and health value. Self-regulation was measured using the Index of Self-Regulation (ISR) (Fleury, 1992). The ISR includes three subscales measuring individual reconditioning, stimulus control, and behavioral monitoring. The ISR contains nine items rated on a scale ranging from 1 to 5 (strongly disagree to strongly agree). Internal consistency estimates range from .73 to .76, with a total scale reliability of .87. Construct validity has been demonstrated through scale convergence with a measure of self-regulation strategies used by individuals in coping with actual or potential health problems.

Regular Physical Activity

Regular physical activity was assessed using a modification of the Minnesota Leisure Time Physical Activity Questionnaire (Folsom, Caspersen, & Taylor,

1985). Participants were asked to respond to self-report questions indexing type and amount of regular physical activity performed per week. Using the compendium of physical activities (Ainsworth et al., 1993) to determine the metabolic equivalent (MET) levels of activity reported, estimates of weekly MET level were calculated as a function of activity type and frequency.

RESULTS

Sample

The sample consisted of 83 African Americans whose ages ranged from 60 to 98 years (mean age: 75). The majority of participants were female (87%), had less than a high school education (68%), were retired (88%), and were single, primarily widowed (80%). Although few of the participants currently smoked cigarettes, 26% used snuff or chewing tobacco. The mean systolic blood pressure for this sample was 152, while the mean diastolic pressure was 76. The mean BMI calculated from participant height and weight was 29. The majority of participants had at least one chronic illness: Seventy-one percent were experiencing arthritis, 57% were hypertensive, and 44% suffered from peripheral vascular disease.

Ninety percent of the sample reported some type of regular physical activity: Forty-two percent performed some type of activity at least one or two times per week, while 37% performed activity five to seven times per week. Types of physical activity reported included walking, swimming, cycling, gardening, and dancing. The usual length of time that the activity was performed was between 10 and 30 minutes. The mean estimated weekly MET level for this sample was 38.4. Thus, it appears that, overall, participants engaged in activity on a fairly regular basis.

Multiple Regression

Multiple regression was used to determine which contextual influences and behavioral change processes were significant predictors of physical activity in this sample. Variables were entered in a stepwise fashion at the .05 level. The variables of social support, cerebrovascular disease and peripheral vascular disease, and motivation appraisal variables including lifestyle reevaluation, goal commitment, and self-monitoring explained 34% of the variance in estimated weekly MET level (see Table 8.1). Behavioral monitoring and lifestyle reevaluation were negatively related to physical activity, perhaps indicating the limits of certain motivational predictors of activity.

DISCUSSION

Among this sample of older African Americans in rural North Carolina, significant predictors of regular physical activity included perceived level of social support, the presence and perception of chronic illness, and commitment to the goal of being physically active. Overall, participants reported higher levels of physical activity than observed in previous studies focusing on older African Americans. This difference may be due to the fact that, in this study, participants were encouraged to respond based on their own conceptions of physical activity and the ways that they took care of themselves.

These findings suggest that intervention strategies based on wellness motivation theory may be most effective when they are tailored to individual goals and acknowledge contextual influences. It is essential that clinicians and researchers examine culturally relevant predictors of behavioral change if they are to develop effective interventions to prevent and reduce the complications of chronic illness. Clinicians may be better able to understand

TABLE 8.1 Multiple Regression Analysis: Significant Predictors of Physical Activity

Variable	Beta
Contextual Influences	
Social support	.48*
Chronic illness–stroke	.27*
Chronic illness–PVD	.34*
Motivation Appraisal	
Reevaluating lifestyle	−.32*
Goal commitment	.43*
Self-regulation	
Behavior monitoring	−.31*

Adj. R^2 = .34
*p < .05

individual strategies and decisions for risk modification if influences specific to the group, family, and community are considered.

Culturally relevant interventions designed to promote physical activity in older, rural-dwelling African Americans need to emphasize the immediate positive aspects of regular physical activity, based on values of caring for family and community, rather than long-term prevention or management of chronic illness. For example, many participants in this study liked to dance as part of their daily routines, such as while folding wash or putting away dishes. While dancing or other nontraditional types of activity may not correspond to current definitions of "activity," these alternative types of activity may be quite effective in preventing chronic illness. Thus, an intervention might stress that dancing makes you feel happy all day, or that walking is a good way of getting out in the fresh air and seeing neighbors. Also, participants in this study expressed strong religious faith, and this was related to the achievement of valued outcomes. Community-based interventions may need to include the support of the church and emphasize that individuals, working with the Lord, can make the most of their health through physical activity.

Cardiovascular nurses may need to broaden their vision to include both the individual and the environment as determinants of preventive efforts. Strategies for behavioral change must be relevant to the individual, given personal and environmental resources. Although supportive others are important throughout the behavior change process, for long-term maintenance of physical activity, the individual must act according to his or her own goals and needs. An expression of personal commitment provides the basis for effective planning. The role of the clinician is to assist the individual to accept the necessity for change and to develop clear objectives.

CONCLUSION

The goals for the prevention of CHD are to develop the best possible therapeutic regimens to modify individual risk factors and enhance adherence to these regimens once they have been established. If nurses are to reduce morbidity and mortality due to coronary heart disease, an awareness of individual motivation to initiate and sustain lifestyle change related to identified risk factors is essential. Clinical and community-based interventions are needed that go beyond the provision of information to address important differences in motivation throughout the process of behavioral change. Through the continued efforts of clinicians and researchers, more effective interventions may be designed to enhance motivation in risk reduction for those at greatest risk for chronic illness—the elderly, poor, and minorities.

ACKNOWLEDGMENT

This research was funded by NIH, NINR grant # P30 NR03962 to the Center for Research on Chronic Illness, University of North Carolina at Chapel Hill, School of Nursing.

REFERENCES

Ainsworth, B. E., Haskell, W. L., Leon, A. S., Jacobs, D. R., Montoye, H. J., Sallis, J. F., & Paffenbarger, R. S. (1993). Compendium of physical activities: Classification of energy costs of human physical activities. *Medicine and Science in Sports and Exercise, 25,* 71–80.

American Heart Association. (1993). *Heart and stroke facts statistics.* Dallas: Author.

Arroll, B., & Beaglehole, R. (1992). Does physical activity lower blood pressure: A critical review of clinical trials. *Journal of Clinical Epidemiology, 45,* 439–447.

Bandura, A. (1989). Regulation of cognitive processes through perceived self-efficacy. *Developmental Psychology, 25,* 729–735.

Broman, C. (1995). Leisure-time physical activity in an African-American population. *Journal of Behavioral Medicine, 18,* 341–353.

Carver, C. S., & Scheier, M. F. (1982). Control theory: A useful conceptual framework for personality-social, clinical, and health psychology. *Psychological Bulletin, 92,* 111–135.

D'Andrade, R. G. (1990). Some propositions about the relations between culture and human cognition. In J. W. Stigler, R. A. Shweder, & G. Herdt (Eds.), *Cultural psychology: Essays on comparative human development* (pp. 65–129). Cambridge: Cambridge University Press.

Ewart, C. (1991). Social action theory for a public health psychology. *American Psychologist, 9,* 931–946.

Fleury, J. (1991). Empowering potential: A theory of wellness motivation. *Nursing Research, 40,* 286–291.

Fleury, J. (1992). The application of motivational theory to cardiovascular risk reduction. *Image, 3,* 229–239.

Fleury, J. (1994). The index of readiness: Development and psychometric characteristics. *Journal of Nursing Measurement, 2,* 143–154.

Fleury, J. (1996). Theoretical relevance of wellness motivation theory. *Nursing Research, 45,* 277–283.

Folsom, A. R., Caspersen, C. J., & Taylor, H. L. (1985). Leisure time physical activity and its relationship to coronary risk factors in a population-based sample: The Minnesota Heart Survey. *American Journal of Epidemiology, 121,* 570–579.

Hooker, K., & Kaus, C. R. (1992). Possible selves and health behaviors in later life. *Journal of Aging and Health, 4,* 390–411.

King, A. C. (1995). Community intervention for promotion of physical activity and fitness. *Exercise in Sport Science, 19,* 211–260.

Lewis, C. E., Raczynski, J. M., Heath, G. W., Hilyer, J. C., Jr., & Cutter, G. R. (1993). Promoting physical activity in low-income African American communities: The PARR Project. *Ethnicity and Disease, 3,* 106–118.

Macera, C. A., Heath, G. W., Eaker, E. D., Croft, J. B., Yeager, K. K., & Wheeler, F. C. (1993). Leisure-time physical activity and high-density lipoprotein cholesterol in a biracial community sample. *Ethnicity and Disease, 3,* 152–157.

Marcus, H., & Nurius, P. (1986). Possible selves. *American Psychologist, 41,* 954–969.

Miller, T. D., Balady, G. J., & Fletcher, G. F. (1997). Exercise and its role in the prevention and rehabilitation of cardiovascular disease. *Annals of Behavioral Medicine, 19,* 220–229.

Murdaugh, C. (1982). *Instrument development to assess specific psychological variables explaining individuals differences in preventive behaviors for coronary artery disease.* Doctoral dissertation, University of Arizona, Tucson.

National Center for Health Statistics. (1996). *Health, United States, 1995.* Hyattsville, MD: U.S. Public Health Service.

Pate, R., Pratt, M., Blair, S., Haskell, W. L., Macera, C. A., Bouchard, C., Buchner, D., Ettinger, W., Heal, G. W., & King, A. C. (1995). Physical activity and public health—A recommendation from the Centers for Disease Control and Prevention and the American College of Sports Medicine. *Journal of the American Medical Association, 273,* 402–407.

Reker, G., Peacock, E., & Wong, P. (1987). Meaning and purpose in life and well-being: A life-span perspective. *Journal of Gerontology, 42,* 44–49.

Tilden, V. P., Nelson, C. A., & May, B. A. (1990). The IPRI Inventory: Development and psychometric characteristics. *Nursing Research, 39,* 337–343.

U.S. Department of Health and Human Services (USDHHS). (1995). Proceedings from the Healthy People 2000 midpoint review. *Healthy People 2000 Midpoint Review.*

U.S. Department of Health and Human Services. (USDHHS). (1996). *Physical activity and health: A report of the Surgeon General.* Atlanta: USDHHS Centers for Disease Control and Prevention, National Center for Chronic Disease Prevention and Health Promotion.

[9]

Maintenance of Regular Physical Activity in Working Women

Barbara J. Speck

There is growing evidence that regular physical activity reduces morbidity and mortality from cardiovascular disease (Blair et al., 1995; Haskell et al., 1992; Manson et al., 1999) and decreases risk for osteoporosis, diabetes, and some types of cancer (Bernstein, Henderson, Hanisch, Sullivan-Halley, & Ross, 1994; Manson et al., 1991; Snow-Harter & Marcus, 1991); it is also associated with better mental health (Brown et al., 1995). The *Healthy People 2010* goals are for at least 30% of the population age 18 and older to engage in regular moderate physical activity, preferably daily, and for at least 80% to engage in some leisure-time physical activity (U.S. Department of Health and Human Services, USDHHS, 2000).

Although the benefits of regular physical activity are well known, cross-sectional surveys indicate that levels of physical activity remain low. In the 1988 national Behavioral Risk Factor Surveillance System (BRFSS), 58.7% of women reported a sedentary lifestyle (irregular activity or no leisure-time activity) (Yeager & Macera, 1994), and 58.5% were sedentary in 1991 (Centers for Disease Control and Prevention, CDCP, 1993). In the 1992 BRFSS, 30.2% of women reported no leisure-time activity, and 42.7% reported irregular activity (CDCP, 1995).

Further, more than 50% of those who begin programs of physical activity do not continue (Dishman, 1982, 1988). Researchers have identified some characteristics of the individual, the environment, and the activity itself that predict initiation of physical activity (Gatch & Kendzierski, 1990; Perusse, Tremblay, LeBlanc, & Bouchard, 1989; Sallis et al., 1989; Volden, Langemo, Adamson, & Oechsle, 1990). Reported barriers to activity include lack of motivation and lack of time due to work commitments and family obligations (Eaton et al., 1993; Lutter et al., 1998; Nies, Vollman, & Cook, 1998). However, there is less information on maintenance of regular physical activity, and the majority of the studies on maintenance have involved a time-limited, prescribed exercise program (e.g., Gillis & Perry, 1991; McAuley, 1992; McAuley, Bane, & Mihalko, 1995). The purpose of this study, therefore, was to identify factors associated with maintenance of regular physical activity in working women as a basis for development of interventions to help women incorporate this important health behavior into their lifestyle.

The conceptual framework developed for the study combined variables from Self-Efficacy Theory (Bandura, 1986) with individual, social, and environmental variables that have been significantly associated with physical activity (Speck, 1997). The variables examined as antecedent variables or predictors of activity were psychological (self-efficacy, outcome expectation, value expectancy), social environmental (perceived barriers to regular physical activity, friend support, family support, socioeconomic status, marital status, number of children at home), physiologic (blood pressure [BP], body mass index [BMI], percent body fat, age), and physical activity (current level of activity, type of physical activity, length of current level, past experiences). Change variables were defined as antecedent variables that could change over time (self-efficacy, outcome expectation, value expectancy, perceived barriers, friend support, family support, BMI, percent body fat, BP, current level of physical activity); change variables were examined to see if they predicted activity maintenance (see Figure 9.1).

METHODS

The study design was longitudinal, descriptive, and correlational. Data were collected at baseline and at 26 weeks by self-report questionnaires and direct measurement of physiologic parameters. In addition, subjects kept a daily record of their physical activity during the 26 weeks between the two data collection points.

Sample and Setting

Women were recruited from four occupational sites in central North Carolina: a research institute, an insurance corporation, a hospital, and a univer-

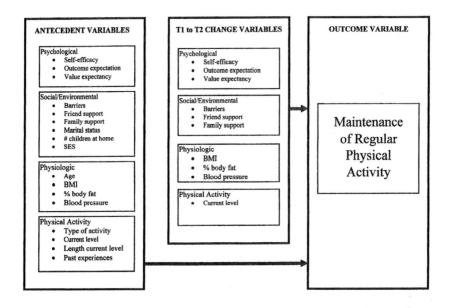

FIGURE 9.1 Conceptual framework for maintenance of regular physical activity.

sity. To be included, women had to be working outside the home and currently engaged in self-selected regular physical activity of at least moderate intensity. The criterion of working was used so that potential leisure time, and therefore time for physical activity, would be equitable across the sample. Moderate-intensity physical activity was defined as activity that is performed at 3 to 6 metabolic equivalent (MET) units, which is equivalent to brisk walking at 3 to 4 miles per hour (Ainsworth et al., 1993; Pate et al., 1995).

Variables and Their Measurement

Psychological Characteristics

The self-efficacy instrument used in the study was an adaptation of the Self-Efficacy for Exercise Behaviors Scales developed by Sallis, Pinski, Grossman, Patterson, and Nader (1988). In their instrument, responses are on a 5-

point Likert scale with three anchor points ("I know I can do it," "Maybe I can do it," and "I know I cannot do it") and an additional response option for "Does not apply." Using factor analysis, Sallis and colleagues identified two factors with Cronbach's alphas of .83 and .85. Test-retest reliability was .68 for each factor. Criterion validity was determined with a one-item question, "Is there any physical activity that you perform at least 20 minutes, three times a week, which is vigorous enough to make you breathe hard and sweat?" This item was significantly correlated with the scale ($p < .001$).

In the current study, a 4-point Likert scale was used instead of a 5-point Likert scale, but with a descriptor for each response ("I know I can," "Maybe I can," "Maybe I cannot," "I know I cannot"). The response option "Does not apply" was also given. Cronbach's alpha for the total scale in this study was .83.

Outcome expectation was measured by the 19-item expected outcomes scale of the Expected Outcomes and Barriers for Habitual Physical Activity questionnaire. This questionnaire was tested with a work site sample of 968 by Steinhardt and Dishman (1989), who reported that factor analysis yielded five factors with a total explained variance of 65%. Cronbach's alpha for the total scale in the current study was .87.

Because there is no instrument that measures value expectancy for regular physical activity, items from the Expected Outcomes for Habitual Physical Activity Scale (Steinhardt & Dishman, 1989) were used to develop a Value to Me of Regular Physical Activity Scale. A 5-point Likert scale was used to determine the value subjects placed on each of the 19 outcomes. Cronbach's alpha for the value expectancy total scale was .88.

Social/Environmental Characteristics

Perceived barriers to maintaining regular physical activity were measured by the 15-item barriers scale of the Expected Outcomes and Barriers for Habitual Physical Activity questionnaire (Steinhardt & Dishman, 1989), along with one additional item, concern for safety. Cronbach's alpha for the 15 items of the barriers scale was .79, and it increased to .81 with the addition of the safety item.

Friend and family support was measured by asking the number of times per week a family member (1) encouraged the subject to exercise and (2) offered to exercise with the subject, and the number of times per week a friend (3) encouraged the subject to exercise and (4) offered to exercise with the subject. This format is similar to one used by Sallis and associates (Sallis et al., 1989, 1990; Sallis, Hovell, Hoffstetter, & Barrington, 1992). The four possible responses to this question were 0 times, 1 to 2 times, 3 to 4 times, or 5 to 7 times per week. The mean number of times per week a friend or family member encouraged or offered to be physically active with the subject was calculated, and for each set of two items (referring to friends or family) a summed score was calculated.

Demographic variables were also measured. Educational level was used as a proxy variable for socioeconomic status. Age, marital status, and the number and ages of children at home were determined by self-report.

Physiologic Characteristics

Weight was measured to the nearest 0.1 kg using a balance beam scale with the subjects' clothes on and shoes off. Height was measured to the nearest 0.1 cm using a stadiometer (Perspective Enterprises, Kalamazoo, MI) with subjects shoeless, standing erect with heels at the base of the stadiometer. BMI was calculated by dividing weight by height squared (kg/m^2).

Percent body fat was estimated using generalized equations for predicting body density from age and the sum of three skinfolds obtained at the following three sites: triceps, suprailiac, and midthigh (Jackson, Pollock, & Ward, 1980). All skinfold measurements were obtained using a Lange skinfold caliper (Cambridge Scientific Industries, Cambridge, MD). The measures were taken three times at each site and averaged. Cross-validation studies comparing body composition as estimated using skinfold measurements and as determined hydrostatically with different samples have shown that the regression equations are valid for predicting body density in women (Jackson et al., 1980). Percent body fat was calculated from body density using Siri's equation (Durnin & Womersley, 1974).

Blood pressure was measured using American Heart Association (AHA) guidelines (USDHHS, 1993) with the subject seated for 5 minutes and her arm at heart level. Three readings were taken 2 minutes apart; the first reading was discarded. The mean values for systolic and diastolic pressure from the second and third blood pressure readings were used in the analyses.

Physical Activity

Current level of physical activity was assessed by a 7-day recall questionnaire. This questionnaire, developed by Sallis and colleagues (1985), includes both work and leisure activities. Reported activities are classified by their MET units. One MET is the energy expenditure of approximately 1 kilocalorie per kg of body weight per hour, or an oxygen uptake of 3.5 ml per kg per minute (Lakka et al., 1994). The questionnaire was tested on 2,126 adults (53% female), and 64 persons completed a retest at 2 weeks. Pearson correlations were high for vigorous ($r = .83$, $p < .001$) and moderate ($r =$

.75, $p < .001$) activities (Sallis et al., 1985). The 7-day recall was originally designed to be administered as an interview, but in this study it was completed by participants.

Subjects were asked to identify their current types of physical activity from a list of eight activities (e.g., aerobic exercise, walking, jogging) or to write in activities if theirs were not listed. Subjects were then classified as participating in physical activity, in exercise, or in a combination of the two. Physical activity was defined as any bodily movement produced by skeletal muscles that results in energy expenditure, and exercise was defined as a subcategory of physical activity involving, in addition to the above, planned structured and repetitive movements with the objective to improve or maintain physical fitness (Caspersen, Powell, & Christenson, 1985).

The subject's past experience with regular physical activity was assessed by asking the number of times a regular physical activity program (either a formal exercise program like structured aerobic classes or informal physical activities like neighborhood or mall walking) had been started and then stopped. The responses were grouped into three categories—never, once or twice, and more than two times. The questions were derived from Sallis and associates (1989, 1992).

Subjects kept records of their daily physical activities (type and duration) during the 26 weeks of the study. Maintenance of regular physical activity, the outcome variable, was calculated from these daily records. Regular physical activity was defined as at least moderate-intensity physical activity for 30 minutes or more per session for at least 3 days per week, or an accumulated 30 minutes per day, in not less than 10-minute segments, for a minimum of 5 days per week. The number of days and the amount of time a subject was physically active each week were used to determine whether she met the definition of regular physical activity for that week. Maintenance of regular physical activity was operationalized as the percentage of weeks in the 26-week period that the subject met the definition of regular physical activity. For example, if a subject was active for 13 weeks of the 26 weeks in the study she would receive a score of .50 (50%).

Procedures

Written informed consent was obtained from subjects prior to data collection. Incentives to participate included a 12-month calendar, two free lunches at data collection points, refreshments at physiologic data collection, and feedback on height, weight, and blood pressure. As an additional incentive, five Sony Walkman cassette AM/FM sports radios were given in a random drawing from the list of subjects who completed the study.

Questionnaire and physiologic data were collected at baseline (time 1) and at 26 weeks (time 2). Questionnaires were administered during lunch time, and physiologic data were collected afterwards in a private conference or seminar room. At the completion of time 1 physiologic data collection, subjects were given a calendar on which to record the days they engaged in physical activity for at least 10 continuous minutes per day for the following 26 weeks. Subjects received written and verbal instructions on recording activities. They were told to cross through a day when they did not participate in physical activity for at least 10 minutes. For days on which they were physically active, they wrote in the minutes and types of physical activity. To simplify recording, common types of physical activity were given two-letter abbreviations (for example, walking = WA), and these were included with the calendar instructions; subjects wrote in other activities not designated with an abbreviation. At the end of each calendar month, each subject received a letter from the investigator with a self-addressed stamped envelope to send the calendar page for that month to the investigator.

RESULTS

The initial sample included 132 women; however, because of missing data on 10 subjects, only 122 subjects made up the final sample. The 10 subjects who were not included were similar to the final sample in most demographic variables; however, a higher proportion of subjects with incomplete data (44.5%) had household incomes less than $40,000 than the final sample (29%). Subject ages ranged from 20 to 62 years (mean age = 39.9, SD = 9.2). The majority (64%) had annual family incomes between $20,000 and $59,999, and 68% were college graduates.

Physical activities were self-selected, and each subject could report one or more. Walking was reported by the highest percentage of women (76.2%). Other activities reported were aerobics (36.1%), jogging (33.6%), exercises at a health fitness club (28.7%), use of home exercise equipment (25.4%), biking outside (19.7%), and swimming (12.3%). Physical activities reported by less than 10% of subjects included dancing, gardening, tennis, weight lifting, and yard work.

Eighteen antecedent variables were entered into a multiple regression equation to predict physical activity maintenance. These variables were self-efficacy, outcome expectation, value expectancy, perceived barriers, friend support, family support, type of physical activity, marital status, number of children in the home, educational level, age, BMI, systolic BP, current level of physical activity, length of current level of physical activity, number of times started and stopped a formal or informal program of physical activity, and past experience with organized sports. The full model with 18 variables significantly predicted maintenance of regular physical activity ($F(18,81) = 2.42$, $p = .004$), with an R^2 of .349.

Although the full model significantly predicted maintenance, the majority of the 18 variables did not contribute significantly to the prediction. To find a more parsimonious model, backward elimination techniques were used to remove nonsignificant variables. The final model was significant ($F(5,94) = 8.28$, $p = .0001$), with an R^2 of .305. The 13 variables eliminated explained less than 5% of the variance in maintenance. The 5 variables that remained in the reduced model are shown in Table 9.1. Older age, higher self-efficacy, more friend support, less family support, and fewer times of starting and stopping an informal program of physical activity predicted maintenance. Friend support contributed most to the prediction of maintenance.

Nine change variables plus the five antecedent variables from the model above were then entered into a regression equation to see if the change variables increased the prediction of maintenance. This model was significant ($F(14,82) = 3.33$, $p = .0003$), with an R^2 of .363. Again, not all variables contributed significantly to the prediction. Backward elimination techniques were used to determine which variables significantly predicted maintenance; the five antecedent variables shown in Table 9.1 remained in the model and three change variables added to the prediction. This model was significant ($F(8,88) = 5.84$, $p = .0001$), and the R^2 was .347 (see Table 9.2). The significant change variables were a decrease in BMI, an increase in self-efficacy, and an increase in friend support. These change variables improved the prediction of maintenance by explaining an additional 4% of the variance.

TABLE 9.1 Summary of Multiple Regression Analysis for Prediction of Maintenance of Regular Physical Activity ($N = 100$)

Variable	B	$SE\ B$	β
Age	0.01	0.00	0.29
Self-efficacy	0.17	0.06	0.24
Family Support	−0.04	0.01	−0.40
Friend Support	0.06	0.02	0.53
Informal exercise	−0.08	0.03	−0.21

Test of model: $R^2 = .305$ ($F(5,94) = 8.28$, $p = .0001$).
Note: B = Unstandardized regression coefficient; $SE\ B$ = Standard error of B; β = Standardized coefficient.

TABLE 9.2 Summary of Multiple Regression Analysis for Prediction of Maintenance of Regular Physical Activity with Five Antecedent Variables and Three Change Variables ($N = 100$)[a]

Variable	B	$SE\ B$	β
Age	0.01	0.00	0.21
Self-efficacy	0.17	0.06	0.25
Family support	−0.03	0.01	−0.33
Friend support	0.05	0.02	0.48
Informal exercise	−0.08	0.03	−0.22
Change in BMI	−0.06	0.03	−0.18
Change in self-efficacy	0.18	0.07	0.26
Change in friend support	0.02	0.01	0.20

[a]Four subjects who became pregnant during the study were deleted from analyses that included time 2 physiologic variables

B = Unstandardized regression coefficient; $SE\ B$ = Standard error of B; β = Standardized coefficient.

Test of model: $R^2 = .347$ (F (8,88) = 5.84, $p = .0001$).

DISCUSSION

Antecedent variables that predicted maintenance of regular physical activity were age, self-efficacy, family support, friend support, and number of times started and stopped informal exercise programs. Other studies have also shown self-efficacy to be positively associated with both initiation and maintenance of regular physical activity (e.g., Conn, 1998; McAuley, 1992; Sallis et al., 1989, 1990; Stetson, Rahn, Dubbert, Wilner, & Mercury, 1997). Similarly, age has been shown to be significant in other studies: Cross-sectional national surveys found that younger women reported higher physical activity levels (CDCP, 1995; CDCP, 1993). However, although in the national surveys physical activity levels decreased as women aged, the greatest decrease was in the 65 and older age group; none of the subjects in this study were older than 62 years.

Friend support and family support reflected the number of times friends and family either encouraged or offered to be physically active with the subject. Friend support was positively correlated with maintenance of regular physical activity, but family support was negatively correlated with maintenance. That is, as family support increased, maintenance decreased. This was an interesting finding, because a majority of the subjects were married (64%), and 41% had children (from age 1 to 34) living in their home. Friend support has also been found by others to predict vigorous physical activity (Sallis et al., 1989); but in contrast to this study, family support was a significant predictor in a community study of walking for exercise (Hovell et al., 1989). It may be that the emotional tone, and thus the consequences, of family and friend support differ; perhaps friend support is positive and helpful, whereas family support might be negative, like nagging. Another possibility is that family members may be resentful when a wife or mother takes time from her busy schedule to engage in physical activity. Additional information on different types of social support would help to clarify this.

Women who had started and stopped an informal program of regular physical activity less often maintained regular activity more. An important component of any intervention for maintenance may be assisting women to begin informal programs of self-selected physical activity so that they can incorporate the physical activity into their lifestyle and reduce the number of times they quit a program.

Three change variables (decreased BMI, increased self-efficacy, and increased friend support) increased the prediction of maintenance of regular physical activity by 4%. A decrease in BMI was predictive of maintenance. Losing weight could have been a psychological incentive for subjects to continue regular physical activity. An increase in self-efficacy was also predictive of maintenance. Sallis and colleagues (1992) also found increases in self-efficacy for regular physical activity to predict maintenance of activity. The positive effect of an increase in friend support suggests the importance of this kind of social support in maintenance.

The requirement of recording daily physical activity could have influenced the activity level of some women in the study. One subject told the investigator that when she saw on her calendar she had not been physically active for several days, she "had to get some exercise so that week would not have all X's." Another subject said that one night she exercised before bed when she saw the calendar, so she "would not have to put down another X." Because of these comments, questions were added to the time 2 questionnaire to determine if subjects thought their participation in the study influenced their pattern of physical activity. Almost half of the subjects felt that participation in the study and recording their activities increased their physical activity. This is an important finding, because daily record keeping is a simple and inexpensive intervention.

The significant benefits for those who engage in regular physical activity are well known. Health care professionals need to increase their inclusion of physical activity assessment and counseling in their practice inclusion. One study of physicians found that in an estimated 40 million visits, only 23.0% of men and 17.5% of women were counseled regarding physical activity (CDCP, 1998). In a study of nurse practitioners and family physicians, between 40% and 75% "always or frequently" encouraged regular exercise in their pediatric patients (Jessup & Harrell, 1996). One *Healthy People 2000* (USDHHS, 1990) goal was that at least 50% of primary care providers would assess and counsel their clients regarding regular physical activity. Clinicians can also develop interventions to increase levels of physical activity in individual patients. Interventions that increase physical activity, self-efficacy, and social support mechanisms may be most effective. All clinicians should stress the importance of moderate-level regular physical activity as part of a healthy lifestyle.

ACKNOWLEDGMENTS

This research was partially supported by a Traineeship Award from the University of North Carolina Center for Health Promotion and Disease Prevention's Cooperative Agreement Number U48/CCU409660, funded by the Centers for Disease Control and Prevention.

REFERENCES

Ainsworth, B. E., Haskell, W. H., Leon, A. S., Jacobs, D. R., Montoye, H. J., Sallis, J. F., & Paffenbarger, R. S. (1993). Compendium of physical activities: Classification of energy costs of human physical activities. *Medicine and Science in Sports and Exercise, 25*, 71–80.

Bandura, A. (1986). *Social learning theory.* Englewood Cliffs, NJ: Prentice Hall.

Bernstein, L., Henderson, B. E., Hanish, R., Sullivan-Halley, J., & Ross, R. K. (1994). Physical exercise and reduced risk of breast cancer in young women. *Journal of the National Cancer Institute, 86*, 1403–1408.

Blair, S. N., Kohl, H. W., Barlow, C. E., Paffenbarger, R. S., Gibbons, L. W., & Macera, C. A. (1995). Changes in physical fitness and all-cause mortality: A prospective study of healthy and unhealthy men. *Journal of the American Medical Association, 273*, 1093–1098.

Brown, D. R., Wans, Y., Ward, A., Ebbeling, C. B., Fortlage, L., Puleo, E., Benson, H., & Rippe, J. M. (1995). Chronic psychological effects of exercise and exercise plus cognitive strategies. *Medicine and Science in Sports and Exercise, 27*, 765–775.

Caspersen, C. J., Powell, K. E., & Christenson, G. M. (1985). Physical activity, exercise, and physical fitness: Definitions and distinctions for health-related research. *Public Health Reports, 100*, 126–131

Centers for Disease Control and Prevention, CDCP. (1993). Prevalence of sedentary lifestyle—Behavioral Risk Factor Surveillance System, United States, 1991. *Morbidity and Mortality Weekly Report, 42*, 577–579.

Centers for Disease Control and Prevention, CDCP. (1995). Prevalence of recommended levels of physical activity among women—Behavioral Risk Factor Surveillance System, 1992. *Morbidity and Mortality Weekly Report, 44*, 105–113.

Centers for Disease Control and Prevention, CDCP. (1998). Missed opportunities in preventive counseling for cardiovascular disease, United States, 1995. *Morbidity and Mortality Weekly Report, 47,* 91–95.

Conn, V. S. (1998). Older adults and exercise: Path analysis of self-efficacy related constructs. *Nursing Research, 47,* 180–189.

Dishman, R. K. (1982). Compliance/adherence in health-related exercise. *Health Psychology, 1,* 237–267.

Dishman, R. K. (1988). *Exercise adherence: Its impact on public health.* Champaign, IL: Human Kinetics.

Durnin, J. V. G. A., & Womersley, J. (1974). Body fat assessed from total body density and its estimation from skinfold thickness: Measurements on 481 men and women aged from 16 to 72 years. *British Journal of Nutrition, 32,* 77–97.

Eaton, C. B., Reynes, J., Assaf, A. R., Feldman, H., Lasater, T., & Carleton, R. A. (1993). Predicting physical activity change in men and women in two New England communities. *American Journal of Preventive Medicine, 9*(4), 209–219.

Gatch, C. L., & Kendzierski, D. (1990). Predicting exercise intentions: Theory of planned behavior. *Research Quarterly for Exercise and Sport, 61*(1), 100–102.

Gillis, A., & Perry, A. (1991). The relationships between physical activity and health-promoting behaviors in mid-life women. *Journal of Advanced Nursing, 16,* 299–310.

Haskell, W. L., Leon, A. S., Caspersen, C. J., Froelicher, V. F., Hagberg, J. M., Harlan, W., Holloszy, J. O., Regensteiner, J. G., Thompson, P. D., Washburn, R. A., & Wilson, P. W. F. (1992). CV benefits and assessment of activity and fitness in adults. *Medicine and Science in Sports and Exercise, 24,* S201–S220.

Hovell, M. F., Sallis, J. F., Hofstetter, C. R., Spry, V. M., Faucher, P., & Caspersen, C. J. (1989). Identifying correlates of walking for exercise: An epidemiologic prerequisite for physical activity promotion. *Preventive Medicine, 18,* 856–866.

Jackson, A. S., Pollock, M. L., & Ward, A. (1980). Generalized equations for predicting body density in women. *Medicine and Science in Sports and Exercise, 12,* 175–182.

Jessup, A. N., & Harrell, J. S. (1996). Promotion of cardiovascular health in children by nurse practitioners and physicians in family practice. *Journal of the American Academy of Nurse Practitioners, 8,* 467–475.

Lakka, T. A., Venalainen, J. M., Rauramaa, R., Salonen, R., Tuomilehto, J., & Salonen, R. (1994). Relationship of leisure-time physical activity and cardiorespiratory fitness to the risk of acute myocardial infarction in men. *New England Journal of Medicine, 330,* 1549–1554.

Lutter, J. M., Simons-Morton, D. G., Kriska, A. M., Freedson, P. S., Shangold, M. M., Bauer, K. M., & Marcus, B. H. (1998). Promoting physical activity among women throughout the lifespan: Barriers and interventions. *Women's Health Issues, 8*(2), 80–89.

Manson, J. E., Hu, F., Rich-Edwards, J. W., Colditz, G. A., Stampfer, M. J., Willett, W. C., Speizer, F. E., & Hennekens, C. H. (1999). A prospective study of walking as compared with vigorous exercise in the prevention of coronary heart disease in women. *New England Journal of Medicine, 341,* 650–658.

Manson, J. E., Rimm, E. B., Stampfer, M. J., Colditz, G. A., Willett, W. C., Krolewski, A. S., Rosner, B., Hennekens, C. H., & Speizer, F. E. (1991). Physical activity and incidence of non-insulin-dependent diabetes mellitus in women. *The Lancet*, *338*, 774–778.

McAuley, E. (1992). The role of efficacy cognitions in the prediction of exercise behavior in middle-aged adults. *Journal of Behavioral Medicine, 15*(1), 65–88.

McAuley, E., Bane, S. M., & Mihalko, S. L. (1995). Exercise in middle-aged adults: Self-efficacy and self-presentational outcomes. *Preventive Medicine, 24*(4), 319–328.

Nies, M. A., Vollman, M., & Cook, T. (1998). Facilitators, barriers, and strategies for exercise in European American women in the community. *Public Health Nursing, 15*, 263–272.

Pate, R. R., Pratt, M., Blair, S. N., Haskell, W. L., Macera, C. A., Bouchard, C., Buchner, D., Ettinger, W., Heath, G. W., King, A. C., Kriska, A., Leon, A. S., Marcus, B. H., Morris, J., Paffenbarger, R. S., Patrick, K., Pollock, M. L., Rippe, J. M., Sallis, J., & Wilmore, J. H. (1995). Physical activity and public health: A recommendation from the Centers for Disease Control and Prevention and the American College of Sports Medicine. *Journal of the American Medical Association, 273*, 402–407.

Perusse, L., Tremblay, A., LeBlanc, C., & Bouchard, C. (1989). Genetic and environmental influences on level of habitual activity participation. *American Journal of Epidemiology, 129*, 1012–1022.

Sallis, J. F., Haskell, W. L., Wood, P. D., Fortmann, S. P., Rogers, T., Blair, S. N., & Paffenbarger, R. S. (1985). Physical activity assessment methods in 5-city project. *American Journal of Epidemiology, 121*(1), 91–106.

Sallis, J. F., Hovell, M. F., Hoffstetter, C. R., & Barrington, E. (1992). Explanation of vigorous physical activity during two years using social learning variables. *Social Science and Medicine, 34*, 25–32.

Sallis, J. F., Hovell, M. F., Hoffstetter, C. R., Elder, J. P., Faucher, P., Spry, V. M., Barrington, E., & Hackley, M. (1990). Lifetime history of relapse from exercise. *Addictive Behaviors, 15*, 573–579.

Sallis, J. F., Hovell, M. F., Hoffstetter, C. R., Faucher, P., Elder, J. P., Blanchard, J., Caspersen, C. J., Powell, K. E., & Christenson, G. M. (1989). A multivariate study of determinants of vigorous exercise in a community sample. *Preventive Medicine, 18*, 20–34.

Sallis, J. F., Pinski, R. B., Grossman, R. M., Patterson, R. L., & Nader, P. R. (1988). The development of self-efficacy scales for health-related diet and exercise behaviors. *Health Education Research, 3*, 283–292.

Snow-Harter, C., & Marcus, R. (1991). Exercise, bone mineral density, and osteoporosis. In J. O. Holloszy (Ed.), *Exercise and sport sciences reviews* (vol. 19, pp. 351–388). Baltimore: Williams & Wilkins.

Speck, B. J. (1997). *Maintenance of regular physical activity in working women.* Unpublished doctoral dissertation, University of North Carolina, Chapel Hill.

Steinhardt, M. A., & Dishman, R. K. (1989). Reliability and validity of expected outcomes and barriers for habitual physical activity. *Journal of Occupational Medicine, 31*(6), 536–546.

Stetson, B. A., Rahn, J. M., Dubbert, P. M., Wilner, B. I., & Mercury, M. G. (1997). Prospective evaluation of the effects of stress on exercise adherence in community-residing women. *Health Psychology, 16*(6), 515–520.

U.S. Department of Health and Human Services (USDHHS). (1990). *Healthy people 2000* (USDHHS Pub. No. PHS91-50212). Washington, DC: Government Printing Office.

U.S. Department of Health and Human Services (USDHHS). (2000). *Healthy people 2010.* Washington, DC: ODPHP.

U.S. Department of Health and Human Services (USDHHS). (1993). *Fifth report of the Joint National Committee on Detection, Evaluation, and Treatment of High BP* (USDHHS Pub. No. NIH 93-1008). Bethesda, MD: Author.

U.S. Department of Health and Human Services (USDHHS). (1997). *Healthy people 2000 review, 1997* (USDHHS Pub. No. PHS 98-1256). Hyattsville, MD: Government Printing Office.

Volden, C., Langemo, D., Adamson, M., & Oechsle, L. (1990). The relationship of age, gender, and exercise practices to measures of health and self-esteem. *Applied Nursing Research, 3*(1), 20–26.

Yeager, K. K., & Macera, C. A. (1994). Physical activity and health profiles of United States women. *Clinics in Sports Medicine, 13,* 329–335.

[10]

Decreasing Cancer Fatalism among Rural Elders

Barbara D. Powe and Sally Weinrich

African Americans are 30% more likely to die of cancer than Caucasian Americans (American Cancer Society, ACS, 1998). While the incidence of colorectal cancer has declined among Caucasians, the rate has remained constant among African Americans (ACS, 1998). Detection of colorectal cancer in the early, asymptomatic stages is crucial in reducing mortality: Five-year survival approaches 93% when the cancer is found early and treated in its localized stages, but 5-year survival is less than 7% when distant metastases are present at diagnosis (ACS, 1998). The incidence of colorectal cancer increases with age (ACS, 1998; Griffith, 1993; Hansen, 1995; U.S. Preventive Services Task Force, USPSTF, 1996), and colorectal cancer mortality rates are especially high among rural, socioeconomically disadvantaged African-American elders (ACS, 1998; U.S. Department of Health and Human Services, USDHHS, 1990). Yet these elders are less likely than other Americans to participate in colorectal cancer screening programs (Powe, 1995a, 1995b; Underwood, Hoskins, Cummins, Morris, & Williams, 1994; Weinrich, Weinrich, Boyd, Atwood, & Cervanka, 1992).

Increasing participation in colorectal cancer screening is a national priority (USDHHS, 1990). Currently, the ACS (1998) recommends fecal occult blood testing (FOBT) annually after age 50, a digital rectal exam (DRE) annually after age 40, and flexible sigmoidoscopy every 5 years with DRE, or a double contrast barium enema every 5 to 10 years. Fecal occult blood testing (FOBT) is simple and can be completed in the patient's home. The sensitivity and specificity of FOBT for detecting colorectal cancer in asymptomatic persons range from 33% to 97% and from 90% to 99%, respectively (Allison, Tekawa, Ransom, & Adrian, 1996; Ederer, Church, & Mandel, 1997; Griffith, 1993; Lang & Ransohoff, 1994, 1997; St. John, Young, McHutchison, Deacon, & Alexeyeff, 1992). Yet in 1996 the Centers for Disease Control and Prevention (CDC, 1996) found that less than 1% of those surveyed age 50 and above ($N = 128,412$) reported ever participating in FOBT.

Participation in colorectal cancer screening can be influenced by many factors. Barriers to screening that are known to confront rural, socioeconomically disadvantaged African-American elders include cancer fatalism, lack of knowledge of cancer, poverty, and poor access to care (Martin & Henry, 1989; Olsen & Frank-Stromborg, 1993; Powe, 1995b, 1995c, 1997; Underwood & Hoskins, 1994; Weinrich et al., 1992).

Despite awareness of these barriers, successful strategies to increase participation in cancer screening have not been forthcoming. It has been suggested that interventions for rural, disadvantaged African-American elders must be multidimensional and provide information on colorectal cancer in a manner that is culturally appropriate. In particular, interventions must address fatalism, which is believed to be the result of a complex psychological cycle characterized by perceptions of hopelessness, worthlessness, meaninglessness, powerlessness, and social despair (Freeman, 1989; West, 1993). Fatalism has the potential to affect every aspect of the human experience (West, 1993). Cancer fatalism, the belief that death is inevitable when cancer is present, is a situational manifestation of fatalism in which the individual becomes entrapped in a cycle of late cancer diagnosis, limited treatment options, and death. Cancer fatalism is most prevalent among African Americans, females, and persons with low incomes and low educational levels (Freeman, 1989; Powe, 1995a, 1995b; Underwood & Hoskins, 1994). Fatalistic persons are less likely to participate in FOBT (Powe, 1995b).

Spirituality may provide a cultural foundation for addressing fatalistic perceptions. Many rural, disadvantaged African-American elders exhibit a strong faith in God (Powe, 1997). They find meaning in existence through the organized body of thought, experience, and faith that is Christianity (Emblem, 1992; Reed, 1992). Their religious faith provides a source of connection to God and hope in the face of seemingly overwhelming circumstances (Dombeck & Karl, 1987; Dwyer, Clarke, & Miller, 1990; Emblem, 1992; Scandrett, 1994). For these deeply religious rural elders, visits with clergy, interactions with family and friends, personal prayer, and verbalization of beliefs may play a crucial role in enhancing hope, coping abilities, positive health beliefs, positive health care behaviors, and positive health care outcomes (Lincoln & Mamiya, 1990; Lloyd, McConnell, & Zahorik, 1994; Reed, 1992; Scandrett, 1994; Thomas, 1994). Thus inclusion of spirituality in interventions may help to decrease their cancer fatalism.

Interventions to increase the participation of rural, disadvantaged African-American elders in FOBT must also address the lack of knowledge of cancer, low literacy, poor vision, and hearing impairments that are prevalent among this population (Hoskins & Rose, 1989; Powe, 1997; Powe & Johnson, 1995; Rosella, Regan-Kubinski, & Albrecht, 1994). Rural, disadvantaged African-American elders have less knowledge of colorectal cancer than other Americans (Weinrich et al., 1992), and elders with less knowledge have been found to be more fatalistic (Powe, 1995c, 1997) and less likely to participate in FOBT (Powe, 1995b; Weinrich et al., 1992).

Videotaped interventions have been effective in enhancing learning and short-term retention among patients with low literacy levels, decreased vision, and decreased hearing (Chang & Hirsch, 1994; Meade, 1996). The ACS's video (*Colorectal Cancer: The Cancer that No One Talks About*) has been used as an educational tool to increase participation in FOBT among rural disadvantaged elders. However, African-American elders who view the ACS video still have less knowledge of colorectal cancer than Caucasian elders, are still fatalistic, and still participate less in FOBT (Powe, 1995a; Weinrich, Weinrich, Boyd, Johnson, & Frank-Stromborg, 1992). This study, therefore, evaluated the effectiveness of a new 20-minute video entitled *Telling the Story . . . To Live Is God's Will,* which was designed to increase participation in cancer screening by addressing cancer fatalism through the spirituality of this population, and by providing information on colorectal cancer using culturally relevant and understandable language.

METHODS

The study used a repeated measures, pretest-posttest design and targeted rural, disadvantaged elders who attended senior citizens centers in a southern state. The majority of those who attend these centers are African-American women. Their average age is 73, their average educational level is less than 8 years, and their average annual income is $6,500. Participants usually attend the centers daily for lunch and other activities. Free transportation is provided for the majority of participants, and participants routinely attend the same center. Therefore, it was possible to randomly select centers for the intervention and control group and select potential participants from these centers. Participants at the centers were eligible for the study if they were ≥ 50 years old and were mentally oriented to date and location.

This age was selected in order to maintain consistency with the ACS recommendations for FOBT (ACS, 1998). Individuals who had participated in a colorectal cancer screening program within the previous year were excluded from the study. All participants gave informed consent.

Intervention

The intervention group participants viewed the 20-minute video entitled *Telling the Story . . . To Live Is God's Will.* A critical element in videotaped interventions is video modeling or demonstrating the desired behavior, attitudes, and cognitive effects (Meade, 1996). Therefore, the majority of the participants in the video were African-American and the intervention incorporated the study population's language, dress, food preferences, customs, traditions, attitudes, values, and spiritual belief systems (Landrine & Klonoff, 1994; Rosella et al., 1994).

Telling the Story . . . To Live Is God's Will includes an introduction, three scenes, and a concluding segment. Segments are connected with narration and gospel music. Scene 1 provides an overview of colorectal cancer and cancer screening, and portrays survival after a diagnosis of cancer. The scene depicts a dynamic interaction between two elderly women (Ruth and Naomi) in a senior citizens center. Their discussion centers around Naomi's previous participation in colorectal cancer screening, the diagnosis of her colorectal cancer in its early stages, her survival of the cancer, and her encouragement to Ruth to participate in FOBT. Scene 2 portrays the interactions of Ruth, her husband, John, and their minister. In the discussion, Ruth and her husband express their fears of cancer and cancer screening to the minister, who alleviates their fears by discussing the importance of caring for one's health from a religious perspective. The scene concludes with Ruth, her husband, and the minister agreeing to attend a colorectal cancer screening program. Scene 3 reinforces the information given earlier on colorectal cancer and depicts Ruth, her husband, the minister, and others at a question-and-answer session in which a nurse discusses colorectal cancer, discusses scriptural support for health care, and encourages FOBT among the group. The nurse models completion of the FOBT using peanut butter and allows a return demonstration by Ruth.

The control group viewed the American Cancer Society's video entitled *Colorectal Cancer: The Cancer No One Talks About.* This video is 13 minutes in length and provides an overview of the prevalence of colorectal cancer, the signs and symptoms of colorectal cancer, and the purposes of FOBT. The video incorporates brief vignettes of persons who have experienced colorectal cancer discussing cancer and the impact the diagnosis had on their lives. The majority of persons portrayed in the video are Caucasian. Following the video, the technique for completing the FOBT was demonstrated to the control group by a research assistant using peanut butter since the technique is not included in the ACS video and this is crucial to accurate use of the FOBT kits.

Instruments

Data were collected before and 7 days after the participants viewed the intervention video or the ACS video, using the Powe Fatalism Inventory and the Colorectal Cancer Knowledge questionnaire. A Demographic Data questionnaire was completed only at the pretest data collection. The researcher and a trained research assistant read the questionnaires to participants as needed during both pretest and posttest data collection visits. Fecal occult blood testing kits were distributed after the video and collected at the posttest.

Powe Fatalism Inventory

The Powe Fatalism Inventory was developed by the researcher (Powe, 1995a) to assess the presence of cancer fatalism. The inventory consists of 15 yes or no questions, with one point added for each yes response and a possible range of scores from 0 to 15. Higher scores indicate higher levels of cancer fatalism. Questions focus on the defining attributes of cancer fatalism, which are fear, pessimism, the inevitability of death, and predetermination (Powe, 1995b). Examples of questions on the inventory are "I believe if someone has cancer, it was meant to be" and "I believe if someone has cancer, it is already too late to do anything about it." The inventory has had reliability coefficients ranging from .84 to .89 when used with previous samples from the study population (Powe, 1995a, 1995b, 1997).

Colorectal Cancer Knowledge Questionnaire

The Colorectal Cancer Knowledge questionnaire was developed by Weinrich et al. (1992) to assess knowledge of risk factors, symptoms, and screening recommendations for colorectal cancer. The questionnaire consists of 12 true or false questions, with a possible range of scores from 0 to 12. The questionnaire has had reliability coefficients ranging from .66 to .77 when used with samples from the study population (Powe, 1995c; Weinrich et al., 1992).

Demographic Data Questionnaire

Data on age, education, race, gender, and annual income were collected on each participant. In addition, participants were asked if they had previously been diagnosed with cancer and whether anyone in their family had ever been diagnosed with cancer. Religious affiliation was also determined.

Fecal Occult Blood Testing Kits

Hemoccult II fecal occult blood testing kits (SmithKline, Inc.) were used to determine participation in colorectal cancer screening. These kits allow the participant to collect three separate samples. Hemoccult II kits were distributed at no cost to participants in the intervention and control groups. Participants who returned the kits within 7 days were considered to have participated in colorectal cancer screening. Pictorial posters were left at all sites to remind participants of the time and date to return the kits.

The FOBT kits were analyzed at no cost to participants. A letter summarizing the results of the FOBT was addressed to each participant and mailed to the senior center. This technique was used so that the center's manager would be available to assist individuals with reading and comprehension if needed.

RESULTS

Sample

The sample consisted of 70 participants, 42 in the intervention group and 28 in the control group. The average age of the sample was 75 years, with a range of 52 to 92 years; the average educational level was 6.72 years, with a range of 0 to 16 years. The majority of the sample were African American (90%) and female (86%), and had annual incomes less than $5,000 (81%). Almost three fourths of the sample were Methodist (47%) or Baptist (27%). Only one participant had a family history of colorectal cancer. The majority of the participants (66%) had no family history of cancer and had never been diagnosed with cancer (90%). There were no significant differences between the intervention and control groups except that a greater percentage of the intervention group were African American (98% vs. 79% in control group) and 91% of the intervention group had annual incomes less than $5,000, compared to 68% of the control group.

Cancer Fatalism

It was expected that participants in the intervention group would show a greater decrease in cancer fatalism scores from pretest to posttest than the control group. The intervention group had a mean pretest cancer fatalism score of 9.90 (SD = 4.28), whereas the control group had a mean score of 9.89 (SD = 4.39). At posttest, which occurred 7 days later, the intervention group's mean cancer fatalism score had dropped to 8.5 (SD = 4.20), whereas the control group had a mean score of 9.79 (SD = 5.03) (see Figure 10.1). Analysis of covariance was used to test the change in fatalism cancer scores. Because the intervention and control groups differed on the variables of race and income, these two variables were used as covariates. As expected, the intervention group showed a significantly greater decrease in cancer fatalism scores than the control group ($F(1,65)$ = 9.23; p = .003).

Knowledge of Colorectal Cancer

It was also expected that the intervention group would show a greater increase in knowledge of colorectal cancer than the control group. The intervention group had a mean pretest knowledge score of 7.93 (SD = 1.67), whereas the control group had a mean score of 8.07 (SD = 1.41). At posttest, 7 days later, the intervention group's mean knowledge score had increased to 8.57 (SD = 1.74) and the control group's mean score had

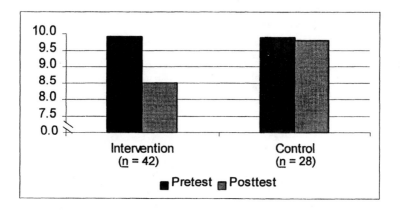

FIGURE 10.1   Mean pretest and posttest cancer fatalism scores for intervention and control groups.

increased to 8.25 ($SD = 1.68$). Analysis of covariance with race and income as covariates was used to test the change in knowledge scores. As expected, the intervention group showed a significantly greater increase in knowledge scores than the control group ($F(1,65) = 3.95$; $p = .044$) (see Figure 10.2).

Participation in FOBT

Finally, it was expected that participation in FOBT would be higher among the intervention group. However, there was no significant difference between the rates of participation of the two groups ($\chi^2 = .50$; $df = 1$; $p = .48$). The majority of both the intervention group (60%) and the control group (68%) participated in FOBT.

DISCUSSION

This study established the effectiveness of a newly developed video intervention, *Telling the Story . . . To Live Is God's Will,* in decreasing cancer fatalism. As in previous studies (Powe, 1995a, 1997; Underwood & Hoskins, 1994), there was a prevailing fatalistic attitude among the sample prior to the intervention. It has been suggested that cancer fatalism develops over time so that hopelessness, meaninglessness, and despair become static (West,

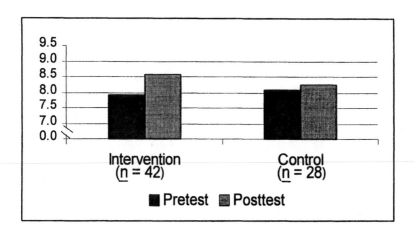

FIGURE 10.2   Mean pretest and posttest knowledge of colorectal cancer scores for intervention and control groups.

1993). Yet 7 days after viewing *Telling the Story . . . To Live Is God's Will,* the level of fatalism was significantly lower in the intervention group than in the control group. This finding suggests that cancer fatalism is a dynamic variable that can be modified.

As in other studies (Powe, 1995c; Weinrich et al., 1992), participants in both the intervention group and the control group lacked information about the signs and symptoms of colorectal cancer and methods of colorectal cancer screening. It has been suggested that when cancer fatalism is high, effective learning may be inhibited (Powe, 1995c; Powe & Johnson, 1995). Yet the group who saw *Telling the Story . . . To Live Is God's Will* were able to increase their knowledge scores; the control group showed only a minimal increase in knowledge.

Rural, disadvantaged African-American elders have been identified as less likely than other groups to participate in FOBT (Powe, 1995a; Weinrich et al., 1992). Previous studies using samples from the current study population have reported rates of participation in FOBT of <30% even when the ACS video (*Colorectal Cancer: The Cancer No One Talks About*) was shown and testing was offered without cost (Powe, 1995a). However, the African-American elders in the current study had high rates of participation in FOBT. The control group received verbal instructions from the data collector on how to complete the FOBT kit and what foods and medications to avoid while completing the FOBT kits, and this additional information may have contributed to their high rate of participation in FOBT. The intervention group did not receive these additional cues because these areas were addressed in the video *Telling the Story . . . To Live Is God's Will.*

Although *Telling the Story . . . To Live Is God's Will* and the ACS video (*Colorectal Cancer: The Cancer No One Talks About*) both led to high participation in FOBT, *Telling the Story . . . To Live Is God's Will* also decreased cancer fatalism and increased knowledge of colorectal cancer, and thus it has a greater potential for long-term benefits. It may be possible to use the video, *Telling the Story . . . To Live Is God's Will,* in community health care centers to facilitate discussion of colorectal cancer screening issues by health care providers. In addition, it may be beneficial for health care providers to view the video to familiarize themselves with the attitudes and beliefs of some African-American elders so that they can provide culturally appropriate options for patients with these beliefs. Furthermore, clinicians should evaluate the presence of fatalism not only in association with cancer but also in relation to diseases such as hypertension, diabetes, and HIV/AIDS. The next step is to determine if the positive outcomes of this intervention will be supported through replication and to determine if these positive results will be maintained over time.

ACKNOWLEDGMENTS

This research was supported by grants from the Oncology Nursing Foundation, Sigma Theta Tau International, and the NIH-funded Center for Research on Chronic Illness, University of North Carolina at Chapel Hill, School of Nursing (grant #P30NR03962). This chapter is adapted from Powe, B. D., and Weinrich, S. (1999). An intervention to decrease cancer fatalism among rural elders. *Oncology Nursing Forum*, *26*(3), 583–588. Copyright by Oncology Nursing Press, 1999. Printed with permission.

REFERENCES

Allison, J., Tekawa, I., Ransom, L., & Adrian, A. (1996). A comparison of fecal occult blood tests for colorectal cancer screening. *New England Journal of Medicine, 334*(3), 155–159.

American Cancer Society. (1998). *1998 cancer facts and figures.* Atlanta: Author.

Centers for Disease Control. (1996). Trends in cancer screening—United States: 1987 and 1992. *Morbidity and Mortality Weekly Report, 45*(3), 57–61.

Chang, B., & Hirsch, M. (1994). Videotape intervention: Producing videotapes for use in nursing practice and education. *Journal of Continuing Education in Nursing, 25*(6), 263–267.

Dombeck, M., & Karl, J. (1987). Spiritual issues in mental health care. *Journal of Religion and Health, 26,* 183–197.

Dwyer, J., Clarke, L., & Miller, M. (1990). The effect of religious concentration and affiliation on county cancer mortality rates. *Journal of Health and Social Behavior, 31,* 185–202.

Ederer, R., Church, T., & Mandel, J. (1997). Fecal occult blood screening in the Minnesota study: Role of chance detection of lesions. *Journal of the National Cancer Institute, 89*(19), 1423–1428.

Emblem, J. (1992). Religion and spirituality defined according to current use in nursing literature. *Journal of Professional Nursing, 8*(1), 41–47.

Freeman, H. (1989). *Cancer and the socioeconomic disadvantaged.* Atlanta: American Cancer Society.

Griffith, C. J. (1993). Colorectal cancer: Reducing mortality through early detection and treatment. *Physician Assistant, 17*(1), 25–34.

Hansen, C. (1995). Colorectal cancer: A preventable disease. *Physician Assistant, 95*(1), 15–26.

Hoskins, D., & Rose, M. (1989). *Cancer and the poor: A report to the nation.* Atlanta: American Cancer Society.

Landrine, H., & Klonoff, E. (1994). Cultural diversity in causal attributions for illness: The role of the supernatural. *Journal of Behavioral Medicine, 17*(2), 181–193.

Lang, C., & Ransohoff, D. (1994). Fecal occult blood screening for colorectal cancer: Is mortality reduced by chance selection for screening colonoscopy? *Journal of the American Medical Association, 271,* 1011–1013.

Lang, C., & Ransohoff, D. (1997). On the sensitivity of fecal occult blood test screening for colorectal cancer. *Journal of the National Cancer Institute, 89*(19), 1392–1393.

Lincoln, C. E., & Mamiya, L. (1990). *The Black church in the African-American experience.* Durham: Duke University Press.

Lloyd, J., McConnell, P., & Zahorik, P. (1994). Collaborative health education training for African-American health ministers and providers of community services. *Educational Gerontology, 20,* 265–276.

Martin, M., & Henry, M. (1989). Cultural relativity and poverty. *Public Health Nursing, 6*(1), 28–34.

Meade, C. (1996). Producing videotapes for cancer education: Methods and examples. *Oncology Nursing Forum, 23*(5), 837–846.

Olsen, S., & Frank-Stromborg, M. (1993). Cancer prevention and early detection in ethnically diverse populations. *Seminars in Oncology Nursing, 9*(3), 198–209.

Powe, B. D. (1995a). Cancer fatalism among elderly Caucasian and African-Americans. *Oncology Nursing Forum, 22*(9), 1355–1359.

Powe, B. D. (1995b). Fatalism and colorectal cancer screening among elderly African-Americans. *Cancer Nursing, 18*(5), 385–392.

Powe, B. D. (1995c). Perceptions of fatalism among African-Americans: The influence of education, income, and knowledge. *Journal of the National Black Nurses Association, 7*(2), 41–48.

Powe, B. D. (1997). Cancer fatalism . . . Spiritual perspectives. *Journal of Religion and Health, 36*(2), 135–144.

Powe, B. D., & Johnson, A. (1995). Fatalism among African-Americans: Philosophical perspectives. *Journal of Religion and Health, 34*(2), 119–125.

Reed, P. G. (1992). An emerging paradigm for the investigation of spirituality in nursing. *Research in Nursing and Health, 15*(5), 349–357.

Rosella, J., Regan-Kubinski, M., & Albrecht, S. (1994). The need for multi-cultural diversity among health professionals. *Nursing and Health Care, 15,* 242–246.

Scandrett, A. (1994). Religion as a support component in the health behavior of Black Americans. *Journal of Religion and Health,* 123–129.

St. John, D., Young, G., McHutchison, J., Deacon, M., & Alexeyeff, M. (1992). Comparison of the specificity and sensitivity of hemoccult and hemoquant in screening for colorectal neoplasia. *Annals of Internal Medicine, 117,* 376–382.

Thomas, S. B. (1994). The characteristics of northern black churches with community health outreach programs. *American Journal of Public Health, 84*(4), 575–579.

Underwood, S., & Hoskins, D. (1994). Increasing nursing involvement in cancer prevention and control among the economically disadvantaged: The nursing challenge. *Seminars in Oncology Nursing, 10,* 89–95.

Underwood, S., Hoskins, D., Cummins, T., Morris, K., & Williams, A. (1994). Obstacles to cancer care: Focus on the socioeconomically disadvantaged. *Oncology Nursing Forum, 21*(1), 47–52.

U.S. Department of Health and Human Services (USDHHS). (1990). *Healthy people 2000: National health promotion and disease prevention objectives* (DHSS Pub. No. (PHS) 91-50213). Washington, DC: U.S. Government Printing Office.

U.S. Preventive Services Task Force (USPSTF). (1996). *Guide to clinical preventive services* (2nd ed.). Baltimore: Williams & Wilkins.

Weinrich, S., Weinrich, M., Boyd, M., Atwood, J., & Cervanka, B. (1992). Effective approaches for increasing compliance with ACS's screening recommendations in socioeconomically disadvantaged populations. *Second National Conference on Cancer Nursing Research,* Atlanta: American Cancer Society.

Weinrich, S., Weinrich, M., Boyd, M., Johnson, E., & Frank-Stromborg, M. (1992). Knowledge of colorectal cancer among older persons. *Cancer Nursing, 15*(5), 322–330.

Weinrich, S., Weinrich, M., Frank-Stromborg, M., Boyd, M., & Weiss, H. (1993). Using elderly educators to increase colorectal cancer screening. *The Gerontologist, 33*(4), 491–496.

West, C. (1993). *Race matters.* Boston: Beacon Press.

[11]

Early Interventions with Children: A Systems Approach

Rachel Stevens and Peter A. Margolis

Addressing the adverse health and developmental outcomes of at-risk mothers and their children represents a critical need in our society, as does the prevention of child abuse and neglect. Though good parenting skills are essential to promote the development of children during the critical first years of life, new mothers—especially if they are young and low-income—often have few of these skills and little understanding of child development. A failure to develop good parenting skills is reflected tragically in consequences such as abuse and neglect, foster care, juvenile delinquency, and dysfunctional lives.

The U.S. health care system presents numerous barriers to new mothers living below the poverty level. The care provided is fragmented, with many categorical services designed to address only a subgroup of patients or a specific type of disease. As has often been noted, if McDonald's were run like a health department, they would sell french fries only on Friday and hamburgers on Monday and sodas on Wednesday. Overcoming barriers to care caused by the fragmentation of services must be a central component of any program striving to improve the health promotion care provided to women throughout their pregnancy and during the early years of their children's lives. The Linkages for Prevention project (Margolis et al., 1996) is such a program; it is a system-level intervention designed to overcome barriers to improving the health and developmental outcomes of populations of children. That is to say, the project includes multiple interrelated interventions designed to affect the way health care is organized and delivered at the level of the community, the pediatric practice, and the family. This chapter focuses on the project's approach to improving preventive health care for Medicaid children.

The intervention consists of protocol-guided (Olds et al., 1997) visits to families' homes. A public health nurse from the health department and an early childhood educator from the mental health department make 2 to 4 visits per month. The nurse home visiting is based on the program developed by David Olds and follows his program model, and the early childhood educators follow a child development curriculum. Visits begin when the mother presents for prenatal care and continue through the first year of the child's life. Home visitors use curricula with demonstrated effectiveness in promoting parental and infant health, parenting skills, maternal life-course development, social support, and use of needed health and human services. On average, families receive a visit every 1 to 2 weeks.

The interventions are grounded in several key principles. First, interventions need to have a measurable impact on all children in the community. The long-term goal is for the community to develop a plan to provide the interventions for all eligible women. Second, the interventions are based on evidence (Olds et al., 1997). The traditional public health approach has been to say, "Well, I think this is the best way to do it," or "There's some categorical money coming down; how quickly can we design a program to fit it." To the greatest extent possible, the Linkages project uses interventions with strong evidence to support their effectiveness. In keeping with this principle, the home visiting intervention uses protocols that have been tested extensively through randomized trials and have been demonstrated to be effective (Olds et al., 1997). Third, services should be targeted to a family's risks and should include methods to increase communication among agencies dealing with the family. Lastly, the project includes ongoing evaluation and feedback to ensure continuous improvement in the quality of the services provided.

METHOD

Setting

The Linkages for Prevention project was implemented first as a community-wide effort in Durham, North Carolina. Durham is a medium-sized city with a population of 182,000. It has approximately 3,000 births per year, about half of which are to mothers on Medicaid. Enrollment was conducted through the community health center because that is where the majority of Medicaid women in Durham County seek prenatal care. The intervention was a collaboration between the Departments of Public Health and Mental Health.

Participants

Because our principal funding was through Medicaid, subjects had to be at or below 100% of poverty level. All subjects had to agree to participate in the protocols through the first year of their child's life; of those eligible, 89% agreed to participate. The group included 109 subjects after 17% dropped out or moved out of Durham. The mean age of the subjects was early 20s, the majority had not graduated from high school, and the majority were African American. Most of the women had other children.

Intervention

The project began with a feasibility study to assess what would be required in order to implement the Linkages for Prevention project in a health department. We then worked with Durham County for a year to develop community-level commitment and involvement, with the goal of creating change that would continue beyond the project's funding. During that first year we created a community advisory board that was chaired by the director of Medicaid for the state, with representatives from local community agencies, practices, and county government. Only after the initial groundwork was laid with the community did we begin to test our interventions. Enrollment and data collection for the family-level intervention occurred over a 3-year period.

The project involved a three-tiered intervention strategy. At the community level, interventions were developed to link public health agencies providing similar services such as home visiting and to enhance cooperation and decrease duplication of services. The practice-level intervention provided primary care practices with assistance to improve the organization and delivery of preventive services. The intervention involved assistance to help practices develop "office systems" for preventive care by involving the entire office staff in carrying out this process. A project team comprised of a physician and a health educator helped each practice measure rates of preventive services, analyze problems, and design materials such as flow sheets to improve the delivery of care. The team also helped train staff and implement and monitor system changes.

The family-level intervention was based on the work of David Olds and Harriet Kitzman, which started over 25 years ago in Elmira, New York (Olds & Kitzman, 1992). Olds's initial work focused primarily on impoverished White women in the Appalachian region of New York state. He and his colleagues followed 400 children over 15 years to demonstrate the effectiveness of a home visitation intervention during the first 2 years of life (Olds, Henderson, Tatelbaum, & Chamberline, 1986). More recently, Olds has studied primarily African-American urban southern women in Memphis, Tennessee (Olds et al., 1999). In the New York and Memphis studies, Olds and colleagues found 25% reduction in cigarette smoking during pregnancy among women who smoked cigarettes at registration; 56% fewer hospital emergency room visits where injuries were detected; 79% reduction in rates of child maltreatment among at-risk families from birth through the child's 15th year; 43% reduction in subsequent pregnancy among low-income, unmarried women by first child's fourth birthday (31% reduction through age 15, with two years greater interval between birth of first and second children); 83% increase in the rates of labor force participation by first child's fourth birthday; 30 month reduction in AFDC utilization among low-income, unmarried women by first child's 15th birthday; and 44% reduction in low-income, unmarried mothers' behavioral problems due to alcohol and drug abuse over the 15 years following program enrollment.

Our intervention replicated and augmented the Olds protocols. These protocols are a very detailed program structured to provide intense visits that focus on six domains: maternal health, parental role, parent life development, family and friends, linkages with other health services, and the environment. The program incorporates a strong management information system that provides both intervention and family data.

In our intervention, public health nurses made visits during pregnancy and early infancy and devoted special attention to the mother's and the baby's health, the mother's life, the mother's role as a parent, social support, and use of human services. The specific content of visits was adapted to the needs of each family. Special attention was paid to helping mothers address their own life course development issues (e.g., making plans to return to school or work, family planning).

Our intervention supplemented the Olds protocols by partnering a public health nurse with an early childhood educator. This team approach has enabled us to add additional work on child development and parenting. Thus, in addition to the Olds curriculum and the Linkages Curriculum for Intensive Home Visiting (Margolis et al., 1996), home visitors used parent educational materials, "Partners in Learning" (Sparling, 1996), and the Child Development Health and Safety Project developed by the Injury Prevention Research Center and the Division of Pediatrics, University of North Carolina (Cohen, Sheaffer, Gordon, & Baird, 1996).

Women served by local health departments in North Carolina typically are visited once or twice in their home, and their maternity care coordinators have a caseload of 150. Our intervention nurses carried a caseload of no more than 25, and, on average, families received 33 visits. We sought to link primary care practice interventions and family interventions by encouraging home visitors to identify a nurse in each primary care practice with whom they could communicate about the families' services. We had our intervention nurses go with the mothers for their first visit. The intervention nurses also worked with the office staff to raise their awareness of the way they interacted with Medicaid patients.

To ensure that the home visitors followed the protocols, they received intensive introductory training, followed by ongoing site-based training and evaluation.

We monitored the content covered in home visits by having the intervention nurse self-report on the visits. An outside evaluator interviewed all mothers to validate the content covered. This two-step evaluation confirmed that all the mothers received education in all the fields.

EVALUATION

We are currently evaluating the outcomes of the program at the levels of community, family, and medical practice. As noted earlier, our intervention was based on these principles:

1. To have a measurable impact, needs of *all* children in the community should be considered.
2. Interventions should be based on evidence.
3. Services should be targeted to a family's level of risk.
4. Interventions should include methods to increase communication.
5. Ongoing measurement should be the basis for refining interventions and assessing impact.

Preliminary findings suggest that the intervention was effective in getting these women to use contraception, to reduce smoking, and to improve parenting skills and home safety.

DISCUSSION

The present study extends the work of Olds et al., who recognized the central role that nurses have played in home visitation. The home visiting intervention differs from other programs in its focus on high-risk families, the number of cases per intervention nurse (25 to 30), and the number of family contacts (2 to 4 per month). The home visiting intervention differs from Olds's intervention in several important ways. The nurse is partnered with a childhood educator, and home visiting is incorporated into a three-tiered project addressing the levels of family, community, and pediatric practice. Public health nurses play a central role at all three levels, serving as liaisons between agencies, providers, and the study subjects. Finally, whereas Olds recommends following children for the first 2 years of life, we follow them only for 1 year.

The Linkages project has now expanded from Durham County to 20 counties in North Carolina, and the state is supporting the continued expansion of the program. The objective is to use the intensive home visiting program to assist communities to enhance the services available for pregnant women and for families of children from birth to age two. The long-range goals are to improve perinatal outcomes, enhance child and family development, prevent physical and mental health problems and reduce morbidity and mortality resulting from abuse and neglect. The intent is to achieve these goals through comprehensive, coordinated family-centered services to encourage healthy lifestyles, enhance family functioning and improve the use of cost-effective health care and social services.

We have found that tiered, interrelated interventions that target an entire population of children in a community are feasible. Our work suggests that researchers, in partnership with policy makers, public health leaders, and practicing physicians, can help catalyze meaningful improvement efforts and learn a lot at the same time. Community-based work takes a long time; the present work has been in progress for over 8 years. However, if done well, the investment of time can pay off in improved health for populations of children and mothers. The study has demonstrated that evidence-based community interventions can be beneficial to children and their mothers. The study also reinforces the need to recognize the unique needs and constraints of each community and to tailor evidence-based approaches to fit those needs.

Finally, the study raises important questions for those of us who work for the improvement of maternal and child health. If system-level intervention is feasible and effective, then who is responsible for its implementation and what resources will be required to effect such broad-based change? These questions will need to be addressed if we are to move from concept to application and achieve the potential for gain in the health and development of populations of children.

REFERENCES

Cohen, L. R., Sheaffer, L. G., Gordon, A. N., & Baird, T. L. (1996). *Child development, health, and safety: Educational materials for home visitors and parents.* Gaithersburg, MD: Aspen.

Margolis, P. A., Lannon, C. M., Stevens, R., Harlan, C., Bordley, W. C., Carey, T., Leininger, L., Keyes, L. L., & Earp, J. L. (1996). Linking clinical and public health approaches to improve access to health care for socially disadvantaged mothers and children. *Archives of Pediatric Adolescent Medicine, 150,* 815–821.

Olds, D. L., Eckenrode, J., Henderson, C. R., Jr., Kitzman, H., Powers, J., Cole, R., Sidora, K., Morris, P., Pettit, L. M., & Luckey, D. (1997). Long-term effects of home visitation on maternal life course and child abuse and neglect. *Journal of the American Medical Association, 278*(8), 637–643.

Olds, D. L., Henderson, C. R., Kitzman, H. J., Eckenrode, J. J., Cole, R. E., & Tatelbaum, R. C. (1999). Prenatal and infancy home visitation by nurses: Recent findings. *Future of Children, 9*(1), 190–191.

Olds, D. L., Henderson, C., Tatelbaum, R., & Chamberline, R. (1986). Improving the delivery of prenatal care and outcomes of pregnancy: a randomized trial of nurse home visitation. *Pediatrics, 77*(16), 16–28.

Olds, D. L., & Kitzman, H. (1992). *Home visiting protocols* (Vols. 1 and 2). Unpublished research protocols available from the first author.

Sparling, J. (1996). *Partners for learning.* Chapel Hill: Kaplan Press.

[12]

Development of a Public Health Nurse–Delivered Cholesterol Intervention Program

Thomas C. Keyserling, Alice S. Ammerman, Jan R. Atwood, James D. Hosking, Cristina Krasny, Hany Zayed, and Betty H. Worthy

Residents of the rural South are highly vulnerable to death and disability from cardiovascular disease (Centers for Disease Control and Prevention, 1992). Diet and other behavioral factors are significant contributors to this increased risk, but rural residents often have limited access to health screening and promotion services. In recent years, however, cholesterol screening has been greatly facilitated by the availability of finger-stick cholesterol assessment instruments, and now most Americans, including those in primarily rural states, report they have been screened for high blood cholesterol (Centers for Disease Control and Prevention, 1993). Resources for nutrition services have not increased in proportion to the number of individuals being identified as hypercholesterolemic, raising concerns that screening is conducted with inadequate mechanisms for dietary assessment, counseling, and follow-up.

Public health nutritionists are the most likely sources of dietary counseling in rural areas, but they are in short supply (Haughton, Story, & Keir,

1998). Most nutritionists funded through county health departments are committed to maternal and child health services and largely unavailable for health promotion interventions aimed at chronic disease prevention in adults. Programs are needed that make use of other health care providers to extend the services of nutritionists. Public health nurses exist in greater numbers than most other health professionals serving rural areas (Wright & Jablonowski, 1987) and therefore can substantially extend nutrition services for coronary heart disease (CHD) risk reduction (Pender & Pender, 1987). There are many barriers to the delivery of nutrition services by public health nurses, however, such as lack of time, limited training in nutrition, low self-efficacy regarding lifestyle-change counseling, and inadequate assessment and intervention materials (Wilt, Hubbard, & Thomas, 1990).

This chapter describes the development of a dietary treatment program (the Food for Heart Program) for public health nurses to implement in rural health departments in the South. The intervention is designed to circumvent many of the obstacles common to diet counseling and behavior change. The chapter also presents key descriptive data documenting the need for the intervention.

METHOD

Setting

County health departments were invited to participate provided that the county met the definition of "rural," defined by the Office of Management and Budget as locations that are not metropolitan statistical areas (MSAs). (An MSA is a county or group of contiguous counties with a total population of at least 100,000 or one city with a population of 50,000 or more [Johnson-Webb, Baer, & Gesler, 1997].) An attempt was made to recruit rural counties from each of the three major regions of North Carolina: mountain, piedmont (rolling hills), and coastal plain. Regional nurse consultants from the Division of Community Health, North Carolina Department of Health and Human Services, were contacted to help identify counties with reasonably stable staffing and infrastructure that would facilitate participation. Counties already participating in large-scale health promotion research programs were excluded.

To describe the program and solicit interest among county health departments, study staff made presentations at meetings of health department directors and nursing supervisors. For counties that expressed an interest, a meeting was held at the health department to describe the program in greater detail. The majority of counties contacted chose to participate. Counties choosing not to participate cited the following reasons: staff turnover, vacant positions, or significant staff burden associated with initiating a new health department program.

Eighteen health departments agreed to participate, although one withdrew before enrolling patients. Participating departments were representative of the geographic diversity of North Carolina, with three from the coastal plain, six from the piedmont, and eight from the Appalachian Mountains. According to 1990 U.S. Census data (U.S. Census Bureau, 1997), the average population in the counties represented by these departments was 46,850 (range: 7,196–110,605), with 82% White, 16% African American, and 1% American Indian. Median family income was $16,754.

Local health departments were responsible for recruiting nurses to participate in the program; the majority of these nurses were adult health or general clinic nurses. The nursing supervisors at each site were asked to identify one nurse as the study's on-site coordinator to serve as a liaison with research office personnel.

Patients

Health department staff were instructed to screen a sufficient number of patients considered candidates for CHD risk factor modification in order to identify 30 with high cholesterol during a 3-month enrollment period. Patients were screened from a variety of settings, including primary care clinics, health screening clinics, and occupational settings. Inclusion criteria required that patients be between the ages of 20 and 70 years (inclusive), plan to reside in the community for a year, be accessible by phone, and have registered a total cholesterol level of greater than 180 mg/dL if checked within the past year. Exclusion criteria included severe medical conditions such that preventive measures for CHD were not a priority; acute, self-limiting medical conditions (patient was eligible for screening 3 or more weeks after improvement); inability to speak or comprehend English; and active treatment for hypercholesterolemia, defined as taking lipid-lowering medication or more than two diet counseling sessions by a health professional within the past 6 months.

Risk factors and blood lipids were assessed to determine eligibility, following the guidelines of the Adult Treatment Panel II of the National Cholesterol Education Program (National Cholesterol Education Program Adult Treatment Panel II, 1993). The following risk factors were recorded by the enrolling nurse: age, gender, family history of premature CHD, cigarette smoking, hypertension, diabetes, and known CHD. Risk attributed to high-density lipoprotein cholesterol (HDL-C) (defined as a level < 35 mg/dL) was assessed at the time of the first lipid panel.

Screening blood work included a fasting lipid panel and a thyrotropin level. If the triglycerides were greater than 500 mg/dL, the patient was excluded because low-density lipoprotein cholesterol (LDL-C) could not be calculated reliably using the Friedewald formula (DeLong, DeLong, Wood, Lippel, & Rifkind, 1986). If the thyrotropin was more than two times the upper limit of normal, the patient was excluded for hypothyroidism. Patients were enrolled if their LDL-C was ≥ 160 mg/dL, 130 to 159 mg/dL with two or more risk factors, or more than 100 mg/dL with known CHD. About 2 weeks after each blood test, participants were sent letters reporting their total cholesterol level, and their nurses received the results of all study blood tests. Enrollment was completed during a 10-month period.

Baseline Characteristics of Enrolled Patients

Participating health departments screened 781 subjects. Of these, 468 met all eligibility criteria and participated in the study. The average number of participants per health department was 27.5. The sample was largely female (71%), older (mean age: 55), and predominantly White (80%); almost three quarters were high school graduates. Participants were at relatively high risk for CHD: One third reported a positive family history, 20% were current smokers, 40% had a history of hypertension, and more than 20% had low HDL-C. The majority of participants (59%) had two or more CHD risk factors, and about 10% had known CHD at the time of screening (defined as either prior myocardial infarction, coronary artery bypass graft surgery, percutaneous transluminal coronary angioplasty, or angina). Although more than three quarters of participants reported a cholesterol check during the preceding year, only 11% reported receiving counseling for high cholesterol from a doctor, nurse, or nutritionist during the preceding 6 months.

The mountain area of North Carolina is geographically distinct from the other two regions and has different historical, cultural, and economic characteristics, so participants from the mountain counties were compared to those in the rest of the state on all baseline variables. Except for a difference in the percentage of participants by race (95% White in the mountains vs. 67% in the piedmont and coastal plain, $p = .0002$), there were no other differences noted (data not shown).

Food for Heart Program Design and Rationale

The Food for Heart Program (FFHP) is a dietary assessment and counseling program targeting lower literacy and income patients in the southeastern

United States. Originally developed for primary care physicians practicing in community health centers, it has been adapted for a broader variety of health professionals with limited training in nutrition counseling for chronic disease prevention (Ammerman et al., 1992, 1993). The FFHP is designed to facilitate counseling by health care professionals (in this case, public health nurses), taking into consideration their preexisting knowledge and attitudes about diet counseling along with organizational barriers such as limited time and lack of appropriate educational materials. The program also addresses patient knowledge and attitudes, as well as environmental barriers likely to be faced by lower income patients, such as culturally insensitive and costly dietary recommendations. The FFHP is structured to increase both patient and counselor confidence by being culturally sensitive and clinically feasible and by incorporating sound behavior change theory.

Dietary Risk Assessment

The FFHP intervention is initiated and guided by a dietary risk assessment (DRA) instrument developed for the program. The design and validation of the DRA have been described in detail elsewhere (Ammerman et al., 1991). In brief, the DRA is intended to meet six specific criteria: (1) ease of administration and scoring, (2) relevance to the diet of the target population, (3) identification of positive as well as problematic dietary behaviors, (4) emphasis on food rather than nutrient-based results, (5) identification of misconceptions and attitudes that may serve as barriers to dietary change, and (6) accurate ranking of individuals by dietary atherogenic risk. The DRA was validated against a more rigorous but less efficient dietary assessment method in a sample of 42 low-income individuals. The total DRA score was correlated with results from three 24-hour recalls entered into a Keys equation, which predicts the cholesterol-raising potential of the diet (Keys, Anderson, & Grande, 1959). The DRA compared favorably with the more complex method in assessing the level of dietary atherogenic risk ($r = .60$, $p < .001$) (Ammerman et al., 1991).

The DRA can be administered and scored by a nonnutritionist in 10 to 15 minutes. Foods included in the assessment were selected on the basis of their contribution to saturated fat in the diet of African Americans and cholesterol in the diet of all Americans (Block, Dresser, Hartman, & Carroll, 1985). Additional questions address southern food preparation practices such as seasoning vegetables with meat fat. The DRA scoring system facilitates rapid identification of positive as well as negative dietary habits. The instrument quantifies the degree of excessive or inadequate consumption of specific *foods* rather than *nutrients*, using shaded columns that categorize the responses to food frequency questions as "significant problem," "needs work," and "doing well." The DRA permits efficient counseling by tailoring advice to the individual's dietary habits.

All foods included in the DRA are grouped in four categories, each on a separate page: (1) meats; (2) dairy; (3) side dishes, desserts, snacks; and (4) spreads, salad dressing, oils. An additional page focuses on diabetes and weight control for those patients needing guidance in these areas. A simple score is calculated for each category and scores are used to rank the categories in descending order by contribution to dietary risk, so that the most atherogenic dietary practices are addressed first. The DRA also includes supplemental attitude and barrier questions important to behavior change.

Table 12.1 shows DRA scores for the study population, with a higher score reflecting a higher intake of atherogenic foods. In the gender-specific analysis, males had a higher score for meat consumption than females. There was a marked difference in reported behaviors between non-Whites and Whites, with non-Whites reporting higher scores for meats, side dishes, and oils. The total score for non-Whites was 26.1, compared to 21.5 for Whites ($p = .0003$).

More than 70% of participants reported minimal to modest intake of red meat products. Portion size for meats appeared to be relatively large, however, with 45% noting portion size greater than 3 oz. A majority of the participants ate poultry regularly and reported that the chicken was not fried and they did not eat the skin. Only 20% reported eating fish two or more times a week (and usually the fish was fried). Half of the participants reported occasionally eating dried peas and beans instead of meat, and about three quarters reported regular consumption of peanut butter.

In the category of side dishes, desserts, and snacks, participants reported inadequate consumption of fruits and vegetables and overconsumption of

TABLE 12.1 Dietary Risk Assessment Scores

Food Category	Female	Male	p	Non-White	White	p
Meats	9.3	10.6	.03	11.5	9.2	.0002
Side dishes, desserts, snacks	7.8	7.9	.82	8.6	7.6	.027
Dairy, eggs	1.8	2.1	.16	2.1	1.9	.32
Spreads, salad dressings, oils	3.1	3.0	.53	3.9	2.9	.0012
Total score	22.0	23.5	.22	26.1	21.5	.0003

sweets. More than half reported consuming fruits and vegetables one time per day or less. In addition, only a third of the participants reported frequent consumption of complex carbohydrates (rice, potatoes, noodles, and bread).

The reported consumption of high-fat dairy products and eggs was very low. Eighty percent reported consumption of whole milk zero to one time per week, 71% reported eating cheese zero to two times per week, 82% reported consumption of ice cream zero to one time per week, and 76% reported eating zero to two eggs per week. For spreads, salad dressings, and oils, 87% reported consumption of margarine, compared to 8% who reported consumption of butter; few participants (9%) reported consumption of more than two pats a day of either. Vegetable oil was clearly preferred for frying at home, and about half of the participants used vegetable shortening for baking; however, one third seasoned vegetables with butter, fatback, side meat, or bacon.

Structured Dietary Treatment

Few existing educational materials focus on fat and cholesterol reduction for a low-income, southern population. Therefore, we developed new materials, relying heavily on the book *Teaching Patients with Low Literacy Skills* (Doak, Doak, & Root, 1985), recommendations from staff members of the North Carolina Agricultural Extension Service, and pilot testing in the target population. A single illustrated page of recommendations (tip sheet) was developed to correspond with each of the DRA food and attitude assessment pages. Tip sheets and individual tips are color and number coded with the DRA and provide specific behavior change strategies. Readability of the materials is at about the fifth- or sixth-grade level (McLaughlin, 1969). Stop sign symbols are used to flag foods that should be eaten infrequently, and realistic food illustrations are included. Where appropriate, regional terminology is used, and southern eating practices are targeted both for behavior change and for reinforcement of positive practices.

Supplemental educational pamphlets include "Good Food for Your Heart," a simplified explanation of diet and heart disease; a "Heart Helper" pamphlet given to a support person identified by the patient and offering suggestions on how to assist and encourage someone who is trying to change his or her diet; and a "Fast Food Facts" pamphlet with practical suggestions on eating sensibly at fast food restaurants. Each patient is also given a cookbook titled *Food for Heart Southern Style Recipes*, which includes 74 simple, low-cost recipes compiled from several well respected sources. The book builds on positive regional aspects of the diet like greens, fish, chicken, and dried peas and beans. Additional recipes suggest ingredient substitutions to lower the fat and cholesterol content of traditional southern foods such as biscuits and cornbread. Recipes in the cookbook are referenced by number on the tip sheets, so that, for example, when the recommendation to eat less fried chicken is made, the nurse can quickly direct the patient to alternate chicken recipes. To circumvent economic barriers, FFHP materials suggest "stretching" meats with less expensive and less atherogenic starches such as potatoes and rice. Suggestions for sensible, low-cost fast-food meals are offered, such as two small plain hamburgers instead of one deluxe burger, which is more expensive and much higher in saturated fat and cholesterol.

To increase the likelihood of patient and thus counselor success, the FFHP is based on behavior change theory (Eraker, Kirscht, & Becker, 1984). Behavior change recommendations are broken into small, achievable steps, and specific strategies are recommended to make the changes more palatable. Nurses are encouraged to negotiate with the patient on the selection of two goals to accomplish before the next visit. These goals are then marked on the DRA for monitoring by the nurse and on the tip sheet as a reminder for the patient. To direct counseling toward improving patient self-efficacy, the FFHP dietary risk assessment and educational materials identify and reinforce positive behaviors and make it easier to spot small but important improvements.

Monitoring and Follow-up

Nurses may become discouraged with dietary counseling efforts, in part because progress is difficult to monitor. Patients may feel less motivated if the counselor appears to have lost interest in their dietary change efforts. For these reasons, the FFHP treatment folder serves as both a prompt and a flow sheet or monitoring system. DRA results can either be filed in the patient's medical record under a specially labeled tabbed divider or in a separate treatment folder placed in the chart. A system of recording dietary behaviors and goals with dates and appropriately placed checkmarks limits the amount of time required for charting and makes it easy to monitor progress at subsequent visits. Monitoring and follow-up are also possible using a mail and telephone system; portions of the DRA results and educational materials are sent to the patient and then discussed by phone.

DISCUSSION

Residents of the rural South are at high risk for CHD and are frequently identified as having high blood cholesterol. Reducing their cholesterol would decrease their CHD risk, but resources for nutrition counseling in rural areas are often limited, raising concerns that hypercholesterolemic individuals may not receive adequate dietary assessment and follow-up. In order to increase the availability of high-quality nutrition counseling for high blood cholesterol, the authors developed a program for use by public health nurses that is designed to circumvent many of the obstacles common to dietary counseling. Incorporating features of behavior change theory and designed to be feasible in a typical clinical setting, this program provides public health nurses with techniques and strategies to counsel patients about diet and heart disease even if their training in nutrition is limited.

This chapter has described the assessment and treatment program designed for use by public health nurses, and baseline data on a southern rural population at risk for hypercholesterolemia. In this study, self-reported dietary data were notable for the relatively modest intake of foods highest in saturated fat and cholesterol. For example, over 80% of the participants reported minimal to modest intake of hamburger, beef, and pork. Major dietary problems identified included inadequate consumption of fruits and vegetables, only modest intake of complex carbohydrates, and excessive consumption of sweets. Non-Whites had substantially higher (more atherogenic) scores for meats; side dishes, desserts, and snacks; spreads, salad dressings, oils; and substantially higher total scores. Whether these differences represent different dietary patterns or self-reporting practices cannot be determined from these data.

ACKNOWLEDGMENTS

This work was supported in part by grant NRO3042 from the National Institute of Nursing Research, National Institutes of Health, Bethesda, Maryland. We are indebted to the health departments' staff and study participants whose generous cooperation made this study possible. This chapter is adapted from Keyserling, T. C., Ammerman, A. S., Atwood, J. R., Hosking, J. D., Krasny, C., Zayed., H., & Worthy, B. H. (1999). A cholesterol intervention program for public health nurses in the rural Southeast: Description of the intervention, study design, and baseline results. *Public Health Nursing*, *16*(3), 156–167. Copyright by Blackwell Science, Inc., 1999. Printed with permission.

REFERENCES

Ammerman, A. S., DeVellis, R. F., Carey, T. S., Keyserling, T. C., Strogatz, D. S., Haines, P. S., Simpson, R. J., Jr., & Siscovick, D. S. (1993). Physician-based diet counseling for cholesterol reduction: Current practices, determinants, and strategies for improvement. *Preventive Medicine, 22*(1), 96–109.

Ammerman, A. S., DeVellis, B. M., Haines, P. S., Keyserling, T. C., Carey, T. S., DeVellis, R. F., & Simpson, R. J., Jr. (1992). Nutrition education for cardiovascular disease prevention among low-income populations: Description and pilot evaluation of a physician-based model. *Patient Education and Counseling, 19*(1), 5–18.

Ammerman, A. S., Haines, R. S., DeVellis, R. F., Strogatz, D. S., Keyserling, T. C., Simpson, R. J., Jr., & Siscovick, D. S. (1991). A brief dietary assessment to guide cholesterol reduction in low-income individuals: Design and validation. *Journal of the American Dietetic Association, 91*(11), 1385–1390.

Block, G., Dresser, C. M., Hartman, A. M., & Carroll, M. D. (1985). Nutrient sources in the American diet: Quantitative data from the NHANES II survey. II. Macronutrients and fats. *American Journal of Epidemiology, 122*(1), 27–40.

Centers for Disease Control and Prevention. (1992). Trends in ischemic heart disease mortality—United States, 1980–1988. *Morbidity and Mortality Weekly Report, 41*(30), 548–549, 556.

Centers for Disease Control and Prevention. (1993). State-specific changes in cholesterol screening-behavioral risk factor surveillance system, 1988–1991. *Morbidity and Mortality Weekly Report, 42*(34), 663–667.

DeLong, D. M., DeLong, E. R., Wood, P. D., Lippel, K., & Rifkind, B. M. (1986). A comparison of methods for the estimation of plasma low- and very low-density lipoprotein cholesterol. The Lipid Research Clinics Prevalence Study. *Journal of the American Medical Association, 256*(17), 2372–2377.

Doak, C. C., Doak, L. G., & Root, J. H. (1985). *Teaching patients with low literacy skills.* Philadelphia: Lippincott.

Eraker, S. A., Kirscht, J. P., & Becker, M. H. (1984). Understanding and improving patient compliance. *Annals of Internal Medicine, 100*, 258–268.

Haughton, B., Story, M., & Keir, B. (1998). Profile of public health nutrition personnel: Challenges for population/system focused roles and state-level monitoring. *Journal of the American Dietetic Association, 98*(6), 664–670.

Johnson-Webb, K. D., Baer, L. D., & Gesler, W. M. (1997). What is rural? Issues and considerations. *Journal of Rural Health, 13*(3), 253–256.

Keys, A., Anderson, J., & Grande, F. (1959). Serum cholesterol in man: Diet fat and intrinsic responsiveness. *Circulation, 19*, 201–214.

McLaughlin, G. H. (1969). SMOG-grading-a new readability formula. *Journal of Reading, 12*(8), 639–646.

National Cholesterol Education Program Adult Treatment Panel II. (1993). Summary of the second report of the National Cholesterol Education Program (NCEP) expert panel on detection, evaluation, and treatment of high blood cholesterol in adults. *Journal of the American Medical Association, 269*(23), 3015–3023.

Pender, N., & Pender, A. (1987). *Health promotion in nursing practice.* Norwalk, CT: Appleton and Lange.

U.S. Census Bureau. (1997, June). *1990 census of population and housing, summary tape file 1A.* Available: http://www.census.gov/datainap/www/index.html.

Wilt, S., Hubbard, A., & Thomas, A. (1990). Knowledge, attitudes, treatment practices, and health behaviors of nurses regarding blood cholesterol and cardiovascular disease. *Preventive Medicine, 19,* 466–475.
Wright, J. S., & Jablonowski, A. (1987). The rural-urban distribution of health
   professionals in Georgia. *Journal of Rural Health, 3*(1), 53–70.

Part III

THE ILLNESS EXPERIENCE

[13]

Transitions and Challenges: Revival and Uncertainty for Persons Living with HIV or AIDS

Dale E. Brashers, Judith L. Neidig, Linda K. Dobbs, Jane A. Russell, Linda W. Cardillo, and Stephen M. Haas

> The weirdest thing to me now is that I am experiencing stress, because now it looks like I'm going to be living for a long time. You know, I'd said good-bye, and I felt free from all of these responsibilities that had to do with my career, and so on. . . . So, with me it's almost as though the stress had ended when I got really sick because I had reached this coming to terms. I don't think that I felt an enormous amount of emotional stress for a while. But, now it has started back up again, when I've gotten more healthy. And that's the most perverse thing in the world, for what that's worth.
>
> Victor

With the availability of protease inhibitors and potent combination antiretroviral therapies for human immunodeficiency virus (HIV) infection and acquired immune deficiency syndrome (AIDS), a disease once considered uniformly fatal may become a chronic and perhaps even curable illness

141

(Carpenter et al., 1997; Gallo, 1996). For persons with HIV who currently are enjoying dramatically improved health, exciting and clearly welcomed physical changes are accompanied by confusion and uncertainty (Linden, 1996). Especially for persons diagnosed with AIDS before the introduction of these highly effective drugs, the joy of dramatic health renewal is tempered by new concerns about career, finances, social relationships, and identity. This experience has been characterized as the Lazarus syndrome (King, 1997), after Lazarus in the Bible, whom Jesus brought back from death after 4 days in the tomb. Renewed health for many has been a return from the tomb of a swiftly approaching death from HIV infection to the joys and problems of continued life (Gregonis, 1997; Sowell, 1997).

Although the experiences of cancer survivors (e.g., Kennedy, Tellegen, Kennedy, & Havernick, 1976; Lansky, List, & Ritter-Sterr, 1986; see Muzzin, Anderson, Figueredo, & Gudelis, 1994, for a review) and "long-term survivors" of HIV infection (e.g., Barroso, 1996, 1997) have been described, there has been little or no research on the complex psychosocial phenomenon of revival currently unfolding. We use the term *revival* to describe the experience of persons who have lived with the belief that they were dying from HIV infection, but who have come to believe that they can survive due to improved HIV treatments. With effective treatments (Gallo, 1996), prolonged survival may mean high levels of uncertainty for long spans of time for HIV-infected persons (Brashers, Neidig, Reynolds, & Haas, 1998). Uncertainty management interventions therefore are likely to be a vital part of a holistic approach to HIV and AIDS care. As a first step toward developing such interventions, the study reported here explored the uncertainty experiences of HIV-infected individuals who had faced death but now were optimistic about survival because of advances in treatment and care. The study was part of a larger qualitative study of HIV-associated uncertainty.

METHOD

Sample

Data were collected from focus groups conducted to elicit the collective perceptions of adults diagnosed with HIV or AIDS. Recruitment was conducted by one of the researchers at an Adult AIDS Clinical Trials Unit (ACTU) in a large midwestern university. Purposeful sampling (Sandelowski, 1995) was used to recruit and select participants on the basis of their willingness to talk in a small group. Each participant received $40 for participation. Because we hoped to include individuals from throughout the HIV spectrum, the initial sample of 24 was divided evenly into two groups of participants with self-reported CD4 counts >200/mm³ ($n = 12$) and two groups of participants with CD4 counts <200/mm³ ($n = 12$). Although redundant narratives occurred after three group interviews, to increase the participation of women and African Americans, recruitment was continued until six focus groups ($N = 33$) were convened.

We should note that the data presented here are only from individuals whose CD4 counts were less than 200 ($n = 13$) or whose CD4 counts had fallen below 200 but had then risen above 200 ($n = 8$). These were the individuals diagnosed with AIDS; in general, they were the ones who produced the revival narratives, perhaps because they were most likely to have accepted death and experienced revival due to improved treatments. The resulting sample of 21 was 85% male, 67% White (28% African-American, 5% Hispanic), and 81% gay (14% heterosexual, 5% bisexual), closely approximating local AIDS prevalence data. The mean age of the participants was 38 years (range: 26 to 59 years, $SD = 9.6$). Most participants had completed 4 or more years of higher education (62%), and most were unemployed (67%). The mean time since diagnosis was 66 months (range: 6 months to 144 months, $SD = 45.6$). The mean CD4 count was 168 (range: 0 to 490, $SD = 132$).

Data Collection and Analysis

To elicit accounts of uncertainty experiences, participants were asked a variety of open-ended questions meant to stimulate group discussion. Probes and follow-up questions also were included to clarify issues and validate researcher interpretations. The interview schedule for each group contained four major areas: general life experiences since testing positive for HIV, aspects of patients' illness that made them feel uncertain (or have questions), the impact of uncertainty on their lives, and strategies used to manage their uncertainty. Here we report only data on the experiences of revival-associated uncertainty, a predominant issue for many focus group participants.

Before the discussions began, each participant signed an informed consent statement and completed a brief demographic questionnaire. Focus group discussions ranged from 1 1/2 to 2 hours in length and were audiotaped. Latent content analysis (Babbie, 1995) and constant comparative techniques (Lincoln & Guba, 1985; Strauss & Corbin, 1990) were used to analyze interview transcripts. We presented results to several study participants and were told that the analysis was congruent with their revival experiences. Conducting multiple group interviews and verifying participant reactions to revival themes helped to strengthen data credibility.

RESULTS

Participants reported that they had experienced denial and anger upon learning of their HIV-positive status, yet they also eventually accepted the likelihood of their premature death. This acceptance involved changing their perspectives about important issues such as long-range plans, self-identity, and interactions with others. However, while these persons living with HIV or AIDS had been forced to come to terms with the likelihood of an early death, many now had reason to hope for recovery from the disease. With highly active combination drug therapies, they were experiencing increased helper T-cell counts and decreased levels of the HIV virus in their blood stream (Carpenter et al., 1997), strengthening that hope. Almost as a mixed blessing, the prospect of recovery from AIDS brought with it a multitude of new complex issues that were difficult to address. Adam, a focus group participant, spoke of how revival had led to increased anxiety in his life:

> For those of us who've been diagnosed for a long time, we've been planning to die and have quit our careers and given up our assets and now all of a sudden they're saying "you may live." And so now how do I get back into work, still paying for my drugs? So, there's a lot more uncertainty now for me, I think. Because I made my peace a long time ago about the dying issue and now it's "uh-oh." . . . It's a good "uh-oh," but at the same time, when you're financially devastated because of the disease, it's a very scary and uncertain "uh-oh."

For most participants, life priorities, types of financial support and work status, personal relationships, and long-term plans had had to be negotiated when they were diagnosed. The renewed prospect of living required renegotiating many of the realities that participants had come to accept. This renegotiation was a source of uncertainty, and often stress, for participants. Specifically, participants had to renegotiate (1) feelings of hope and future orientation, (2) social roles and identities, (3) interpersonal relations, and (4) the quality of their lives. These themes are elaborated on in the sections below.

Feelings of Hope and Future Orientation

For those living with HIV or AIDS, the possibility for and degree of recovery differ from individual to individual. As a result, many who are living with

HIV or AIDS fear being too hopeful. For those who have come to terms with their own mortality, to hope for recovery may mean reopening themselves to disappointment and new despair. The fear of recurrence of cancer has been called the Damocles syndrome (Koocher & O'Malley, 1981; see also Muzzin et al., 1994). In Greek mythology, "Damocles was invited to dine with a king; however he was seated beneath a sword suspended by a single horsehair. This visual representation is used to depict the tenuousness of happiness" (Quigly, 1989, p. 64). For persons with HIV or AIDS, that tenuousness is particularly salient because of the many possible complications of HIV infection. Many realize that improved health still will mean life with a chronic and possibly life-threatening illness. Feelings of hope and future orientation are thus mixed with uncertainty about the long-term efficacy and safety of medications and ambiguity in the meaning of immune restoration and function.

For our focus group participants, high levels of uncertainty about treatments revolved around a lack of information about the long-term effects of medications. Those taking anti-HIV drugs, either through clinical trials or through prescriptions, realized that most drugs were still being tested, and they questioned the long-term safety and efficacy of the medications. Adam described his uncertainty associated with experimental medications: "The thing we're *not* certain about is ultimately what this drug or drug combination is going to do to us a year from now—we *are* the test." Hugh said, "I'm just not planning. I'm really just trying to deal with today because I don't know what the long-term effects of all these new treatments are going to be yet."

The uncertainty about long-term efficacy centered on the unpredictability of individual responses to the new drug therapies. Hugh noted, "These [protease inhibitors] helped a lot of people. But it's not a miracle, it's not a cure. It doesn't work for everybody." Many knew of unexplained treatment failures, and some worried because of a lack of data on individuals with long-term infections or low CD4 counts. Randy described his concern: "My uncertainty is that they're going to come up with something, this magic bullet, but it's not going to help those of us who are already infected or who have been infected for a long time." Similarly, Clark said:

> I always end up back at, are these new drug therapies gonna work for me? After being infected for so long? You know, you keep hearing about all these great results on people who've just been diagnosed, but they're not telling you how people who've been infected for 12 years are doing because they're not doing so well. That's why they're not telling us.

The potential for development of drug-resistant viruses (see Kuritzkes, 1996) heightened participants' anxiety about the long-term efficacy of medications and the threat of recurrence of HIV replication and progression of the illness. Resistance might mean that certain drugs would only be effective for a limited amount of time. Clark said:

> How are you going to know when [your treatment] has stopped working? When are we going to start drug-resistance testing? So that I'll know, okay, this cocktail doesn't work, I have to switch now to another one. Yeah, it could be, you could wait for 6 months and it could be too late by the time you switch. It's all very confusing.

Fear of being hopeful, then, resulted from uncertainties about the long-term efficacy of treatments. The potential for suboptimal individual response and viral resistance to treatments led participants to question the durability of response. As Ungvarksi (1997) has noted, the next major question to be answered about the new treatments is "Will this last?"

Long-term safety issues were also a source of uncertainty for participants. It was difficult for individuals to discern whether their symptoms were a result of HIV infection or of adverse effects of the medications, heightening their fears about safety. Kent noted:

> And so the other thing is, sure, you live another 40 years—then I'm 72—am I going to get a condition 40 years from now that is related to this that they didn't foresee? Maybe because of these drugs or something, I have a heart condition or something. . . .

Several women expressed concern about the safety of medications because of lack of information on the effects of protease inhibitors on middle-aged and older women. Carol noted: "I really don't like this Crixivan. I think it's too toxic. And I really do think it is playing with my hormones." Alice added:

> There are a lot of women my age who are heading into menopause, and we have no idea how our bodies are going to work. I mean, one month I'm going 28 days. The next month it's 20 days. And then it's 27. There's no rhyme or reason, and the only time I have side effects is during that 10-day period. And I even called Abbott [Abbott Laboratories] to get some feedback and they couldn't even tell me anything.

Thus, many reported feeling grateful that the drugs appeared to be significantly halting HIV replication, yet they remained cautious because of uncertainty about long-term efficacy and safety.

Adding to the uncertainty about long-term efficacy and safety of medications was concern that "restored" immune function might not be effective (e.g., see Voelker, 1997). Participants noted that this uncertainty threatened feelings of hope and future orientation. In the following dialogue, a group of individuals with CD4 counts less than 200 discussed this issue:

Clark:	Is there going to be any immune restoration therapy?
Daniel:	That's what I want to know.
Clark:	And, you know, when are *my* T-cells going to start reproducing?
Miguel:	Or are they good T-cells, or are they bad T-cells?
Clark:	And are these cells even going to work?
Several people:	Yeah; right.
Adam:	Yeah, I mean, just because my viral load went from sky-high to undetectable, what the hell does that really mean? Does it mean that my immune system is any better off? By the way I feel, it's not!

Others also commented on the ambiguity of physiological indicators of health status such as viral load and CD4 counts. Bruce noted:

I was on a protease for three months and my viral load was near undetectable, and then my CD4 counts did nothing, they just stayed around 60, 70, and the doctor called me up and said, "You know, your viral load is almost undetectable." Two days later I was in the hospital with pneumonia. So you spend two days celebrating and then you think, like, "Well, what's up with this?" You know, "What is going on?"

Uncertainty about the functionality of restored immune systems led many to question the meaning of longer survival. Some anticipated that survival might a mean longer period of declining health. For example, as part of the concern about the functionality of restored immune systems, participants raised the issue of whether or not to stop prophylaxis. Adam noted: "I stopped doing one of my PCP prophylaxis. Now I'm having symptoms of PCP or something going on, which they can't diagnose. It's very frustrating, and I don't know whether it's because I stopped this or not." In addition, Clark worried that prophylaxis against the major opportunistic infections today might lead to a longer life with HIV, having to face as yet unknown opportunistic infections:

The uncertainty that's been bothering me lately is prophylaxis. Now that we're surviving [PCP], there are certainly other opportunistic infections out there that we didn't get before because we didn't live long enough. And they're just waiting, lurking, and you get this feeling there's some bug lurking on your shoulder.

Social Roles and Identities

Uncertainty about prospects also came about because of a need to renegotiate roles and identities. Chronic illness can disrupt a person's self-image

(Charmaz, 1994, 1995; Corbin & Strauss, 1988). Persons diagnosed with HIV infection must accept a new identity. Roth and Nelson (1997) note that individuals develop HIV-positive identities in part through their association with HIV-positive communities (e.g., AIDS service organizations or support groups). Other aspects of the HIV-positive identity develop through coming to accept HIV as a terminal illness (Chidwick & Borrill, 1996).

As part of "coming to terms" with an identity of a person with a terminal illness (Corbin & Strauss, 1988), many of the individuals in this study had made end-of-life plans (e.g., securing disability, writing wills, and planning funerals) and had lived their lives with the expectation of dying prematurely (e.g., making viatical settlements and charging credit cards to their limits). Many participants reported coming to terms with the potential for early death. Victor noted:

> I had made all of my funeral arrangements, and I had decided that I was going to die and my partner also, the two of us had gone through all of the stages of dealing with this. I had reached a stage of complacency about it. Lots of really romantic notions of how I was going to pass away, and all of this kind of stuff.

Randy added that the anticipation of an early death affected day-to-day activities:

> When I was first diagnosed, I went through a long period where, you know, I didn't buy any clothes because I figured my weight would change, or I would die and I wouldn't need them. You know, do you buy green bananas? How much time do you have?

For most participants, after accepting death, the prospect of revival led to a need to renegotiate their social roles and personal identity schemas. After having accepted himself as a person with HIV or AIDS in a time when the HIV trajectory was primarily downward, Victor described his own improved health, which included decreased HIV viral load, increased CD4 counts, and remission from Hodgkin's lymphoma, "as close to a medical miracle as I can conceive."

Upon revival, major pressures were reported by participants because of the perceived need to return to work, get off disability, and pay for drugs; yet many expressed concern that their health would be adversely affected by the stress of working. This led to a dilemma for many participants. On the one hand, they wanted to return to their careers, because the "worker role" represented values that many believed important (e.g., independence, self-sufficiency, responsibility, and stability; see Simon, 1997). Becoming "disabled" had been an identity-threatening event (Thoits, 1995) for many

participants. As Rebecca stated, "I was always independent. I don't like being on welfare, going and collecting food stamps, you know." As Neal noted, "I've been on disability, on SSDI (Social Security Disability Insurance), for a year. And yeah, I want to get back into nursing."

Yet, on the other hand, many reported that being on disability had allowed them to make their health care the focus of their lives. Greg and Hugh illustrated this:

Greg: You know, for me the other piece is I know that, after going on disability a couple of years ago—and I was pretty sick when that happened—I've experienced some really good health. One of the big things I attribute that to is the fact I haven't had to deal with the stress of working. What is going to happen if I do go back to work? Am I going to get so stressed out I'm going to end up in the hospital again? You know, I'm healthy because I'm not working.

Hugh: You're healthy because you're taking care of your health.

Greg: . . . right. And that in itself is a full-time job.

Uncertainty created a need to examine the roles that an individual could assume as a person experiencing revival. Managing a new identity often involved dealing with financial and social changes during a time of acute, life-threatening illness. For example, as Hugh noted, revival (i.e., changing to the identity of a person living with a chronic illness rather than a person dying from a terminal illness) led to uncertainty about his ability to pay the debt he had incurred after accepting an early death:

What about that viatical settlement? I mean, what about that vacation I'm taking every other month? I've done all kinds of things planning on my death. And, if I don't die, I owe an awful lot of people an awful lot of money.

Another area of uncertainty for persons experiencing revival involved the diagnosis itself. Many individuals had an AIDS diagnosis solely because their CD4 count had fallen below 200 (by the 1992 CDC definition of AIDS), and they were uncertain of their status when their CD4 count rebounded above 200. Some, such as Victor, would have preferred to no longer be classified as persons with AIDS:

The question that I've got now is that I was diagnosed with AIDS, my CD4 count went down to 40, and I didn't have any other opportunistic infections, but that alone was the diagnosis. Now that it's climbed above 200 again, do I still have AIDS? I want to know this, I want to argue that I don't . . . so, that's a kind of curious little battle.

Similarly, Frank said, "You know, I don't consider myself a person *living* with AIDS. I consider myself as a person *recovering* from AIDS." However, others (e.g., those on SSDI) reported that they might prefer to remain classified as persons with AIDS so that they were not forced off disability and back to work, which they believed might threaten their health.

Although most participants reported stress associated with changes in their roles and identities, not all the experiences of renegotiated identity were stressful. Several members reported that facing one's own mortality was a growth experience. As Victor noted:

> I think that in an important way, I did die, because I am not the same person that I was a couple of years ago. If death is just a really radical change of some sort, that's what has happened to me. And the awareness of death, the awareness of my mortality is with me every moment that I live now. And when I waste time now, I do it on purpose. I still waste time, but I'm just very deliberate and also very carefree about a lot of the things that I do, and I feel like I'm much more spiritual and much more purposeful about what I do with my life. That isn't something that you should have to be laid up in bed to be able to realize; I mean, that's something that we should be taught when we're children or that we should be encouraged to understand from the minute that we're born, but we don't and this has taught that to me. I'm . . . really kind of glad.

Thus, for many participants, the transition from a dying role to the role of a person living with a chronic illness led to uncertainty about how to reenter life. However, some participants experienced transcendence as they faced the new opportunity to live.

Interpersonal Relationships

Revival experiences also involved relational issues for many participants. For example, some participants feared that HIV-associated stigma might be more pronounced with recovery. Many persons with HIV or AIDS have experienced stigmatizing reactions from others (Alonzo & Reynolds, 1995; Crandall & Coleman, 1992; Grossman, 1991), including friends and family. Greg noted, "My parents' idea of support is to call my disease *leukemia.*" Rebecca added, "My family says I have cirrhosis of the liver and lung cancer." These negative reactions increased participants' sensitivity to potential future reactions of family, friends, employers, coworkers, and others as they reentered the workforce. As Adam stated, "You just don't know how people are going to treat you—you know they're going to be treating you differently—you just don't know how that is. And that's, there again, uncertainty."

Because of the uncertainty, Clark argued that keeping one's HIV status private might be necessary for self-protection:

> Yeah, but you have to balance that; there's a time and a place where it's to your personal benefit for people not to know you're HIV positive. I'm always advising people, I mean, if you're working or whatever, hey, if you feel like you have to lie about it, there comes a point when you've got to protect yourself. We're talking about protection. People can make you suffer a great deal.

Participants noted that, as part of revival, there would be increased need to explain or account to others as they moved back into the workforce. This led to uncertainty about the reactions of employers and coworkers. As Thomas suggested, working with individuals on a day-to-day basis would increase the likelihood that he would have to confront issues of HIV-related discrimination:

> I'm trying to figure out whether to go back to work or not, and, for some reason, that's my biggest fear right now. I've got a tattoo and that doesn't bother me. I can walk around town with a tank top, because I guess I'll only see those people once or twice. But I'm going to go into work every day and sit next to these people, and I know some of what these people have already said. And that's just scaring me to death. I mean, my doctor keeps saying don't rush it, you have until May anyway before you actually lose your sick time status and get terminated, so don't rush it. But I feel like I'm ready to go back—that I should be back. But I'm just scared to death of what people are going to say for some reason, and I've never been scared to death about it before, but—maybe it's because before I always thought I was going to get sick and die. But now I know I'm going to have to live with it a lot longer, and, well, forever, in fact, and there is nothing I can do about it.

In addition, according to these participants, simply attempting to return to work after being on disability created a "double stigma." They were not only persons with HIV or AIDS, but also persons who had become disabled. As noted in the following dialogue, this created difficulties for the job search:

Edward: How do you pick up a career after a three-, or four-, or five-year absence? Or longer . . .

Clark: Or longer, yeah.

Miguel: And how do you explain that? I was talking to a friend of mine who is a headhunter the other day, and we were talking very honestly about the fact that after you've been on disability for three or four years, a new employer doesn't look very kindly at that prospect—let alone figuring out why it was that you were on disability. Disability, in general, whether it is a back injury or whether it's a chronic illness, employers just don't look at that very favorably.

Clark responded similarly, adding that his age also was a complicating factor:

That would have been all well and good when you're 25 or 30 years old. I mean, I'm 46 now. I was supposed to be dead 10 years ago. And I've just been hanging around waiting to die. And what do you do? All of a sudden you're 46 years old and you're knocking on doors and saying, "Well, I want to change careers." And they're gonna ask you, like Miguel said, "What have you been doing the last ten years?"

Other interpersonal or relational issues also surfaced in the discussions. For some, revival led to feelings of guilt and unworthiness because many other persons (including friends and partners) had already died from AIDS. Thompson, Nanni, and Levine (1996) have reported that the illness and death of friends, family members, and partners are major sources of stress for HIV-positive individuals. Participants in this study reported survivor guilt as a double bind that resulted from being happy about one's own survival (and potential for revival) and sad about the death of friends and lovers. Participants questioned why they had lived when others died. Many expressed the wish that their friends and lovers could have lived until the new advances in therapy were available. Hugh described his feelings this way:

I have a hard time with friends around me dying. And I carry a lot of guilt because—and I'll use a mutual friend whose death still hurts a lot, our friend, Mark—he was so young when he died. Never got to accomplish as much as he wanted in life. And I've accomplished so much and done so much. I just would want to switch places with some of these people.

Thus, for participants, revival meant having to deal with people on a long-term basis when they had expected many of those relationships to be in the past. In addition, they experienced guilt because of living longer than friends and loved ones.

Changes in Quality of Life

Although HIV disease progression has been associated with declines in scores on quality of life measures (Revicki, Wu, & Murray, 1995; Rizzi, Marchesi, Morrelli, & Avogardi, 1994; Wachtel et al., 1992), it is not clear that revival results in improvement. Concerns about side effects of medications, unforeseen opportunistic illnesses, and living with a chronic disease all were seen by these participants as potential impediments to normal life quality. As Clark noted: "You tell me, 'The good news is you're gonna live. The bad news is you're not going to enjoy the rest of your life.' " Similarly, Wayne said:

> I want to live, you know, it's not that. It's just that I want to live a quality life. So am I going to break out in a rash, or is my blood pressure going to go sky high, if I take this drug?

Bruce added:

> There are other things you're going to get. You know, maybe you're going to live longer and be sick. You know, it's just sort of a chronic illness; I think that's where you're missing the boat. Life's *never* going to be back to where it was; we're *never* going to feel as good as we did before.

Because of the diversity and unpredictability of their symptoms, quality of life issues were a major source of uncertainty for participants. Adam noted, "The hardest thing is to differentiate what symptom is being caused by the drugs you're on, and what symptom is being caused by the virus itself or the infection that's active at the time." These symptoms led to questions about maintaining an acceptable quality of life during prolonged HIV treatment. As Clark noted:

> Yeah, your intestines could take a major beating after a while. How many years can you take these drugs and have an HIV infection? And the HIV can itself affect the intestines, or you can get a parasitic infection, or the drugs can do it. After a while, you don't know what's causing it, you just go from one bout of diarrhea to the next.

Others noted the need for the medical and scientific community to address quality of life issues such as side effects of medications. Adam said:

> Don't you think that physicians now are going to have to change? . . . There are more and more people living with higher T-cells and lower viral loads and the [opportunistic] killers are going to be around less. I mean, they're going to have to start addressing our symptoms that are not being addressed now—like fatigue and the nausea and things that are caused by drugs that we're on.

Finally, some questioned how the cost of expensive medications would affect long-term life quality. Especially for those who were working and were responsible for insurance copayments or drug costs, the prospect of HIV infection as a chronic illness was daunting. As Ian noted:

I think another uncertainty for me is financial. . . . I read about some of these treatments and these protease inhibitors and I think, "Boy, I'd like to be on that." Then I look up the EWP [estimated wholesale price], and "Shit, I can't afford that." You know, I live in a nice house, I drive a nice car, I like to go on vacations a couple of times a year and then I think, with the drugs I'm on, I can afford them and still do this. But if my T-cells start to drop, how far are they going to have to drop before I start giving up some of these luxuries to buy the medications? That's a big uncertainty for me. I think, "Would I rather live ten years having this, what I consider a nice lifestyle, or twenty-five years on Medicaid?" So, yeah, all these new treatments come out and all the newspapers practically tell you it's a cure, these protease inhibitors, but who is going to be able to afford them? And even if you have insurance, I know the behind-the-scenes workings of pharmaceuticals as far as insurance goes, and we can't honestly expect these insurance companies just to pick it up. It would be impossible. I mean, all the premiums for the businesses and every-thing would just go sky high.

Thus, the human and financial constraints of living with a chronic illness all affected life quality. Persons with AIDS wondered, "If I'm getting better, why don't I feel better?"

DISCUSSION

We found that HIV-infected individuals experiencing revival encountered a number of uncertainties that were sources of stress. These included renego-tiating feelings of hope and future orientation, social roles and identities, interpersonal relations, and the quality of their lives. At least in part, their stress was the result of having accepted death and then having that reality change as new treatments provided a basis for optimism. The results of this study have several implications for the care of persons with HIV or AIDS, as well as prevention efforts.

Implications for Care of HIV-Infected Individuals

Health care providers should be aware that improved health can be a source of uncertainty for their clients. Because we expect that persons living with HIV or AIDS will be happy about improvements in their health, we may fail to recognize the stress and anxiety associated with revival. Like Damocles, these individuals enjoy a tenuous happiness: The joy of renewed health is tempered by the threat of relapse. Adjustment requires managing the difficulties associated with life when a *terminal* illness becomes a *chronic* ill-ness.

There is a clear need to develop interventions to assist individuals who are experiencing revival-related uncertainty and stress. Persons living with HIV or AIDS have needed to restructure (or "reconstruct," see Barroso, 1997; Sowell, 1997; Sowell, Phillips, & Grier, 1998) many aspects of their lives. Sowell (1997) noted that, due to renewed health and the Lazarus syndrome, "reconstruction case management" is needed to help individuals; and advocacy programs, support services, "back-to-work" and career counseling, and peer support are key ingredients of such case management.

Information and instruction in information-seeking skills should be provided these individuals to reduce stress-provoking uncertainty. To help manage their lives, persons living with HIV need information about HIV illness, the health care system, and the social and financial systems affecting them. Individuals experiencing revival who are concerned about the long-term efficacy and safety of drugs may want regular updates from results of clinical trials. That information should be easily accessible. Eakes (1993) found that provision of timely and understandable information mediated chronic sorrow in individuals with cancer, and she suggested that nurses (and other health care providers) need to interpret and explain information to patients. Linn, Monnig, Cain, and Usoh (1993) found that a sense of "coherence" was needed by persons with HIV or AIDS; they concluded that "a necessary part of helping people cope with the stress of HIV infection is to provide information about what to expect, which is realistic, but which still allows them to maintain optimism and a feeling that their life is under control" (p. 31; see also Weitz, 1989).

Our study participants described symptom management as an important new HIV research priority. Extended life spans are not without cost. Persons with HIV disease now must cope with lifelong drug regimens that may have very uncomfortable side effects (nausea, diarrhea, neuropathy). As a result, effective symptom control will be increasingly important for longer periods of time. Although the need to prevent or manage the symptoms of HIV disease and treatment is well recognized (Ropka, 1994; Zeller, Swanson, & Cohen, 1993), little research has been done on this. Clinicians have borrowed symptom management approaches used by other patient populations, and patients have shared their personal strategies with their peers, but the effectiveness of these approaches has not been studied (Zeller et al., 1993). Nurses can play a critical role in HIV symptom management research and patient education aimed at improving the quality of life.

Finally, individuals with HIV may need counseling or stress management training (McCain, Zeller, Cella, Urbanski, & Novak, 1996) to help them deal with stigmatizing reactions or rejection from others, survivor guilt, and diminished quality of life, and to manage uncertainty that cannot be reduced. As HIV disease becomes a chronic illness, learning to live with chronic uncertainty (see Mishel, 1990, 1993, 1997) may be a necessary adaptive coping mechanism for these individuals.

Implications for Prevention and Education

Our findings also have implications for prevention and education. Some research indicates that gay men are paying less attention to safe sex because of media messages that triple drug cocktails with protease inhibitors are "the cure" for HIV or AIDS (Dilley, Woods, & McFarland, 1997). This poses a real threat to prevention efforts. Some individuals have said they will engage in risky sex because they believe the new drug combinations offer both a therapeutic and a prophylactic remedy for HIV infection. These individuals need to know that life on the new drug cocktails is not the same as life without infection. Severe stressors are associated with complicated drug regimens, the side effects of medications, the unknown long-term efficacy and safety of drugs, and the financial consequences of long-term reliance on the medications. Prevention and education efforts need to reinforce that life with an HIV infection and antiretroviral medications is complicated and uncertain. Although some individuals report adapting to chronic uncertainty, most still are dealing with a multitude of unresolved issues. Issues of drug failure and drug resistance complicate the ability to predict sustained response ("Guidelines shed new light," 1997). As Bradley-Springer (1997) notes:

> All in all, treatment optimism must be tempered with medical and social reality: treatment will not be available or effective for all of those who need it, no one is claiming a cure, and prevention must still play a pivotal role in an overall approach to the epidemic. (p. 87)

CONCLUSION

Improved treatments have brought optimism for many individuals with HIV or AIDS, but that hope is tempered by many unanswered questions and sources of uncertainty that may affect a person's ability to successfully reconstruct his or her life. The phenomenon of revival appears to be most pronounced among individuals who experienced a definite downward trajectory in their illness (as evidenced by CD4 counts falling below 200) prior to the advent of potent therapies and who now are experiencing recovery. The phenomenon may be different for individuals who are diagnosed early (when their immune system is still relatively intact). For both groups, uncertainty may result from cycles of viral response and rebound, or when new issues arise (such as concerns about HIV reservoirs; see Perelson et al., 1997). Thus, continued work to understand the uncertainty experiences of those individuals with HIV or AIDS is needed.

Finally, as noted earlier, not all the experiences associated with revival were stressful for participants in this study. As one might expect, revival was a source of renewed hope and optimism for many. Researchers have termed the phenomenon of finding positive meaning in one's negative experiences "transcendence" (Mellors, Riley, & Erlen, 1997). Others have noted that periods of extreme stress can still be marked by positive affect (Folkman, 1997), perhaps because people are able to focus on positive meaningful events that occur in those times (Folkman, Moskowitz, Ozer, & Park, 1997). As Alan noted, the potential for revival due to protease inhibitors was an important second chance for him:

> Well, this seems to me at times to be sort of pie in the sky, but I think that, especially with the introduction of protease inhibitors, this presents an opportunity, of course, that just never existed before. And I've been thinking about that cliché, "I wish I could go back to when I was 18 and know what I know now." Well, to an extent, that's what I feel like now. And I haven't tried protease inhibitors, I don't know if they will work for me at all, but part of me feels like, I *can* go back to 18 and know what I know now. Because, the bigger thing that this has taught me is to . . . I keep thinking of that scene from Scrooge where he runs out into the street, and it's sunny, and it's like, "I got a second chance at life," you know, that whole scene. And it makes me think, now I can stop living like the rat race millions, now I live in the here and now, now I don't have to be so fixated on dying, now I can stop projecting into the future, now I can just be happy in the here and now and live the life I want to live. And if that is the lesson that's come out of all this, great. I certainly wouldn't want to think that I had to go through this to learn this, but if anything this wonderful has come out of it, then so much the better.

ACKNOWLEDGMENTS

We gratefully acknowledge support for this research from the National Institute of Nursing Research (1R29NR04376), the National Institute of Allergy and Infectious Diseases (Adult AIDS Clinical Trials Group #AI25924, R. J. Fass), and The Ohio State University College of Social and Behavioral Sciences. We also wish to thank the men and women who participated in this study and to acknowledge Marie Garland, William McCartney, Sally Nemeth, and Angela Swary for their help with data collection and transcription. This chapter is adapted from Brashers, D. E., Neidig, J. L., Cardillo,

L. W., Dobbs, L. K., Russell, J. A., & Haas, S. M. (1999). In an important way I did die: Uncertainty and revival in persons living with HIV and AIDS. *AIDS Care, 11*, 201–219. Copyright 1999 by Taylor and Francis Ltd. Printed with permission.

REFERENCES

Alonzo, A. A., & Reynolds, N. R. (1995). Stigma, HIV, and AIDS: An exploration and elaboration of a stigma trajectory. *Social Science and Medicine, 3*, 303–315.

Babbie, E. R. (1995). *The practice of social research* (7th ed.). Belmont, CA: Wadsworth.

Babrow, A. S., Kasch, C. R., & Ford, L. A. (1998). The many meanings of "uncertainty" in illness: Toward a systematic accounting. *Health Communication, 10*, 1–24.

Barroso, J. (1996). Focusing on living: Attitudinal approaches of long-term survivors of AIDS. *Issues in Mental Health Nursing, 17*, 395–407.

Barroso, J. (1997). Reconstructing my life: Becoming a long-term survivor of AIDS. *Qualitative Health Research, 7*, 57–74.

Bradley-Springer, L. (1997). Prevention versus treatment: An ongoing dilemma. *Journal of the Association of Nurses in AIDS Care, 8*, 87–88, 94.

Brashers, D. E., Neidig, J. L., Reynolds, N. R., & Haas, S. (1998). Uncertainty in illness across the HIV/AIDS trajectory. *Journal of the Association of Nurses in AIDS Care, 9*, 66–77.

Carpenter, C. C., Fischl, M. A., Hammer, S. M., Hirsch, M. S., Jacobsen, D. M., Katzenstein, D. A., Montaner, J. S., Richman, D. D., Saag, M. S., Schooley, R. T., Thompson, M., Vella, S., Yeni, P. G., & Volberding, P. A. (1997). Antiretroviral therapy for HIV infection in 1997: Recommendations of an International AIDS Society-USA panel. *Journal of the American Medical Association, 277*, 1962–1969.

Charmaz, K. (1994). Identity dilemmas of chronically ill men. *The Sociological Quarterly, 35*, 269–288.

Charmaz, K. (1995). Identity dilemmas of chronically ill men. In D. Sabo & D. F. Gordon (Eds.), *Men's health and illness: Gender, power, and the body* (pp. 266–291). Thousand Oaks, CA: Sage.

Chidwick, A., & Borrill, J. (1996). Dealing with a life–threatening diagnosis: The experience of people with the human immunodeficiency virus. *AIDS Care, 8*, 271–284.

Corbin, J. M., & Strauss, A. (1988). *Unending work and care: Managing chronic illness at home*. San Francisco: Jossey-Bass.

Crandall, C., & Coleman, R. (1992). AIDS-related stigmatization and the disruption of social relationships. *Journal of Social and Personal Relationships, 9*, 163–177.

Dilley, J. W., Woods, W. J., & McFarland, W. (1997). Are advances in treatment changing views about high-risk sex? *New England Journal of Medicine, 337*, 501.

Eakes, G. G. (1993). Chronic sorrow: A response to living with cancer. *Oncology Nursing Forum, 20*, 1327–1334.

Folkman, S. (1997). Positive psychological states and coping with severe stress. *Social Science and Medicine, 45*, 1207–1221.

Folkman, S., Moskowitz, J. T., Ozer, E. M., & Park, C. L. (1997). Positive meaningful events and coping in the context of HIV/AIDS. In B. H. Gottlieb (Ed.), *Coping with chronic illness* (pp. 293–314). New York: Plenum.

Gallo, R. C. (1996). AIDS as a clinically curable disease: The growing optimism. *AIDS Patient Care and STDs, 10*, 7–9.

Gregonis, R. (1997). Magic Johnson and Lazarus: The new syndromes. *Journal of the Association of Nurses in AIDS Care, 8*, 75–76.

Grossman, A. H. (1991). Gay men and HIV/AIDS: Understanding the double stigma. *Journal of the Association of Nurses in AIDS Care, 2*(4), 28–32.

Guidelines shed new light on identifying failed regimens. (1997). *AIDS Alert, 12*(8), 87–88.

Kennedy, B. J., Tellegen, A., Kennedy, S., & Havernick, N. (1976). Psychological response of patients cured of advanced cancer. *Cancer, 38*, 2184–2191.

King, M. (1997, November 28). "Lazarus Syndrome" perpetuates a new crisis. *Washington Blade*, p. 31.

Koocher, G. P., & O'Malley, J. E. (1981). *The Damocles syndrome: Psychosocial consequences of surviving childhood cancer.* New York: McGraw-Hill.

Kuritzkes, D. R. (1996). Clinical significance of drug resistance in HIV-1 infection. *AIDS, 10*(Suppl. 5), S27–S31.

Lansky, S. B., List, M. A., & Ritter-Sterr, C. (1986). Psychosocial consequences of cure. *Cancer, 58*, 529–533.

Lincoln, Y., & Guba, E. (1985). *Naturalistic inquiry.* Beverly Hills, CA: Sage.

Linden, P. (1996, November–December). "What if I live?" PLWH/As begin coping with a future they thought they had lost. *Positively Aware*, 14–15.

Linn, J. G., Monnig, R. L., Cain, V. A., & Usoh, D. (1993). Stage of illness, level of HIV symptoms, sense of coherence, and psychological functioning in clients of community-based AIDS counseling centers. *Journal of the Association of Nurses in AIDS Care, 4*, 24–32.

McCain, N. L., Zeller, J. M., Cella, D. F., Urbanski, P. A., & Novak, R. M. (1996). The influence of stress management training in HIV disease. *Nursing Research, 45*, 246–253.

Mellors, M. P., Riley, T. A., & Erlen, J. A. (1997). HIV, self-transcendence, and quality of life. *Journal of the Association of Nurses in AIDS Care, 8*, 59–69.

Mishel, M. H. (1990). Reconceptualization of the uncertainty in illness theory. *Image: Journal of Nursing Scholarship, 22*, 256–262.

Mishel, M. H. (1993). Living with chronic illness: Living with uncertainty. In S. G. Funk, E. M. Tornquist, M. T. Champagne, & R. A. Weise (Eds.), *Key aspects of caring for the chronically ill: Hospital and home* (pp. 46–58). New York: Springer.

Mishel, M. H. (1997). Uncertainty in chronic illness. *Annual Review of Nursing Research, 15*, 57–80.

Muzzin, L. J., Anderson, N. J., Figueredo, A. T., & Gudelis, S. O. (1994). The experience of cancer. *Social Science and Medicine, 38*, 1201–1208.

Perelson, A. S., Essunger, P., Cao, Y., Vesanen, M., Hurley, A., Saksela, K., Markowitz, M., & Ho, D. D. (1997). Decay characteristics of HIV-1–infected compartments during combination therapy. *Nature, 387*, 188–191.

Quigly, K. M. (1989). The adult cancer survivors: Psychosocial consequences of cure. *Seminars in Oncology Nursing, 5,* 63–69.

Revicki, D. A., Wu, A. W., & Murray, M. I. (1995). Changes in clinical status, health status, and health utility outcomes in HIV-infected patients. *Medical Care, 33,* AS173–AS182.

Rizzi, M., Marchesi, S., Morrelli, E., & Avogardi, M. (1994). Quality of life in PWAs: Evaluation of the Medical Outcomes Study Instrument. *AIDS Patient Care, 8,* 265–268.

Ropka, M. (1994). HIV symptom management. In W. Holzemer & C. Portillo (Eds.), *Proceedings of HIV/AIDS Nursing Care Summit* (pp. 137–142). Washington, DC: American Academy of Nursing.

Roth, N. L., & Nelson, M. S. (1997). HIV diagnosis rituals and identity narratives. *AIDS Care, 9,* 161–179.

Sandelowski, M. (1995). Sample size in qualitative research. *Research in Nursing and Health, 18,* 179–183.

Simon, R. W. (1997). The meanings individuals attach to role identities and their implications for mental health. *Journal of Health and Social Behavior, 38,* 256–274.

Sowell, R. L. (1997). Reconstruction case management. *Journal of the Association of Nurses in AIDS Care, 8,* 43–45.

Sowell, R. L., Phillips, K. D., & Grier, J. (1998). Restructuring life to face the future: The perspective of men after a positive response to protease inhibitor therapy. *AIDS Patient Care and STDs, 12*(1), 33–42.

Strauss, A., & Corbin, J. M. (1990). *Basics of qualitative research: Grounded theory procedures and techniques.* Newbury Park, CA: Sage.

Thoits, P. A. (1995). Identity-relevant events and psychological symptoms: A cautionary tale. *Journal of Health and Social Behavior, 36,* 72–82.

Thompson, S. C., Nanni, C., & Levine, A. (1996). The stressors and stress of being HIV positive. *AIDS Care, 8,* 5–14.

Ungvarski, P. J. (1997). HIV/AIDS: New knowledge, new treatments, and the challenges for nursing. *Journal of the Association of Nurses in AIDS Care, 8,* 5–6.

Voelker, R. (1997). Physicians face new contradictions in HIV care. *Journal of the American Medical Association, 277,* 1504–1505.

Wachtel, T., Piette, J., Mor, V., Stein, M., Fleishman, J., & Carpenter, C. (1992). Quality of life in persons with human immunodeficiency virus infection: Measurement by the Medical Outcomes Study Instrument. *Annals of Internal Medicine, 116,* 129–137.

Weitz, R. (1989). Uncertainty and the lives of persons with AIDS. *Journal of Health and Social Behavior, 30,* 270–281.

Zeller, J. M., Swanson, B., & Cohen, F. L. (1993). Suggestions for clinical nursing research: Symptom management in AIDS patients. *Journal of the Association of Nurses in AIDS Care, 4*(3), 13–17.

[14]

Heart Failure: Living with Uncertainty

Charlene A. Winters

With improvements in diagnostic and treatment modalities for heart disease, the number of patients surviving an acute cardiac event has steadily increased, with a concomitant increase in the prevalence of heart failure. Thus, heart failure is now a major public health problem in the United States (Kannel, Ho, & Thom, 1994; National Heart, Lung and Blood Institute, NHLBI, 1996; Yamani & Massie, 1993). Nearly 5 million individuals in the United States have heart failure, and 400,000 new cases occur each year (American Heart Association, AHA, 1997).

Uncertainty is a major source of stress for individuals with chronic heart disease (Strauss et al., 1984), yet little is known about the uncertainty experienced by persons with heart failure. According to Mishel (1981, 1983, 1984, 1988, 1990a; Mishel, Hostetter, King, & Graham, 1984), uncertainty in illness results from the perceived ambiguity of the illness, lack of information about the diagnosis and seriousness of the illness, complex treatment options and a complex system of care, and the unpredictability of the course of the disease. Uncertainty is thought to be moderated by familiarity of symptoms and events, the individual's ability to process the information given, and the resources available to the individual to assist in interpreting illness related events. Mishel (1990a) has also proposed that individuals who experience continual uncertainty may revise their view of life to include uncertainty as an inescapable part of living and an opportunity for growth and change. Thus, uncertainty once evaluated as a threat can now be accepted as an opportunity. This new view of life is thought to be facilitated by friends, family, and health care providers who share the individual's point of view.

Researchers have reported a strong relationship between high uncertainty and stress, emotional distress, mood disturbance, anxiety (Christman et al., 1988; Hawthorne & Hixon, 1994; Mishel, 1984; Webster & Christman, 1988), poor quality of life (Braden, 1990a, 1990b; Hawthorne & Hixon, 1994; Padilla, Mishel, & Grant, 1992), and poor psychosocial adjustment to illness (Christman, 1990; Mishel & Braden, 1987; Mishel et al., 1984; Mishel & Sorenson, 1991). Uncertainty is not related to gender (Hawthorne & Hixon, 1994), marital status, age, or employment status (Christman et al., 1988; Mishel, 1984; Webster & Christman, 1988). Level of education has been inconsistently associated with uncertainty (Christman et al., 1988; Mishel, 1984; Patterson & Faux, 1993).

Most of the studies of uncertainty in persons with heart disease have involved individuals experiencing an acute phase of the illness or its treatment; few have included individuals with heart failure (Hawthorne & Hixon, 1994; Winters, 1997). The purpose of this study was therefore to explore the experience of uncertainty for men and women with heart failure, and thus to extend our understanding of uncertainty in chronic illness.

METHOD

In this descriptive exploratory study, data were collected over a 4-month period and included demographic and clinical data, audiotaped interviews, field notes, and the Community Form of the Mishel Uncertainty in Illness Scale (MUIS-C).

Sample

The purposive sample consisted of 15 men and 7 women recruited from the offices of three cardiologists practicing in an urban area of a rural western state. Individuals were included in the study if they were 18 years of age or older, English speaking, and diagnosed with New York Heart Association (NYHA) Class I, II, III, or IV (mild to severe) heart failure (NYHA Criteria Committee, 1994) from any etiology. Individuals with significant comorbidities were excluded from participation. At the time of the interview, the majority of the participants were classified as NYHA Functional Class II ($n = 11$) or Class III ($n = 8$) heart failure. The mean number of years with heart failure was 7 (range 1 to 21 years). The most common etiology of CHF was coronary heart disease (35%) and the most commonly reported symptoms were fatigue and shortness of breath (45%). Most participants were 70–79 years old, but ages ranged from 38 to 88 years. Most were male (67%) and married (77%) and all but 3 were retired. Participants in the study closely matched the profile of individuals with heart failure reported in the literature (AHA, 1997; Ho, Pinsky, Kannel, & Levy, 1993; Moser, 1996; Oka, 1996).

Procedure

Three cardiologists were asked to identify and approach patients from their practice for potential inclusion in the study. The investigator telephoned those individuals who expressed an interest in participating, to explain the study and schedule an interview. Seventeen in-person and five telephone interviews were conducted. Of the 17 in-person interviews, 3 were conducted in a conference room arranged by the investigator, and 14 were done in the home of the participant. Prior to starting the interview, informed written consent was obtained from each participant. When interviews were done by phone, the consent and questionnaire were mailed to the participant prior to the interview. It was made clear to each participant that the researcher was not an employee of the referring physician and a decision to participate in the study would not affect the medical care he or she received. Interviews lasted from 1 to 2 hours; all were audiotaped.

During the semi-structured interview, participants were asked to describe their experience with heart disease and heart failure and to discuss any uncertainties they might have experienced. Additional questions were posed to elicit further information, clarify what was said, and confirm or refute conclusions being drawn from the ongoing analysis. The Mishel Uncertainty in Illness Scale-Community Form (MUIS-C) was completed at the end of the interview, following directions provided in the scale manual (Mishel, 1990b). The MUIS-C is a 23-item Likert-format scale (strongly agree to strongly disagree), which is designed to measure perceived uncertainty in illness (Mishel, 1990b). Possible uncertainty scores range from 23, indicating a low level of uncertainty, to 115, reflecting a high degree of illness uncertainty. Based on data from eight samples, coefficient alpha scores for the MUIS-C are reported in the moderate to high range (.75 to .90) (Mishel, 1990b). Total uncertainty scores were derived for each participant. Internal consistency reliability (Chronbach's alpha) for this sample was .70. Demographic and clinical data were collected from the participant during the interview and from the medical record after the interview was completed, and recorded on a structured data collection sheet.

Data Analysis and Management

The audiotaped interviews were transcribed verbatim. The transcribed interviews and field notes were then coded and analyzed for common themes using the methods described by Miles and Huberman (1994). The topical codes (first-level codes) were reduced to reflect similar topics, renamed with interpretive codes, and displayed in a matrix according to NYHA class. Displaying the data in this manner facilitated further grouping of codes and development of initial themes. Techniques established for maintaining rigor in naturalistic inquiry (Lincoln & Guba, 1985; Miles & Huberman, 1994) were used to ensure trustworthiness (validity and reliability) during the collection and analysis of the qualitative data.

Quantitative data were analyzed to determine item frequencies and measures of central tendency. The data from the uncertainty scale were then reviewed to identify areas of uncertainty, and this information was combined with the interview data to gain a fuller view of the uncertainty experience.

RESULTS

Overview

The uncertainty described by participants in this study was primarily related to new or changing symptoms and treatment, trying to stay well, and the quality of their life and death. Uncertainty increased when symptoms or treatments changed, information was incomplete, or a sense of control over illness was lost; when patients dwelled on their illness or thought about the future; and when they were unable to distinguish illness symptoms from changes that occurred as a result of aging. Greater uncertainty was noted during the initial diagnostic period and while waiting for test results. Whether the heart failure was a result of new-onset heart disease or followed a long history of cardiac illness and treatment, the uncertainty of heart failure was marked by fear of the unknown.

Uncertainty was reduced by open communication with physicians and nurses, faith in health care providers and the treatments they prescribed, spirituality, understanding of symptoms and treatment outcomes, symptom stability, hope for a better future, the ability to provide self-care, and other coping measures. The three major themes and subthemes used to describe the uncertainty experience are displayed in Table 14.1.

The findings derived from the interview data were supported by scores on the uncertainty scale. Total uncertainty scores for these participants ranged from 39 to 66 (possible range = 23 to 115), with a mean score (M) of 54.9 (SD = 7.7). The mean uncertainty score fell between the mean scores reported by Mishel (1990b) for patients following coronary artery bypass surgery (M = 60) and for patients postmyocardial infarction (M = 49). The item that received the highest rating from participants (indicating greatest uncertainty) was uncertainty about whether or not the physician would find anything else wrong with them (M = 3.59 on the 1–5 scale). Participants also indicated that they were not sure what was going to happen to them (M = 3.18) or how bad their symptoms would become (M = 2.77). As expected, participants demonstrated the least uncertainty (M = 1.45) about their diagnosis, strongly disagreeing with the statement "I don't know what is wrong with me."

Uncertainty Themes

Three themes describe these participants' experience with heart failure: recognition and response, trying to stay well, and looking forward.

TABLE 14.1 Themes and Sub-themes of Uncertainty

Themes and Sub-themes

Recognition and Response: Symptoms and Treatment

- New or changing symptoms/treatment
- Cause of symptoms: age vs. illness
- Self care vs. health care

Trying to Stay Well: A Shared Responsibility

- Vigilance
- Cautious trust of provider
- Staying well

Looking Forward: Quality of Life and Death

- Death awareness
- Living with the illness
- The importance of activity
- Healthy within Illness

Recognition and Response: Symptoms and Treatment

The first theme refers to the manner in which participants recognized and responded to their symptoms and treatments. Participants experienced uncertainty when symptoms first occurred or symptoms or treatments changed, and when they thought about their future. This finding was corroborated by the responses of participants to the uncertainty scale. As noted above, MUIS-C scores were highest for items related to knowing whether anything else wrong would be found, what else would happen to them, and how bad their symptoms would become.

Like other persons with heart disease (Johnson & Morse, 1990; Winters, 1997), the participants in this study had been unsure about the nature of their initial symptoms and had tried to "gut it out" before seeking medical attention. Their inability to recognize symptoms as cardiac related was due in part to the absence of chest pain or to the initial diagnosis of fatigue and shortness of breath as respiratory illness. Some had attributed their fatigue and dyspnea with exertion to the aging process. Participants became less uncertain about their illness when symptoms were accurately identified and stable, and the diagnosis was confirmed. Uncertainty arose again when participants did not know what to expect from new treatments or when symptoms changed.

Following the diagnosis of heart failure, participants were more likely to attribute changes in their symptoms to their illness, but many continued their "wait and see" approach to seeking health care. As in other studies, both before and after the diagnosis of heart failure, the decision to seek health care was influenced by participants' experience with illness (Cohen, 1993; Winters, 1997), their ability to maintain activities of daily living (Winters, 1997), the advice of family members (Dempsey, Dracup, & Moser, 1995), the ability to distinguish changes due to age from changes due to illness (Clark, Janz, Dodge, & Garrity, 1994; Stanley, 1997; Tresch, 1997), and the desire to care for oneself (Clark et al., 1994; Winters, 1997). Consistent with the findings of several other researchers, the degree to which symptoms were anticipated, familiar, and understood influenced participants' uncertainty and response to uncertainty (Hilton, 1988; Mishel & Braden, 1988; Mishel et al., 1984; Searle & Jeffrey, 1994; Winters, 1997).

Trying to Stay Well: A Shared Responsibility

The feeling of being out of control and the desire to gain control have been found in patients with chronic heart disease (Winters, 1997), myocardial infarction (MI) (Johnson & Morse, 1990), breast cancer (Nelson, 1996), and coronary artery bypass surgery (CAB) (King & Jensen, 1994). The theme trying to stay well reflects our participants' strong desire to stay well and share responsibility for their care with their physician. Participants were vigilant in monitoring their care, asked questions of their physician, read the lay and professional literature about heart failure, suggested the use of alternative therapies, and adjusted their medications when needed. Such vigilance is not uncommon in chronic illness (Cohen, 1993; Strauss et al., 1984) and, like information seeking, is a strategy used to cope with uncertainty (Mishel, 1988). Through their vigilance, these participants were able to gain a sense of control and mastery over their illness.

Participants trusted in their physician "or they wouldn't be there," yet they demonstrated caution, questioning prescribed treatments, adding alternative therapies to their treatment regime, and asking God to "watch over them and their physician." Similar behaviors have been identified in others with chronic illness (King & Jensen, 1994; Winters, 1997). Because the physician can provide information about the causes and consequences of symptoms, confirm symptom importance, and diagnose illness, the relationship between the patient and the physician may reduce or prevent uncertainty (Mishel, 1988, 1993; Mishel & Braden, 1988). In this study, a trusting relationship was facilitated by frank dialogue between the physician and the patient and further enhanced when the participants perceived the nurse and the physician to be "saying the same thing" and "working from the same page."

Looking Forward: Quality of Life and Death

The third major theme reflects participants' uncertainty about their future health, the quality of their life, and the circumstances of their death. Their uncertainties about how bad their symptoms would become, what else might happen, and whether additional problems would be diagnosed were clear during the interview and in their high scores on the MUIS-C. Although participants indicated on the MUIS-C that they were uncertain about what was going to happen to them, they made it clear during the interview that they knew they were going to die. What they were uncertain about was when and how death would occur. This uncertainty about the circumstances of their death appeared to provide participants an opportunity to hope and wonder about the future and was therefore viewed positively by participants.

Quality of life was critical to participants in this study, and the ability to remain active and independent played an important role in evaluating quality of life. Because illness and "getting older" were seen as a part of life, participants' view of a quality life included illness and a gradual decline in functioning. "I'm not 20 years old anymore" and "You have to expect changes" were common statements by participants. Manageable symptoms, the ability to remain active, and the ability to "do what I want to do" were equated with health and wellness. In order to stay active, participants prioritized their activities and adjusted their activity levels to accommodate their fatigue and dyspnea. Inability to be active was considered untenable by all participants and was identified as "worse than death" by some. Although the ability to see health within illness (Jensen & Allen, 1993; Moch, 1989; Sim, 1990; Simmons, 1989; Winters, 1997) and to equate activity with health is not new (McWilliams, Stewart, Brown, Desai, & Coderre, 1996), these participants add new depth to the idea.

Participants saw no choice for themselves but to accept their heart failure and learn to live with it. They looked to the future, maintained a positive attitude, tried not to dwell on their illness, kept busy, ignored their symptoms, sought advice from their health care providers, and sought support from their faith, family, and friends. They appraised uncertainty as an inescapable part of life, and it prompted them to reevaluate their life and reorder priorities. They took an active role in their care, lived one day at a time, hoped for improved symptoms and treatments, and tried to "live life to the fullest."

Some of these same strategies have been used by women adjusting to MI (Johnson & Morse, 1990), families of children adjusting to cancer (Cohen, 1993), older women managing heart disease (Clark et al., 1994), men and women with chronic heart disease (Winters, 1997), and women living with breast cancer (Nelson, 1996).

Symptom fluctuation appeared to be a major determinant of illness uncertainty. The highest uncertainty score (MUIS-C = 66) was recorded by a man with an 8-year history of heart failure and decreasing left ventricular ejection fraction. In the 9 months preceding his participation in this study, he had a "mild stroke" and underwent angioplasty (PTCA), and at the time of the interview, he had NYHA Class III failure. Of the participants with the lowest uncertainty scores (MUIS-C = 39), one was a woman whose Class IV failure had recently stabilized; she saw her life as "good" and looked forward to further improvement with the addition of new treatments. The other was a man with an improving ejection fraction after valve repair. The two participants diagnosed with heart failure within the past year were experiencing more stable symptoms following the initiation of treatment; they demonstrated a moderate amount of uncertainty (MUIS-C = 48 and 54).

Participants identified their family members, friends, and health care providers as sources of emotional and physical support. Family members supported the participants' view that life was uncertain and encouraged them to "live life to the fullest." Health care providers supported this view with their honest and direct discussions of current health status and prognosis. Although physicians and nurses encouraged hope for improvements in treatment and symptoms, they also realistically portrayed the uncertain future.

Isolation is common for individuals living in rural areas, and isolation is thought to promote uncertainty (Mishel, 1990a). Several participants in this study lived alone, in small towns or out of town, putting them at risk for social isolation. Yet these participants described reliance on neighbors and church members and frequent phone calls and visits with their out-of-area children. Some of the participants also thought that "talking with other people with heart failure" would be helpful.

IMPLICATIONS FOR PRACTICE

These persons with heart failure recognized uncertainty as a normal part of life and illness. Their responses to uncertainty were summed up by one 68-year-old participant who said, "I plan to keep on breathing. Enjoy myself. What do you do when you get old? What are you supposed to do? I'm going to keep on living. That's all I can think of to do." Uncertainty fluctuated and was influenced by changes in illness symptoms and treatment, past illness experiences, and an unknown future. Thus, education about cardiac symptoms, expected treatment outcomes, and physiologic changes associated with aging may reduce uncertainty for patients such as these. Education should begin upon diagnosis of the cardiac condition and continue throughout the treatment period. Helping persons newly diagnosed with heart failure to accept the unpredictabilities of life and illness may be useful. Also, ongoing assistance in interpreting symptoms is required, suggesting a need for follow-up of heart failure patients. Education should also support individuals' involvement in their care.

The ability to remain active influenced these participants' quality of life. Illness was equated with a decline in activity and the need for hospitalization. Clearly, independence in daily activities, daily physical activity, and individual efforts to achieve potential should be supported.

The support of family members, friends, and neighbors was an important aspect of living with heart failure. Sharing ideas and opinions about their illness with other people diagnosed with heart failure was also seen as a useful strategy to deal with uncertainty. Family members should be included in all aspects of health care, and participation in formal and informal support groups should be encouraged. Connecting rural dwellers to others with heart failure via telephone, electronic mail, or the Internet is an option worth exploring.

ACKNOWLEDGMENTS

This chapter is adapted from Winters, C. A. (1999). Heart failure: Living with uncertainty. *Progress in Cardiovascular Nursing, 14*(3), 85–91. Copyright by Le Jacq Communications 1999. Printed with permission.

REFERENCES

American Heart Association (AHA). (1997). *1997 heart and stroke facts.* Dallas: Author.

Braden, C. J. (1990a). Learned self-help response to chronic illness experience: A test of three alternative learning theories. *Scholarly Inquiry for Nursing Practice, 4,* 23–41.

Braden, C. J. (1990b). A test of the self-help model: Learned response to chronic illness experience. *Nursing Research, 39,* 42–47.

Christman, N. J. (1990). Uncertainty and adjustment during radiotherapy. *Nursing Research, 39,* 17–20.

Christman, N. J., McConnell, E. A., Pfeiffer, C., Webster, K. K., Schmitt, M., & Ries, J. (1988). Uncertainty, coping, and distress following myocardial infarction: Transition from hospital to home. *Research in Nursing and Health, 11,* 71–82.

Clark, N. M., Janz, N. K., Dodge, J. A., & Garrity, C. R. (1994). Managing heart disease: A study of the experiences of older women. *Journal of the American Medical Women's Association, 49*(6), 202–206.

Cohen, M. H. (1993). The unknown and the unknowable—Managing sustained uncertainty. *Western Journal of Nursing Research, 15*(1), 77–96.

Dempsey, S. J., Dracup, K., & Moser, D. K. (1995). Women's decision to seek care for symptoms of acute myocardial infarction. *Heart and Lung, 24*(6), 444–456.

Hawthorne, M. H., & Hixon, M. E. (1994). Functional status, mood disturbance and quality of life in patients with heart failure. *Progress in Cardiovascular Nursing, 9,* 22–32.

Hilton, B. A. (1988). The phenomenon of uncertainty in women with breast cancer. *Issues in Mental Health Nursing, 9,* 217–238.

Ho, K. K., Pinsky, J. L., Kannel, W. B., & Levy, D. (1993). The epidemiology of heart failure: The Framingham study. *Journal of the American College of Cardiology, 22*(4 Suppl. A), 6–13.

Jensen, L., & Allen, M. (1993). Wellness: The dialectic of illness. *Image: Journal of Nursing Scholarship, 25*(3), 221–224.

Johnson, J. L., & Morse, J. M. (1990). Regaining control: The process of adjustment after myocardial infarction. *Heart and Lung, 19,* 126–135.

Kannel, W. B., Ho, K., & Thom, T. (1994). Changing epidemiological features of cardiac failure. *British Heart Journal, 72*(2 Suppl.), S3–9.

King, K. M., & Jensen, L. (1994). Preserving the self: Women having cardiac surgery. *Heart and Lung, 23*(2), 99–105.

Lincoln, Y. S., & Guba, E. G. (1985). *Naturalistic inquiry.* Beverly Hills, CA: Sage.

McWilliams, C. L., Stewart, M., Brown, J. B., Desai, K., & Coderre, P. (1996). Creating health with chronic illness. *Advances in Nursing Science, 18*(3), 1–15.

Miles, M. B., & Huberman, A. M. (1994) *Qualitative data analysis* (2nd ed.). Thousand Oaks, CA: Sage.

Mishel, M. H. (1981). The measurement of uncertainty in illness. *Nursing Research, 30*(5), 258–263.

Mishel, M. H. (1983). Adjusting the fit: Development of uncertainty scales for specific clinical populations. *Western Journal of Nursing Research, 5,* 357–370.

Mishel, M. H. (1984). Perceived uncertainty and stress in illness. *Research in Nursing and Health, 7,* 163–171.

Mishel, M. H. (1988). Uncertainty in illness. *Image: Journal of Nursing Scholarship, 20*(4), 225–232.

Mishel, M. H. (1990a). Reconceptualization of the uncertainty in illness theory. *Image: Journal of Nursing Scholarship, 22*(4), 256–262.

Mishel, M. H. (1990b). *Uncertainty in illness scales manual.* Chapel Hill, NC: Author.

Mishel, M. H. (1993). Living with chronic illness: Living with uncertainty. In S. G. Funk, E. M. Tornquist, M. T. Champagne, & R. A. Wiese, (Eds.), *Key aspects of caring for the chronically ill: Hospital and home* (pp. 46–58). New York: Springer.

Mishel, M. H., & Braden, C. J. (1987). Uncertainty a mediator between support and adjustment. *Western Journal of Nursing Research, 9*(1), 43–57.

Mishel, M. H., & Braden, C. J. (1988). Finding meaning: Antecedents of uncertainty in illness. *Nursing Research, 37*(2), 98–103, 127.

Mishel, M. H., Hostetter, T., King, B., & Graham, V. (1984). Predictors of psychosocial adjustment in patients newly diagnosed with gynecological cancer. *Cancer Nursing, 7,* 291–299.

Mishel, M. H., & Sorenson, D. S. (1991). Coping with uncertainty in gynecological cancer: A test of the mediating function of mastery and coping. *Nursing Research 40,* 167–171.

Moch, S. D. (1989). Health within illness: Concept evolution and practice possibilities. *Advances in Nursing Science, 11*(4), 23–31.

Moser, D. K. (1996). Maximizing therapy in the advanced heart failure patient. *Journal of Cardiovascular Nursing, 10*(2), 58–70.

National Heart, Lung and Blood Institute (NHLBI). (1996). *Congestive heart failure in the United States: A new epidemic.* Available: nih.gov/institutes/NHLBI.

Nelson, J. P. (1996). Struggling to gain meaning: Living with the uncertainty of breast cancer. *Advances in Nursing Science, 18*(3), 59–76.

New York Heart Association (NYHA) Criteria Committee. (1994). *Nomenclature and criteria for diagnosis of diseases of the heart and great vessels* (9th ed.). Boston: Little, Brown.

Oka, R. K. (1996). Physiologic changes in heart failure: What's new. *Journal of Cardiovascular Nursing, 10*(2), 11–28.

Padilla, G. V., Mishel, M. H., & Grant, M. M. (1992). Uncertainty, appraisal and quality of life. *Quality of Life Research, 1,* 155–165.

Patterson, C., & Faux, S. A. (1993). Uncertainty and appraisal in patients diagnosed with abdominal aortic aneurysms. *Canadian Journal of Cardiovascular Nursing, 4*(1), 4–10.

Searle, C., & Jeffrey, J. (1994). Uncertainty and quality of life of adults hospitalized with life-threatening ventricular arrhythmias. *Canadian Journal of Cardiovascular Nursing, 5*(3), 15–23.

Sim, J. (1990). The concept of health. *Physiotherapy, 76*(7), 423–428.

Simmons, S. J. (1989). Health: A concept analysis. *International Journal of Nursing Studies, 26*(2), 155–161.

Stanley, M. (1997). Current trends in the clinical management of an old enemy: Congestive heart failure in the elderly. *AACN Clinical Issues, 8*(4), 616–626.

Strauss, A. L., Corbin, J., Fagererhaugh, S., Glaser, B. G., Maines, D., Suczek, B., & Weiner, C. L. (1984). *Chronic illness and the quality of life* (2nd ed.). St. Louis: Mosby.

Tresch, D. D. (1997). The clinical diagnosis of heart failure in older patients. *Journal of the American Geriatric Society, 45*, 1128–1133.

Webster, K. K., & Christman, N. J. (1988). Perceived uncertainty and coping post myocardial infarction. *Western Journal of Nursing Research, 10*(4), 384–400.

Winters, C. A. (1997). Living with chronic heart disease: A pilot study. *The Qualitative Report, 3*(4). Available: http://www.nova.edu/ssss/QR/QR3-4/winters.html.

Yamani, M., & Massie, B. M. (1993). Congestive heart failure: Insights from epidemiology, implications for treatment. *Mayo Clinic Proceedings, 68*(1), 1214–1218.

[15]

Self-Care Decision Making in Clients with Diabetes and Hypertension

JoAnne Weiss

Diabetes and hypertension affect millions of Americans. Frequently the diseases coexist, and when other risk factors such as dyslipidemia and obesity are also present, cardiovascular, cerebrovascular, and renal diseases are more likely (Karam, 1992). Following recommended guidelines on dietary intake and exercise, proper use of prescribed medications, and smoking cessation are essential to prevent disease complications. However, more than 50% of those with diabetes (Karam, 1992) and even more of those with hypertension (Massie & Sokolow, 1992) do not make such self-care choices. The result is increased morbidity and mortality for individuals as well as the expenditure of millions of health care dollars. If the threat of increased illness and even death does not capture the attention of these clients and influence their decision-making processes, the question is, what will? Health care professionals struggle with this question daily.

The root of the problem, often termed nonadherence, is a concern not only for health care providers, but also for clients and the nation. Adherence is defined as the extent to which a person's behavior coincides with medical or health advice (Haynes, Taylor, & Sackett, 1979). Most studies of clients with diabetes and/or hypertension identify nonadherence as a problem and point to the benefits of adhering to health recommendations, but few show effective ways of accomplishing this. Adherence is complex, and adherence research has produced inconclusive and even contradictory findings (Pfister-Minogue, 1993). Although theoretical models have been helpful in explaining and predicting behaviors, they have not been very effective in bringing about change.

The effectiveness of health programs appears to depend on the willingness of individuals to accept responsibility for initiating and sustaining health behaviors (Fleury, 1992). The term *self-care* suggests this. The way that people form perceptions and make decisions about self-care could be an important missing link in understanding adherence and nonadherence and in improving client outcomes. However, little research has examined self-care decision making in clients with diabetes or hypertension. This grounded-theory study, therefore, was undertaken to explain how clients think about adherence to professional advice.

METHOD

English-speaking adults diagnosed with both diabetes and hypertension were invited to participate by health care providers, acquaintances, and ministers, particularly of African-American churches, who had been provided written materials about the research. Invitations to participate in the study were also placed in churches and health care providers' offices.

Twenty-one clients were interviewed: 13 females (11 Caucasian and 2 African-American) and 8 males (6 Caucasian and 2 African-American). Clients ranged in age from 24 to 75 years, and their economic status ranged from indigent to affluent. All participants were taking oral medications for hypertension. Most had type 2, adult onset diabetes; 7 of the women and 4 of the men were taking insulin, 9 were taking oral medications, and 1 controlled his diabetes by diet alone. Many participants had complications associated with these diseases: Three had known cardiovascular disease; 4 were aware of renal disease, 1 had received a kidney transplant, and 1 was on dialysis and hoping to improve enough for a kidney transplant. As a result of complications of diabetes, one participant had had both lower extremities amputated and another had lost several toes. Some participants had experienced episodes of transient vision loss, but none were blind.

Data Collection and Analysis

Data were collected through unstructured interviews with clients that lasted from 1 to 2 hours and were audio-recorded and transcribed verbatim. To add a broader perspective, three health care providers who cared for clients with diabetes and hypertension were also interviewed: one physician (nephrologist) and two primary care nurse practitioners. Most client interviews occurred in clients' homes; interviews with providers occurred in their offices. Follow-up interviews to confirm and expand the initial interviews were conducted with both clients and providers. In keeping with the grounded theory method, data were collected, coded, and analyzed concurrently; the ongoing analysis guided decisions about further data collection and analysis.

Credibility of the research was enhanced by discussing the findings with colleagues (peer review) and study participants (member checks) (Lincoln & Guba, 1985). Dependability was confirmed by providing a clear audit trail encompassing all of the decisions made during data analysis (Beck, 1993).

RESULTS

These persons with diabetes and hypertension described being bombarded by warnings about their diseases and their present and future vulnerability. The warnings were broader than an urging of caution. Warnings began at the time of diagnosis and continued throughout the individuals' lives. Warnings varied in intensity and were both external, coming from outside sources such as health care providers, family, friends, and/or the media, and internal, originating within the individual.

External warnings, usually based on physical signs or objective evidence detected by health care providers, generally came in the form of instructions, admonitions, and, occasionally, threats. Initially, warnings from health care providers came in the form of instructions. The most common instructions/warnings centered on the need for a healthy diet, regular exercise, proper use of prescribed medications, and smoking cessation. Admonitions and threats became more frequent when initial instructions/ warnings were not heeded. The client's health status often influenced the quantity and quality of these external warnings. Because diabetes and hypertension generally do not cause any symptoms until complications occur, the impact of the warnings varied.

> I feel so good. Why do I feel so good, and you tell me I'm so sick? Okay, that's what it basically comes down to. . . . [The doctor says,] "Well, how do you feel?" I say, "I feel great, but I'm sure that damn lab work's gonna be bad. . . . He says, "Yeah, you're right."

Usually warnings originated from within clients in the form of physical symptoms. The most dramatic symptoms these clients experienced were related to diabetes, in particular blood sugar highs and lows.

> I've been out and all of a sudden started getting the shakes. And I've been in the supermarket where I've had to have something to eat right now because I thought I was gonna lose it. And people could see my physical condition, that there was something wrong, and wanted to get me help. . . .

Other symptoms included vision loss and neuropathic pain related to complications from the diabetes. Symptoms related to high blood pressure were more vague. Because they could feel bodily changes, clients tended to pay more attention to warnings caused by symptoms. These symptoms/ warnings were usually the basis for seeking either initial or continued treatment. Symptoms also tended to have more impact in promoting positive self-care choices. "That [vision loss] scared the hell out of me, to be perfectly blunt. Boy, I walked, I did everything, watched my diet, took my food, cut it in half, lost weight." For this participant the warning was, "An out-and-out siren! . . . I don't want to go blind."

Personal Theorizing

Clients responded to warnings by evaluating their meaning and relevance in order to decide on appropriate self-care choices. This process, called personal theorizing, was the method the individuals used to make sense of their health, and it provided the basis for their self-care choices.

> I didn't take it [diabetes] serious[ly] because I didn't feel anything wrong. I thought they [the doctors] were just kidding at how serious it could be. . . . I knew . . . that you probably can lose your eyes, and you probably can lose your legs, but I feel great, it's not happening to me. But you take advantage of it; you eat the sugar.

Personal theorizing was an ongoing process of thinking about realities in order to explain or prescribe self-care. The purposes of personal theorizing were not only to sort, review, and analyze data for explanations and personal relevance, but also to determine the most appropriate self-care choices. This complex process lasted only a few moments for some, but much longer for others.

Model of Self-Care Decision Making

The Model of Self-Care Decision Making (Figure 15.1) illustrates the process of personal theorizing. This model has four components: cost-benefit

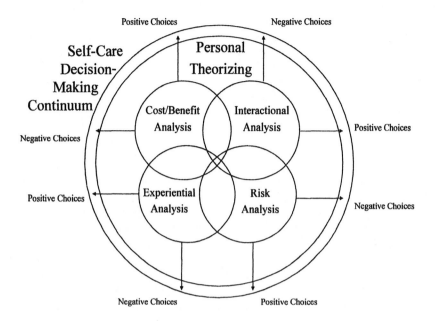

FIGURE 15.1   Model of self-care decision making.

analysis, interactional analysis, experiential analysis, and risk analysis. When subjects received warnings, they considered the costs and benefits (cost/benefit analysis), the influence of other people (interactional analysis), the influence of previous experiences (experiential analysis), and/or the potential risks of loss related to their diseases (risk analysis) to determine the significance of the warnings and to make self-care choices. At times analysis involved primarily one component; at other times it involved several or all the components.

Cost/Benefit Analysis

Cost/benefit analysis was used by most subjects to determine which self-care choices to make. In response to warnings received, subjects weighed the costs and benefits of various choices. This weighing was unique for each individual, although there were some common features. As noted earlier, most external warnings centered on choices about diet, exercise, body size, insulin use, the use of other medications, blood sugar testing, and cessation of smoking. When subjects weighed the costs and benefits of these choices, they frequently found that the costs of making health-promoting decisions were quite high. These costs were physical, psychological, social, financial, and temporal.

> I love fruit, and if I eat any fruit at all my sugar goes sky-high. In a matter of minutes it goes sky-high. And to restrict yourself from all these . . . pleasures of different foods is . . . hard to live with.

Interactional Analysis

Interactional analysis involved evaluation of interactions with health care providers, significant others, acquaintances, and strangers. External warnings came through interactions with these individuals. When an interaction was relevant for self-care decision making, subjects evaluated it just as they evaluated costs and benefits. That is, they analyzed interactions to determine their meaning, value, and influence. They reflected not only on what was said to them, but also on who was speaking and how they felt about what was said. At times self-care choices were based solely on interactional analysis. The most significant interactions for self-care decision making took place between subjects and health care providers and/or significant others. Occasionally interactions with acquaintances and strangers also were influential. The influence of interactions with health care providers was determined primarily by respect, trust, feelings of collegiality, and the provider's style of presentation. Most influential was a feeling of mutual respect. One participant noted his feelings about provider respect:

> It's important to me that they respect me. . . . That's how they get my respect, by respecting me, just like I get their respect by respecting them. And if they're not willing to do that, then I'm not interested in participating.

Experiential Analysis

Experiential analysis occurred as subjects reviewed their relevant personal history (historical analysis); looked at themselves, assessing their own strengths and weaknesses (personality analysis); and compared their personal experiences with the experiences of others (comparative analysis). Often they spent a great deal of time analyzing their experiences to try to derive meaning from them and find direction for future choices. Previous warnings, responses to those warnings, actions taken, and the outcomes of those actions were considered. Subjects wanted to know if their previous choices could explain their present health status. Personal theories of health, illness, and appropriate treatment were formed and revised through this process. Subjects thus took a retrospective view in order to develop explanations and find direction for self-care decision making.

By analyzing their previous history and personality, and by comparing their experiences to those of others, these subjects seemed to be working toward a definition of themselves. Often they developed explanations for their present health status and decision making; this, in turn, provided direction for future decisions. When subjects saw the connections among their choices, their history, their personality, their similarities to others, and their present health problems, health-promoting decisions were more likely.

Risk Analysis

Risk analysis occurred when subjects considered potential risks to their health due to diabetes and hypertension. During cost/benefit analysis and interactional analysis, subjects analyzed their present circumstances to make self-care choices. During experiential analysis, they evaluated past decision making. In risk analysis, future health was considered prior to making self-care decisions.

Responses to risks varied from fear to appreciation, and from total disregard to being overwhelmed. These responses also varied from subject to subject, and within each subject from time to time. Positive or health-promoting self-care choices were most likely when risks were feared, and least likely when risks were ignored or considered overwhelming.

> That [near blindness] played a big part in [my] really knowing that I needed to stick with my diet . . . and to go straight instead of . . . maybe one month do good and the next month not do good because I know that this could happen again. . . . I would say that it played a big part in [my] . . . wanting to . . . stay on my diet and do different things like that.

DISCUSSION

People with diabetes and hypertension often do not follow their health care providers' recommendations. Both providers and clients find this frustrating and frequently do not understand why adherence is so difficult. Often providers label clients as either adherent or nonadherent based on physical examinations. If clients are consistently overweight, with elevated blood sugars and/or blood pressures, they are labeled nonadherent. This judgment is naive and oversimplistic. As this study shows, clients receive many warnings daily, process them, and make choices based on this process. Appreciating this from clients' perspectives gives insight into the struggles they often face. For example, saying no to a bowl of ice cream may be a significant positive choice for a client, but if the provider sees only the narrow picture of the client's consistently elevated blood sugar, he or she will miss the significance of the choice. The Model of Self-Care Decision-Making (MSCDM) explains the basic process of personal theorizing. Understanding this process, which may or may not result in health-promoting choices, can broaden our perspective from a limited provider view of adherence (following the rules) to a broader client view of responsibility for self-care (determining the rules). The model shows the complexity of the process that clients use in making the numerous self-care choices required during the course of a single day.

The Model of Self-Care Decision-Making has some similarities to yet differs from traditional behavior change models. Traditional models predict behavior based on client perceptions related to health, illness, the environment, and expectations of others, as well as personal capabilities, benefits, and barriers to action. Unfortunately, although these models identify influential perceptions, they provide little insight into how these perceptions are formed. The MSCDM is a helpful adjunct to these models since it provides insight into how clients form perceptions, reason, and make decisions (Chenitz & Swanson, 1986). For example, benefits and barriers are often determined during cost/benefit analysis, whereas perceptions of personal capabilities or self-efficacy are often formed during historical analysis and/or personality assessments. The MSCDM provides an understanding of the cognitive process involved in decision making from the client's viewpoint; further, this model can be useful for predicting behavior. Thus, the MSCDM provides a new perspective on the self-care decision making of clients by showing how clients think about the choices they make and what components they analyze to inform their decision making.

Self-care decision making begins with, but is not determined by, the warnings clients receive (often from health care providers). The process of personal theorizing in response to warnings determines the decisions. Thus, encouraging positive self-care decision making probably involves influencing the analytical process.

During cost/benefit analysis, clients evaluate the costs and benefits of various self-care choices. Often, from the client's perspective, the costs outweigh the benefits, although providers focus only on the benefits. To promote positive self-care decision making, it is important to listen carefully and appropriately address client concerns about costs, whether physical, psychological, social, or financial. Although emphasizing benefits may be helpful, exploring with clients both the costs and the benefits may be more effective.

The manner in which clients are treated by providers (mutual respect and trust) and the importance of the interaction to the client may be as significant in encouraging health promoting choices as the information providers give. Sensitivity to client responses to warnings during provider/ client interactions is essential. Further, significant family members may need to be encouraged to participate in client health care management plans.

During experiential analysis clients review their previous history, appraise their personality, and compare their experiences with those of others. In this process they develop explanations, make connections between past experiences and present reality, and find direction for self-care choices. Often providers are unaware of the influence of clients' previous experiences. Becoming aware of these may be important in helping clients to make health-promoting choices. For example, if clients believe that because they have never been in a diabetic coma, the disease is not that serious (as several subjects in this study believed), their choices may be less health promoting. If clients do not associate serious infections and the loss of toes, feet, and limbs with their diabetes (several in this study did not), health care providers need to explain the connections. Perhaps statistical and/or graphic examples, not as fear-generating warnings but as instructional interventions, may be effective.

Risk analysis involves examining future health expectations. Concerns include loss of present health status, independence, and/or life. These risks may be ignored, appreciated without fear, feared, or considered overwhelming. Often health care providers try to promote adherence to health care directives by instilling fear in clients. Rather than simply communicating their own analysis of risks, providers need to ask clients how they view the future and recognize which risks are most important to them. If the risk of loss of independence is of more concern than the risk of loss of life, fear of falling may inhibit exercise and therefore weight loss choices. If risks are overwhelming to clients, an underlying depression may need attention. Examining risks with clients in terms of potential personal loss may be more helpful than warnings. Providing accurate information that clients can use during risk analysis is probably also beneficial.

Perhaps it is time to retire the term *adherence*. The real issue is not adherence behavior but self-care decision making. Health care providers generally give clients directives to follow and evaluate them as well as their health status in terms of adherence to these directives. This process simply does not work. Many clients are concerned about following providers' directives, but the choices they should make to best care for themselves are of greater concern. Eating a healthy diet and performing other positive behaviors can only occur when clients own their behavior and execute the necessary lifestyle changes. Clients must be empowered to make the best possible self-care choices for their health. Empowerment begins by giving the responsibility to clients.

Rather than spending time warning, admonishing, and/or threatening clients, more time should be taken to listen to clients' self-care decision making, as a basis for teaching. Subjects in this study had received a great deal of information about living with diabetes and hypertension. Some used the information; others did not. The MSCDM sheds light on why this is the case, and thus can lead to more effective interventions for clients with chronic diseases such as diabetes and hypertension.

REFERENCES

Beck, C. T. (1993). Qualitative research: The evaluation of its creditability, fittingness, and auditability. *Western Journal of Nursing Research, 15,* 263–266.

Chenitz, W. C., & Swanson, J. M. (1986). Qualitative research using grounded theory. In W. C. Chenitz & J. M. Swanson (Eds.), *From practice to grounded theory* (pp. 3–15). Menlo Park, CA: Addison-Wesley.

Fleury, J. (1992). The application of motivational theory to cardiovascular risk reduction. *Image, 24,* 229–239.

Haynes, R. B., Taylor, D. W., & Sackett, D. L. (Eds.). (1979). *Compliance in health care.* Baltimore: Johns Hopkins University Press.

Hutchinson, S. A. (1993). Grounded theory: The method. In P. L. Munhall & C. O. Boyd (Eds.), *Nursing research: A qualitative perspective* (pp. 180–212). New York: National League for Nursing Press.

Karam, J. H. (1992). Diabetes mellitus, hypoglycemia, and lipoprotein disorders. In S. A. Schroeder, L. W. Tierney, S. J. McPhee, M. A. Papadakis, & M. A. Krupp (Eds.), *Current medical diagnosis and treatment* (pp. 900–945). Norwalk, CT: Appleton & Lange.

Lincoln, Y. S., & Guba, E. G. (1985). *Naturalistic inquiry.* Beverly Hills, CA: Sage.

Massie, B. M., & Sokolow, M. (1992). Cardiovascular disease. In S. A. Schroeder, L. W. Tierney, S. J. McPhee, M. A. Papadakis, & M. A. Krupp (Eds.), *Current medical diagnosis and treatment* (pp. 257–356). Norwalk, CT: Appleton & Lange.

Pfister-Minogue, K. (1993). Enhancing patient compliance: A guide for nurses. *Geriatric Nursing, 14*(3), 124–132.

[16]

"Just Worn Out": A Qualitative Study of HIV-related Fatigue

Julie Barroso

Although deaths from HIV infection have dropped dramatically in the United States, patients are still dealing with significant symptoms that interfere with their ability to lead full, productive lives. Fatigue is the most frequent and debilitating complaint of HIV-positive people, with an incidence ranging from 20% to 60% (Breitbart, McDonald, Rosenfeld, Monkman, & Passik, 1998; Cunningham et al., 1998; Walker, McGown, Jantos, & Anson, 1997). It is widely accepted that the fatigue is related to HIV infection, since most of the people who suffer from it are young, have no comorbid conditions, and report developing this fatigue after becoming infected with HIV. HIV-related fatigue is associated with significantly poorer physical functioning and is a strong predictor of both limitations of daily activity and disability days (Breitbart et al., 1998; Cleary et al., 1993; O'Dell, Hubert, Lubeck, & O'Driscoll, 1998). People with HIV have been shown to exhibit declines in functioning over a 1-year period that were related not only to increasing disease severity, but also to reports of fatigue and poor self-rated health (Fleishman & Crystal, 1998).

Fatigue has also been found to be an important common denominator in the development of physical limitations and disability in ambulatory men with advanced HIV illness (Ferrando et al., 1998). Darko, McCutchan, Kripke, Gillin, and Golshan (1992) found that fatigue was a significantly greater problem for seropositive patients than for seronegative comparison subjects, and interfered more with activities such as employment and driving. The HIV-infected patients were significantly more likely to be unemployed, to feel fatigued more hours of the day, to sleep more, to nap more, and to have diminished midmorning alertness. Seropositive women have reported that fatigue resulted in lack of stamina, frequent absenteeism, and poorer quality work; they were afraid they might lose their jobs as a result (Semple et al., 1993).

A variety of physiologic causes for HIV-related fatigue have been proposed. Some studies have found no relationship between immune functioning, as measured by CD4 count, and fatigue (Breitbart et al., 1998; de Boer, van Dam, Sprangers, Frissen, & Lange, 1993; Ferrando et al., 1998; Perkins et al., 1995; Vlahov et al., 1994); however, Walker and colleagues (1997) found that greater fatigue was associated with lower CD4 counts. Also, Lee, Portillo, and Miramontes (1999) found that in women with HIV, lower CD4 counts were related to more daytime sleep and higher evening and morning fatigue. Darko and associates (1992) found a significant inverse correlation between CD4 count and hours of daily fatigue.

In the only study that has measured both fatigue and HIV viral load, Ferrando and colleagues (1998) found no correlation between fatigue and HIV RNA. Similarly, O'Dell, Meighen, and Riggs (1996) found no significant associations between hemoglobin, hematocrit, albumin, total protein, and fatigue. Nevertheless, anemia, the most common hematologic abnormality in patients with HIV, may be related to fatigue (Groopman, 1998), and there may be endocrine causes of HIV-related fatigue as well (Briggs & Beazlie, 1996; Rondanelli et al., 1997; Schurmeyer, Muller, von zur Muhlen, & Schmidt, 1997; Watson & Jaffe, 1995). Fatigue is a common manifestation of hepatic disorders; thus, abnormal liver function, whether caused by hepatitis or some other entity, could be linked to fatigue (Bartlett, 1996; Koch, Kim, & Friedman, 1998). Another possible physiological cause of fatigue in HIV-positive people is cortisol abnormalities (Abbott, Khoo, Hammer, & Wilkins, 1995; Clerici et al., 1997; Enwonwu, Meeks, & Sawiris, 1996; Norbiato, Galli, Righini, & Moroni, 1994; Piedrola et al., 1996; Rondanelli et al., 1997; Stolarczik, Rubio, Smolyar, Young, & Poretsky, 1998).

Some researchers, pointing to the high rate of depression among seropositive people, speculate that the fatigue seen in HIV disease is psychological. Consistent with this view, Perkins and colleagues (1995) found that increased fatigue was associated with increased depression, but not with HIV disease progression, and they concluded therefore that fatigue in otherwise asymptomatic patients probably has psychological rather than physiological causes. Walker and associates (1997) also found a strong positive correlation between fatigue and depression. In another study, HIV-positive patients with fatigue had significantly greater psychological distress, significantly more depressive symptoms, and greater hopelessness than those without fatigue (Breitbart et al., 1998). The authors of that study, however, concluded that not all fatigued patients with AIDS were depressed, and fatigue was not necessarily a reflection of underlying depression. These findings are similar to those of Ferrando and colleagues (1998), who found that in advanced HIV illness, fatigue was a chronic symptom, which, although associated with depressive symptoms and disorders, was not merely a symptom of depression. They concluded that fatigue in HIV illness may exist with or without a depressive disorder and may require treatment in its own right.

Unfortunately, sorting out the relationship between fatigue and depression is difficult (Hoover et al., 1993; Walker et al., 1997). Depression may cause fatigue, but fatigue may also cause depression. Many of the tools used to measure depression include somatic complaints that are similar to the symptoms of fatigue. Thus, Kalichman, Sikkema, and Somlai (1995) found that the somatic symptoms of depression included in the Beck Depression Inventory were closely associated with a number of AIDS-related diagnoses. These authors recommended that persons who experience HIV-related symptoms be assessed for depression using instruments that do not include somatic symptoms.

Sleep patterns may also affect fatigue in HIV-positive patients. Nocturnal cyclic variations in plasma levels of tumor necrosis factor a (Darko et al., 1995) and interleukin-1 (Darko, Mitler, & Henriksen, 1995) found in HIV-positive subjects may interfere with normal slow wave sleep. The increase in slow wave sleep, along with other changes in the sleep structure noted among seropositive individuals, would result in a subjective experience of poor sleep quality with a feeling during the day that not enough sleep has been achieved, accompanied by a feeling of suboptimal alertness.

Only one qualitative study has looked at HIV-related fatigue. Rose, Pugh, Lears, and Gordon (1998) interviewed 10 participants and identified three concerns involved with the meaning of fatigue for these patients—fatigue as a signal for AIDS; the mental, physical, and social experience of fatigue; and choosing ways to live with fatigue and addiction.

Fatigue in HIV infection is likely to be multifactorial, with cognitive, emotional, and organic components. Because HIV-positive patients can now survive for extended periods, further advances in the management of HIV infection require long-term therapy that recognizes the concerns of the patient about life goals and quality of life (Miles, 1997). Therapy to reduce fatigue could give HIV-positive patients improved vigor and quality of life and reduce societal costs (Darko, Miller, et al., 1995a). Thus, new approaches to managing HIV disease must include strategies that address patient concerns about fatigue. Unfortunately, little research has been done on the experience of fatigue among seropositive individuals. This qualitative study therefore was undertaken to describe comprehensively the experience of HIV-related fatigue.

METHOD

Sample

A descriptive study design was used to elicit in-depth descriptions of the symptom of fatigue. Purposive sampling techniques were used to recruit participants from the Raleigh/Durham/Chapel Hill, North Carolina, area. Flyers were distributed at the infectious diseases clinics of two university-based hospitals, a health department early intervention clinic for people with HIV, and a major AIDS service organization. Participants had to be able to speak and read English, be over the age of 18, and report feeling more fatigue since becoming HIV-positive.

The participants included 1 white female, 9 African-American females, 7 white males, 13 African-American males, and 1 African male who had recently immigrated from Uganda. The mean number of years since diagnosis with HIV was 4.74. The median income was $495/month, and 84% were unemployed. The mean CD4 count was 575, and the mean viral load was 147; these were both obtained via self-report. Therefore, as a group, the 31 participants were relatively healthy immunologically and had decent viral suppression.

Data Collection

Data were collected through interviews conducted over a 3-month period. Each interview began with a statement asking the participant to describe his or her HIV-related fatigue. Then, a series of probes were used. Participants were asked about the temporal qualities of their fatigue: aggravating, alleviating, and associated factors; patterns of fatigue and sleep; and the relationships of fatigue to depression and quality of sleep. The interviews were audiotaped and transcribed verbatim. Interviews ranged in length from 45 minutes to 3 hours, although informants could stop the interview at any time if needed. Participants also reported their most recent CD4 counts and HIV RNA viral load. After the interview, they completed the General Fatigue Scale (Meek & Nail, 1997) and the Beck Depression Inventory II (Beck, Steer, & Brown, 1996). The General Fatigue Scale (GFS) measures intensity, level of distress, and impact of fatigue on activities of daily living. It has seven items and asks respondents to circle the number, on a 1 to 10 scale, which most accurately reflects how they feel about the item. Scores may range from 7 to 70. The authors of the tool report that it is sensitive to change over time and has a Cronbach's alpha of .92. They also provide evidence of concurrent validity (Meek & Nail, 1997). The Beck Depression Inventory II (BDI-II) is a 21-item questionnaire that measures affective, cognitive, and somatic symptoms of depression (Beck et al., 1996). Each item contains a group of statements, ranked by severity, that reflect a specific symptom of depression. Subjects select the statement in each item group that best reflects how they were feeling during the prior week, including that day. Scores range from 0 to 63, with higher scores indicating more depressive symptoms. Coefficient alphas are reported to range from .92 to .93. There is strong evidence of convergent and discriminant validity, and the intercorrelation matrix provides evidence of factorial validity (Beck et al., 1996).

Most of the interviews took place at informants' homes, but a few were conducted in the researcher's office at the participant's request, and two interviews were conducted in a private room at a health department clinic. These alternative arrangements were made to accommodate the participants. Content analysis and constant comparison were used to analyze the transcripts of the interviews.

RESULTS

Participants were first asked to describe their HIV-related fatigue. Their descriptions captured its impact on their daily lives, their relationships with others, and their employment. Many people in the study spoke of needing an entire day to get through the simplest of chores.

> If I get somewhere and sit down, it will take me a good five minutes to get myself to, you know, to just be together. If the clothes are in the dryer, if I put the clothes in to dry, once they finish, I used to . . . stand right up there and just fold them on top of the washer and dryer. But now I have to sit in front of the dryer to do it. Because if I stand there . . . I have to sit down and I just can't stand.

HIV-related fatigue made it difficult for people to fill the roles that were precious to them: being a parent, a grandparent, a partner. There was a sense of social isolation, because the fatigue made it necessary to withdraw from activities with loved ones. One man said:

Before I got sick, I was . . . playing a little baseball, playing a little basketball, playing a little football, always playing with my grandbabies, you know what I mean? I was always doing something. Always doing something, man. I used to scoop my little grandbaby up and take her to the mall or whatever. Take her to Pullen Park and let her go swimming. I was there. You know, we'd go down there and spend all day. But now, I can't even take them to those places anymore. I can't take my grandbabies to go fishing anymore.

HIV-related fatigue was noted by several of the participants as the primary reason for not working; many of them had had to give up jobs they loved and the financial independence that regular employment offered.

I remember it distinctly when I knew I had to go on disability. . . . I was working at the office and I had been up and down having to go to the bathroom—and the building I work in, I think some 2,000 people worked there. It was a humongous office in Charlotte, and my office was right in the middle. So I had to walk a good distance to get to the bathroom, and I had gone several times and the last time on the way there, I just had to stop and lean up against the wall and rest. And at that point I knew that something had to be done. I was not going to be able to continue like that.

There was frustration over the restoration of the immune system but inability to regain their lives due to symptomatology. Life was not the same as before HIV. One participant said:

And they [health care providers] look at pure numbers. I mean, I think because they're so used to the old way of things like T-cells going from 80 down to 60 and then soon after, you die. Now they're saying, "Well, gee, your T-cells are 350 and your viral load is undetectable; you should be feeling wonderful." And so you think to yourself, Well, I'm supposed to be feeling wonderful—what is wrong with me? So you try to push yourself and you just can't do it.

Fatigue affected not only participants' physical being, but their mental state as well. Several people described being unable to think clearly when fatigued:

But I reach a point after about six or six and a half hours after I've gotten up in the morning that it's just like I hit a wall. And it's not only that I'm tired and I know I need to sleep, I don't process well. I really have trouble making the most basic decisions.

Other comments included these: "It's like moving around just makes me tired. . . . I can walk to the bathroom, but when I get in there and sit

down, I feel like I have walked a mile to get there. . . . I am so tired."
"Regardless of how much sleep I'm getting, I'm tired. . . . I'm just drag-
ging . . . it's a place where you are just existing, not really living." "Some
days I just wake up and I don't have any 'get up and go.' And I wonder why."

On the General Fatigue Scale (GFS), 25 of the 31 participants scored
above the mean score of cancer patients at their most fatigued (Meek &
Nail, 1997), indicating fatigue that is interfering significantly with one's life.

The time when the fatigue began varied greatly. For some, fatigue had
been the impetus to get tested for HIV. For some women, the fatigue had
started during pregnancy, which then led them to get tested for HIV. For
other participants, fatigue began after starting antiretroviral medications.
Many reported no detectable patterns to the fatigue and expressed frustration about its lack of predictability ($n = 13$, 42%). Some reported midday
fatigue ($n = 10$, 32%), whereas others reported morning fatigue ($n = 3$,
10%). Still others reported fatigue early in the morning, which recurred
in the evening ($n = 2$, 6%).

Twenty-seven (87%) of the participants were taking highly active antiretroviral therapy, and 32% of those thought that their fatigue might be
related to the antiretroviral medications. Most thought their fatigue was
not related to self-limiting illnesses such as sinusitis and bronchitis; those
with comorbid conditions (asthma, hypertension) said that they had not
suffered from fatigue of this magnitude prior to becoming HIV-positive.
When participants were asked about their best and worst times of the day
as a result of the fatigue, 39% said mornings were best, 19% said afternoons
were best, and 6% said evenings were best. The worst time of the day for
23% was the mornings; 35% said it was the afternoons, and 13% said it
was evenings. (These totals do not add up to 100% because some of the
participants were unable to identify a best and/or worst time of the day as
a result of the fatigue.) Aggravating factors included heat ($n = 11$, 35%)
and stress ($n = 8$, 26%), as well as doing too much, certain foods/alcohol,
medications, and depression. Six participants reported a relationship between fatigue and parenting, including the parenting of grandchildren.

When participants were asked what they thought was causing their fatigue, 65% ($n = 20$) said that HIV was causing it. Other reasons given
included depression ($n = 6$, 19%), medications ($n = 4$, 13%), poor sleep
($n = 2$, 6%), and other illnesses ($n = 2$, 6%); in addition, one participant
each cited stress, guilt, worry, and/or parenting.

Twenty-one participants (68%) reported being depressed, and many
noted that their depression had preceded their HIV infection. Ten were
taking antidepressants, and 48% ($n = 15$) believed there was a relationship
between depression and fatigue. Thirteen of the 31 participants scored in
the moderately to severely depressed range on the Beck Depression Inven-

tory II. General Fatigue Scale scores and BDI-II scores were significantly correlated ($r = .46$, $p = .01$). In an attempt to remove the confounding influence of somatic symptoms on the depression scale, which are also symptoms of fatigue, and to gain a better sense of the relationship between fatigue and depression, an additional analysis was conducted with the somatic items removed from the BDI, leaving only the cognitive/affective items. With the nonsomatic items only, fatigue and depression remained significantly correlated ($r = .45$, $p = .03$). Controlling for antidepressant use (10 of the 31 participants were taking antidepressant medication), there was still a significant correlation between fatigue and depression (partial $r = .42$, $p = .05$). Thus, there appeared to be a relationship between fatigue and depression that was not an artifact of measurement or due to antidepressant use/nonuse.

Participants were also asked if there were changes in their sleep patterns, when they went to sleep at night, when they woke up, the quality of their sleep, and the number of nighttime awakenings. Over half ($n = 17$, 55%) reported that their sleep was of poor quality, and said that they often did not wake up feeling refreshed. Once they went to sleep, their sleep was often interrupted by the need to get up to take antiretroviral medications or to urinate, or by some symptom such as diarrhea or night sweats. Most reported no difficulty falling asleep, but they reported difficulty going back to sleep if awakened for any reason. Many thought that if their sleep improved, they might have less fatigue; others said that even when they got a good night's sleep, they were as tired as before getting any sleep. Several participants believed that depression was causing their sleep problems. Some blamed their poor sleep on fatigue, saying they were too tired at night to sleep. Comments about sleep included these: "I can wake up in the morning and be like I been running somewhere, I am so tired." "Two years ago I could honestly say when I woke up I was refreshed, ready to go to work. I don't feel that way anymore." "Sometimes I just get overwhelmed with it. . . . A lot of times my sleep is not restful," "I can't shut my mind down . . . it seems like more and more I'm getting more and more terrified [of the disease]. . . . Sometimes I feel like if I go to sleep, I might not wake up, so I don't sleep."

DISCUSSION

This study provides some understanding of the fatigue experienced by HIV-positive people. It was startling to find the degree to which fatigue interfered with activities of daily living, relationships, and employment in these seropositive individuals. Fatigue has also been found to interfere with activities of daily living and employment in other studies (e.g., Breitbart et al., 1998; Cunningham et al., 1998; Ferrando et al., 1998; Walker et al., 1997). A large number of participants in the current study reported depression, again as in other studies (e.g., Breitbart et al., 1998; Ferrando et al., 1998; Perkins et al., 1995; Walker et al., 1997). This will be a difficult relationship to sort out, since fatigue can cause depression and depression can cause fatigue. However, for clinicians, the important thing is to screen for depression in seropositive patients who are fatigued and treat them appropriately. Finally, a large number of participants in this study reported problems with sleep, as in the studies conducted by Darko and colleagues (1992; Darko, Miller, et al., 1995; Darko, Mitler, & Henriksen, 1995). Again, clinicians should screen seropositive patients for sleep problems and intervene with a program of sleep hygiene.

Research in this area is still in its infancy, and much more work is needed to get a sense of the physiological and psychological correlates of HIV-related fatigue. Correlates other than depression should be studied, since there may be other psychosocial contributors to HIV-related fatigue, such as anxiety. Further sleep studies in this population would be useful as well. Longitudinal studies would be useful to determine when fatigue begins to play a major role in HIV infection, since the data correlating fatigue with CD4 count or HIV RNA viral loads are conflicting. Research should examine specific biomarkers, particularly those exhibiting a circadian rhythm, and a number of biomarkers at a time, since many of them affect one another in any individual.

Clinicians can help fatigued patients with careful planning of their day's activities. It is also helpful for clinicians to understand the impact of fatigue on many aspects of patients' lives. Clinicians should listen to patients when they complain of symptoms not easily defined by lab values. Clinicians taking care of seropositive people also need to advocate for services such as child care, assistance with activities of daily living, and better treatments that have fewer side effects. Although many patients have benefitted from the scientific advances of the last decade, and HIV has evolved from a fatal illness to a chronic illness, efforts must continue to minimize side effects such as fatigue that affect quality of life.

REFERENCES

Abbott, M., Khoo, S. H., Hammer, M. R., & Wilkins, E. G. L. (1995). Prevalence of cortisol deficiency in late HIV disease. *Journal of Infection, 31,* 1–4.

Bartlett, J. G. (1996). *Medical management of HIV infection.* Glenview, IL: Physicians and Scientists Publishing Co.

Beck, A. T., Steer, R. A., & Brown, G. K. (1996). *BDI-II: Beck Depression Inventory Manual* (2nd ed.). San Antonio, TX: The Psychological Corp.

Breitbart, W., McDonald, M. V., Rosenfeld, B., Monkman, N. D., & Passik, S. (1998). Fatigue in ambulatory AIDS patients. *Journal of Pain and Symptom Management, 15*, 159–167.

Briggs, J. M., & Beazlie, L. H. (1996). Nursing management of symptoms influenced by HIV infection of the endocrine system. *Nursing Clinics of North America, 31*, 845–865.

Cleary, P. D., Fowler, F. J., Weissman, J., Massagli, M. P., Wilson, I., Seage, G. R., Gatsonis, C., & Epstein, A. (1993). Health-related quality of life in persons with acquired immune deficiency syndrome. *Medical Care, 31*, 569–580.

Clerici, M., Trabattoni, D., Piconi, S., Fusi, M. L., Ruzzante, S., Clerici, C., & Villa, M. L. (1997). A possible role for the cortisol/anticortisols imbalance in the progression of human immunodeficiency virus. *Psychoneuroendocrinology, 22*(Suppl. 1), S27–S31.

Cunningham, W. E., Shapiro, M. F., Hays, R. D., Dixon, W. J., Visscher, B. R., George, L., Ettl, M. K., & Beck, K. (1998). Constitutional symptoms and health-related quality of life in patients with symptomatic HIV disease. *American Journal of Medicine, 104*, 129–136.

Darko, D. F., McCutchan, J. A., Kripke, D. F., Gillin, J. C., & Golshan, S. (1992). Fatigue, sleep disturbance, disability, and indices of progression of HIV infection. *American Journal of Psychiatry, 149*, 514–520.

Darko, D. F., Miller, J. C., Gallen, C., White, J., Koziol, J., Brown, S. J., Hayduk, R., Atkinson, J. H., Assmus, J., Munnell, D. T., Naitoh, P., McCutchan, J. A., & Mitler, M. M. (1995). Sleep electroencephalogram delta-frequency amplitude, night plasma levels of tumor necrosis factor a, and human immunodeficiency virus infection. *Proceedings of the National Academy of Science, 92*, 12080–12084.

Darko, D. F., Mitler, M. M., & Henriksen, S. J. (1995). Lentiviral infection, immune response peptides and sleep. *Advances in Neuroimmunology, 5*, 57–77.

de Boer, J. B., van Dam, F. S. A. M., Sprangers, M. A. G., Frissen, P. H. J., & Lange, J. M. A. (1993). Longitudinal study on the quality of life of symptomatic HIV-infected patients on a trial of zidovudine versus zidovudine and interferon-a. *AIDS, 7*, 947–953.

Enwonwu, C. O., Meeks, V. I., & Sawiris, P. G. (1996). Elevated cortisol levels in whole saliva in HIV-infected individuals. *European Journal of Oral Sciences, 104*, 322–324.

Ferrando, S., Evans, S., Goggin, K., Sewell, M., Fishman, B., & Rabkin, J. (1998). Fatigue in HIV illness: Relationship to depression, physical limitations, and disability. *Psychosomatic Medicine, 60*, 759–764.

Fleishman, J. A., & Crystal, S. (1998). Functional status transitions and survival in HIV disease. *Medical Care, 36*, 533–543.

Groopman, J. E. (1998). Fatigue in cancer and HIV/AIDS. *Oncology, 12*, 335–341.

Hoover, D. R., Saah, A. J., Bacellar, H., Murphy, R., Visscher, B., Anderson, R., & Kaslow, R. A. (1993). Signs and symptoms of "asymptomatic" HIV-1 infection in homosexual men. *Journal of Acquired Immune Deficiency Syndromes, 6*, 66–71.

Kalichman, S. C., Sikkema, K. J., & Somlai, A. (1995). Assessing persons with human immunodeficiency virus (HIV) infection using the Beck Depression Inventory: Disease processes and other potential confounds. *Journal of Personality Assessment, 64*(1), 86–100.

Koch, J., Kim, L. S., & Friedman, S. (1998). Gastrointestinal manifestations of HIV disease. In P. T. Cohen, M. A. Sande, & P. A. Volberding (Eds.), *The AIDS knowledge base* (3rd ed.). Available: http://hivinsite.ucsf.edu/akb/1997/05gi/index.html.

Lee, K. A., Portillo, C. J., & Miramontes, H. (1999). The fatigue experience for women with human immunodeficiency virus. *Journal of Obstetric, Gynecologic, and Neonatal Nursing, 28,* 193–200.

Meek, P., & Nail, L. M. (1997, May). *Internal consistency reliability and construct validity of a new measure of cancer treatment related fatigue: The General Fatigue Scale (GFS).* Paper presented at the Oncology Nursing Society Annual Congress, New Orleans.

Miles, S. A. (1997). Introduction. *Journal of Acquired Immune Deficiency Syndrome and Human Retrovirology, 16*(Suppl. 1), S1–S2.

Norbiato, G., Galli, M., Righini, V., & Moroni, M. (1994). The syndrome of acquired glucocorticoid resistance in HIV infection. *Balliere's Clinical Endocrinology and Metabolism, 8,* 777–787.

O'Dell, M. W., Hubert, H. B., Lubeck, D. P., & O'Driscoll, P. (1998). Pre-AIDS physical disability: Data from the AIDS Time-Oriented Health Outcome Study. *Archives of Physical Medicine and Rehabilitation, 79,* 1200–1205.

O'Dell, M. W., Meighen, M., & Riggs, R. V. (1996). Correlates of fatigue in HIV infection prior to AIDS: A pilot study. *Disability and Rehabilitation, 18,* 249–254.

Perkins, D. O., Leserman, J., Stern, R. A., Baum, S. F., Liao, D., Golden, R. N., & Evans, D. L. (1995). Somatic symptoms and HIV infection: Relationship to depressive symptoms and indicators of HIV disease. *American Journal of Psychiatry, 152,* 1776–1781.

Piedrola, G., Casado, J. L., Lopez, E., Moreno, A., Perez-Elias, M. J., & Garcia-Robles, R. (1996). Clinical features of adrenal insufficiency in patients with acquired immunodeficiency syndrome. *Clinical Endocrinology, 45,* 97–101.

Rondanelli, M., Solerte, S. B., Fioravanti, M., Scevola, D., Locatelli, M., Minoli, L., & Ferrari, E. (1997). Circadian secretory pattern of growth hormone, insulin-like growth factor type I, cortisol, adrenocorticotropic hormone, thyroid-stimulating hormone, and prolactin during HIV infection. *AIDS Research and Human Retroviruses, 13,* 1243–1249.

Rose, L., Pugh, L. C., Lears, K., & Gordon, D. L. (1998). The fatigue experience: Persons with HIV infection. *Journal of Advanced Nursing, 28,* 295–304.

Schurmeyer, T. H., Muller, V., von zur Muhlen, A., & Schmidt, R. E. (1997). Thyroid and adrenal function in HIV-infected outpatients. *European Journal of Medical Research, 2,* 220–226.

Semple, S. J., Patterson, T. L., Temoshok, L. R., McCutchan, J. A., Straits-Troster, K. A., Chandler, J. L., & Grant, I. (1993). Identification of psychobiological stressors among HIV-positive women. *Women and Health, 20*(4), 15–36.

Stolarczyk, R., Rubio, S. I., Smolyar, D., Young, I. S., & Poretsky, L. (1998). Twenty-four-hour urinary-free cortisol in patients with acquired immunodeficiency syndrome. *Metabolism, 47,* 690–694.

Vlahov, D., Munoz, A., Solomon, L., Astemborski, J., Lindsay, A., Anderson, J., Galai, N., & Nelson, K. E. (1994). Comparison of clinical manifestations of HIV infection between male and female injecting drug users. *AIDS, 8,* 819–823.

Walker, K., McGown, A., Jantos, M., & Anson, J. (1997). Fatigue, depression, and quality of life in HIV-positive men. *Journal of Psychosocial Nursing, 35*(9), 32–40.

Watson, J., & Jaffe, M. S. (1995). *Nurse's manual of laboratory and diagnostic tests* (2nd ed.). Philadelphia: F. A. Davis Co.

[17]

Maximizing Health for Those with Multiple Sclerosis

Alexa K. Stuifbergen, Anne Seraphine, and Greg Roberts

Recent reports estimate that 49 million Americans live with a chronic disabling condition, including 12 million who are unable to work, go to school, or live independently (Brandt & Pope, 1997; Freudenheim, 1996). As the society ages and chronic disabling conditions increase in prevalence, the emphasis of the health care system on costly high-tech care, cure of disease, and quantity of life has begun to shift (Brandt & Pope, 1997). Health care professionals are now being challenged to consider not only state-of-the-art disease care, but also the rehabilitation and health promotion services that can assist people with chronic disabling conditions to live fuller lives and maximize their health (Freudenheim, 1996; Renwick, Brown, & Nagler, 1996; Stuifbergen, Gordon, & Clark, 1998). However, to date, few studies have examined the health promotion needs or behaviors of persons with chronic disabling conditions.

Health-promoting behaviors involve continuing behavioral, cognitive, and emotional efforts to sustain and improve health and well-being (Pender, 1987). Physical activity, stress management, healthy eating, and cultivation of positive interpersonal relationships can contribute significantly to a subjective sense of wellness, perceived health, functional status, quality of life, and ability to live independently in the community (Lanig, Chase, Butt, Hulse, & Johnson, 1996; Marge, 1988; Roller, 1996; U.S. Department of

Health and Human Services, USDHHS, 1990). Although health-promoting behaviors may not change the course of illness or the barriers and resources existing in an individual's life, they may influence the individual's response to such conditions. For example, regular exercise can change the course of a person's response to illness by minimizing deconditioning and maintaining optimal levels of physical functioning within the limitations imposed by the disease (Rosenthal & Scheinberg, 1990). As the underlying disease and associated disability fluctuate or progress, health-promoting behaviors can nurture the person's overall physical, mental, and social health so that realistic improvement in or maintenance of quality of life is achieved (Holland, 1996).

In this study, persons living with the unpredictable, potentially progressive, and disabling neurological disease of multiple sclerosis (MS) were considered exemplars for study of the process of maximizing health and quality of life in the context of a chronic disabling condition. Although only 350,000 persons in the United States have been diagnosed with MS, it is the third most disabling chronic condition; 70% of the persons who have this disease are disabled (Anderson et al., 1992; Collins, 1993). Persons with MS experience a wide variety of symptoms that may lead to disability, including fatigue, muscle weakness and spasms, numbness, visual disturbances, bladder and bowel problems, pain, and changes in sexual and cognitive functioning.

We sought to explore the health promotion practices of persons with MS and differences in the frequency of health-promoting behaviors related to age, gender, and environmental context. We were also interested in identifying factors and outcomes associated with the frequency of health-promoting behaviors and determining whether such behaviors might mediate the effects of illness-related impairment on quality of life for persons with MS.

METHOD

A large nonprobability sample was recruited for this descriptive correlational study with the assistance of two chapters of the National MS Society in the southwestern United States. One chapter served several large metropolitan areas (population over 1 million), and the second served predominantly rural counties.

A total of 936 persons responded to an informational mailing from the MS Society and ads in rural newspapers about the study by providing their name and address to the investigators and indicating their desire to receive information about the study. A packet containing an informational cover letter, the study instruments, and a stamped, preaddressed envelope was mailed to those expressing an interest in participating. Coded packets allowed follow-up of nonresponders (Stuifbergen & Roberts, 1997).

In all, 834 surveys were returned (89%); 807 were usable, representing 86% of the 936 individuals who asked to receive information about the study (Stuifbergen & Roberts, 1997). Data collection instruments were bound in booklet format and printed in size 14 font to enhance ease of readability. The booklet included the following instruments:

1. *Incapacity Status Scale*—a 16-item measure of impairment due to MS (Kurtzke, 1981) adapted to a self-report format. Each of 16 aspects of personal functioning such as ambulation, vision, and bowel and bladder care are rated on a 5-point scale, with 0 indicating normal functioning and 4 indicating complete inability to perform the activity.

2. *Self-Rated Abilities Scale*—a measure of self-efficacy for health-promoting behaviors (Becker, Stuifbergen, Oh, & Well, 1993). This 28-item scale asks respondents to rate how well they are able to perform each health practice on a 5-point scale, from 0 (not at all) to 4 (completely). Item ratings are summed to yield a total score, and higher scores indicate greater self-efficacy.

3. *Personal Resource Questionnaire*—a 25-item measure of social support (Weinert & Brandt, 1987). Responses are scaled from 1 (strongly disagree) to 7 (strongly agree), with higher scores indicating higher levels of perceived support.

4. *Barriers to Health-Promoting Activities for Disabled Persons Scale*—an 18-item measure of the environmental, interpersonal, and intrapersonal barriers to health behaviors (Becker, Stuifbergen, & Sands, 1991). Responses to potential barriers such as fatigue and lack of money are scaled from 1 (never) to 4 (routinely).

5. *Acceptance of Illness Scale*—a 14-item measure developed by the investigators to indicate the degree of realistic acceptance of MS (Stuifbergen, Seraphine, & Roberts, in press). Respondents are asked to rate statements describing acceptance of MS on a scale ranging from 1 (strongly disagree) to 5 (strongly agree). Higher scores indicate greater acceptance.

6. *Health Promoting Lifestyle Profile II (HPLP-II)*—a 52-item measure of the frequency of health-promoting behaviors (Walker, Sechrist, & Pender, 1995), composed of six subscales (Physical Activity, Spiritual Growth, Health Responsibility, Interpersonal Relations, Nutrition, and Stress Management). Responses are scaled from 1 (never) to 4 (routinely). Because the six subscales do not have an equal number

of items, the average item subscale scores (total subscale score divided by the number of items) for the HPLP-II are computed to allow comparison of scores across subscales. Higher scores indicate that the behavior or group of behaviors is practiced more frequently.

7. *Center for Epidemiological Studies Depression Scale (CESD-10)*—a measure of depressive symptoms (Andresen, Malmgren, Carter, & Patrick, 1994). Respondents are asked to indicate how often in the past week they have experienced each of the 10 descriptions of depressive symptoms (e.g., "I felt that everything I did was an effort") on a scale from 0 (rarely or none of the time) to 3 (most or all of the time). Responses are summed to form a scale from 0 to 30; higher scores indicate more depressive symptoms.

8. *Quality of Life Index, MS version*—a 72-item measure of the person's satisfaction with important life domains (Ferrans & Powers, 1985). Part 1 includes 36 items that measure satisfaction with various domains of life on a 6-point scale ranging from 1 (very dissatisfied) to 6 (very satisfied). Part 2 measures the importance of the same items on a scale ranging from 1 (very unimportant) to 6 (very important). Total quality of life scores are calculated by weighting each satisfaction response with its paired importance response. Combinations of high satisfaction/high importance responses produce the highest scores.

All instruments had acceptable reliability estimates when used in this study. Means and standard deviations are provided in Tables 17.1 and 17.2.

RESULTS

The average age of the 807 participants was 48 ($SD = 10.6$). Most were Anglo (93%) and female (80%). Their average number of years of education was 14.25, 94% had completed high school, and 36% had completed college. Most respondents were married (71%) and not presently in the labor force (63%). Almost half (45%) reported relapsing remitting MS. Benign sensory MS, characterized by sensory symptoms and little or no long-term disability, was reported by 13%. About one third (36%) reported chronic progressive MS, and 6% reported severe progressive MS. The average time since diagnosis was 10.9 years. Slightly more than half of the respondents (52%) rated their health as good or excellent.

The sample for this study was similar to the population of persons with MS in the United States. Using National Health Interview Survey data, Minden, Marder, Harrold, and Dor (1993) reported that among those with MS, 73% were female, 95% were Caucasian, 85% were married, 82% had

TABLE 17.1 Means and Standard Deviations for Study Variables

Variable	Measure	Mean	(SD)	Range	Possible range
Severity of illness	Incapacity Status Scale	17.94	(8.70)	1–48	0–64
Self-efficacy	Self-Rated Abilities for Health Practices	78.42	(19.07)	11–112	0–112
Resources	Personal Resource Questionnaire	137.25	(23.34)	58–175	25–175
Barriers	Barriers to Health-Promoting Activities for Disabled Persons Scale	33.20	(8.13)	18–66	18–72
Acceptance	Acceptance of Illness Scale	36.03	(5.87)	14–62	14–70
Depression	CESD-10	10.75	(6.60)	0–30	0–30
Quality of life	Quality of Life Index	19.59	(5.04)	2.45–29.51	0–36

completed high school, and 71% were not in the labor force. In our sample, 71% had been diagnosed for more than 5 years, compared to a population estimate of 67%. The national sample had somewhat less favorable health appraisals, as only 44% rated their health good or excellent (Stuifbergen, Seraphine & Roberts, 2000).

Health Promotion Practices of Persons with MS

The Health Promoting Lifestyle Profile II (HPLP-II) (Walker et al., 1995) was used to assess the frequency with which individuals reported engaging in activities to improve their health and well-being. Overall, these respondents scored highest on the subscales of interpersonal relations (mean 3.04) and spiritual growth (mean 2.97) and lowest on physical activity (mean 1.88) (see Table 17.2). Examination of individual items on the HPLP-II indicated that the most frequently reported behaviors were the following (the percentage of respondents reporting that they often or routinely practiced the behavior is given in parentheses):

- Find it easy to show concern for others (87%)
- Am aware of what is important to me in life (85%)
- Maintain meaningful and fulfilling interpersonal relationships (79%)

TABLE 17.2   Comparison of Average Health Promoting Lifestyle Profile II Subscale Scores for Sample with MS and the Comparison Group

Health Promoting Life-style Profile II Subscale	MS Group ($n = 807$)		Comparison Group ($n = 712$)		t
	Mean	(SD)	Mean	(SD)	
Interpersonal relationships	3.04	(.55)	2.99	(.58)	1.72
Spiritual growth	2.97	(.64)	3.08	(.54)	−3.59*
Stress management	2.70	(.58)	2.61	(.55)	3.09*
Nutrition	2.56	(.60)	2.60	(.59)	−1.31
Health responsibility	2.47	(.56)	2.49	(.64)	−0.65
Physical activity	1.88	(.66)	2.34	(.71)	−13.08**
Total	2.60	(.43)	2.69	(.45)	−3.98*

*$p < .01$
**$p < .001$

- Believe my life has purpose (76%)
- Accept those things in my life that I cannot change (74%)
- Look forward to the future (72%)
- Question health professionals in order to understand their instructions (71%).

The practices reported least frequently were:

- Check my pulse when exercising (10%)
- Attend educational programs on personal health care (12%)
- Spend time with close friends (19%)
- Exercise vigorously for 20 or more minutes 3 times per week (22%)
- Eat 6–11 servings of bread, cereal, rice, and pasta per day (22%)
- Take part in light to moderate activity (22%)
- Practice relaxation or meditation (32%)
- Get exercise during usual daily activities (35%).

Scores on the HPLP-II subscales from this sample were compared to a group of 712 community-residing adults using t tests (Table 17.2). Persons with MS scored significantly lower on the subscales measuring physical activity ($t (1517) = -13.08$, $p < .001$) and spiritual growth ($t (1517) = -3.59$,

$p < .01$), but higher on the stress management subscale (t (1517) = 3.09, $p < .01$) (Walker & Hill-Polrecky, 1996).

Within this sample of persons with MS, there were significant differences in the HPLP-II scores by gender (Hotellings T^2(6, 800) = .043, $p < .001$), environmental context (Hotellings T^2 (6, 800) = .021, $p < .01$), and age group (Wilks' lambda (12, 1598) = .874, $p < .001$). Women scored significantly higher than men on the nutrition (F (1, 805) = 7.36, $p < .01$) and interpersonal relationships subscales (F (1, 805) = 18.63, $p < .001$). Persons living in metropolitan areas scored significantly higher on the physical activity subscale than those in nonmetropolitan areas (F (1, 805) = 5.99, $p < .05$). Older persons (over age 60) scored significantly higher on the stress management (F (2, 804) = 34.77, $p < .001$), nutrition (F (2, 804) = 13.83, $p < .001$), and health responsibility (F (2, 804) = 3.65, $p < .05$) subscales than younger (age 18–45) persons.

Factors Associated with Health-Promoting Behaviors

A number of variables were examined to determine if they were significantly related to the reported frequency of health-promoting behaviors. There were significant (p < .05) but weak associations with age ($r = .15$), education ($r = .18$), economic resources ($r = .30$), and illness-related impairment ($r = -.18$). Those reporting more frequent health-promoting behaviors tended to be older, have more years of education, perceive their economic resources more positively, and have less illness-related impairment.

Attitudinal variables were much stronger predictors of health-promoting behaviors. More frequent health-promoting behaviors were associated with higher scores on self-efficacy ($r = .69$), social support ($r = .58$), and acceptance of illness ($r = .42$), and lower scores on the measure of barriers ($r = -.39$). Those who reported more frequent health-promoting behaviors also reported fewer depressive symptoms ($r = -.48$) and perceived their quality of life more positively ($r = .52$).

Structural equation modeling (SEM) was used to analyze the possibility that health-promoting behaviors mediate the negative effects of illness-related impairment on quality of life. An explanatory model refined in earlier qualitative and quantitative work (Stuifbergen & Rogers, 1997) was assessed and modified using LISREL-8 (Joreskog & Sorbom, 1996). The 786 participants in the sample between the ages of 18 and 70 were selected for testing of the model because the health appraisals of this group differed widely from the appraisals of older (over age 70) participants (Roberts & Stuifbergen, 1998), and we wanted to avoid confounding the effects of aging and disability on the variables of interest. The resulting model (see

Figure 17.1) reflects the hypothesized relationships of severity of illness-related impairment, antecedent variables (resources, barriers, self-efficacy, and acceptance), health-promoting behaviors, and quality of life. Because, as hypothesized, the indirect effects of severity of illness on quality of life were significant, the mediation of health-promoting behaviors and other antecedent variables was supported. In fact, the magnitude of the coefficient (an indicator of the strength of the effect) of the direct path between severity and quality of life was only −.18, a value smaller than many of the indirect path coefficients. The refined model in Figure 17.1 had adequate fit, with χ^2 (8, N = 786) = 77.00, p < .05; Goodness of Fit Index (GFI) = .962, Incremental Fix Index (IFI) = .982, Comparative Fit Index (CFI) = .982. As shown in this figure, all specified paths, except the path between barriers and acceptance, differed significantly from 0. The proposed model explained 66% of the variance in quality of life scores (Stuifbergen, Seraphine, & Roberts, 2000).

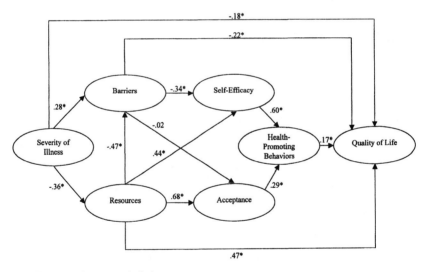

All parameter estimates are standardized.
*p < .01

FIGURE 17.1   Final model of quality of life in persons with multiple sclerosis.

Adapted from Stuifbergen, A., Seraphine, A., & Roberts, G. (2000). An explanatory model of health promotion and quality of life in chronic disabling conditions. *Nursing Research, 49*(3), 122–129. Copyright by Lippincott, Williams & Wilkins. Printed with permission.

DISCUSSION

This study provides important descriptive data on a large sample of community-residing individuals with the chronic disabling condition of multiple sclerosis. However, it also has limitations that must be considered when interpreting the findings. Data were obtained from a convenience sample recruited primarily through the National MS Society; the sample included very few minority respondents. However, the impressive response rate (89%) of those identifying themselves as potential participants suggests that health promotion is an important area of interest for persons with chronic and disabling conditions. Of course, it is possible that those with MS who do not identify themselves to the National MS Society may have different attitudes and behaviors (Stuifbergen & Roberts, 1997). A second possible limitation is the fact that the data were self-reported, and there is a possibility of bias in this type of data on health practices. However, these respondents had a wide range of scores with an approximately normal distribution.

Multiple roles in family, work and community, sociocultural values that derive from ethnicity and class, and personal beliefs and attitudes related to health have all been cited as important influences on health promotion. This study suggests that the experience of living with a chronic disabling condition also affects the behaviors used to maintain and promote health. Although it is not surprising that persons with fatigue and weakness and with balance and coordination difficulties have low scores on physical activity, this finding should be of concern to health care professionals. In the general population, physical activity is inversely associated with morbidity and mortality from several chronic diseases that become more frequent with increasing age (Blair et al., 1989). The impact of inactivity, especially when compounded by the physical changes of aging, may be even more significant for individuals with MS, who are already experiencing physical limitations. Therefore, it would be useful to develop programs of adaptive activity for such individuals.

Indeed, the strong relationships among daily activity, functional ability, and perceived health observed here and in earlier studies of persons with MS (Stuifbergen, 1997) highlight the importance of encouraging persons with MS to maximize activity in their daily lives. It has been suggested that improved fitness may not only improve the physical capacity needed for activities of daily living, but may also maximize the benefits of costly medical therapies such as interferon-B (Stuifbergen, 1997). Activity need not be in the form of structured exercise. Any form of physical activity—gardening, vacuuming, dancing—can bring beneficial short- and long-term effects. However, to maximize safety, recommendations must consider the individual's disability and disease activity and follow careful assessment of coordination, balance and trunk stability, muscle tone, and usual physical activity.

Although in this study subjects with MS scored significantly lower on physical activity and spiritual growth than a comparison group of community-residing adults, they scored significantly higher on stress management. Perhaps health care professionals should try to capitalize on areas of strength when developing programs to enhance health promotion for persons with MS. For example, individuals already engaging in stress management activities might be attracted to the stress-reducing benefits of stretching exercises and programs that incorporate both mind and body activities such as yoga and tai-chi.

The explanatory model tested in this study indicates that quality of life is the outcome of a complex interplay between contextual factors (severity of illness), antecedent variables, and health-promoting behaviors. The path coefficients in Figure 17.1 suggest areas that would be fruitful targets for interventions to enhance quality of life for persons with chronic disabling conditions. For example, interventions to enhance social support, decrease barriers to health promotion, and increase self-efficacy for health-promoting behaviors could increase health-promoting behaviors and improve quality of life. The investigators are presently testing the effects of such an intervention in a randomized clinical trial with a sample of women with MS (R01HD35047). Preliminary findings suggest that the intervention is effective in improving both health-promoting behaviors and quality of life.

Severity of illness and its associated disability are key determinants of the quality of life of persons with chronic disabling conditions. The findings of this study suggest that some effects of severity of illness may be mediated by intervening variables. Nurses and other health care professionals are often frustrated by the limited impact they have on the progressive course of chronic disabling conditions. Yet, although the trajectory of illness may continue downhill and over time can be expected to have increasing negative effects on quality of life, strengthening mediating variables such as resources and health-promoting behaviors may help to maintain and perhaps even enhance quality of life.

Thus, while state-of-the-art disease-directed care and treatment should be pursued, this study suggests that attention should also be directed to maximizing health-promoting behaviors. The continuing increases in the number of persons with chronic disabling conditions make it imperative to explore strategies to help these persons identify and maximize their resources, develop their self-efficacy for health behaviors, and enhance physical activity, nutrition, stress management, and spiritual growth in order to maintain quality of life.

ACKNOWLEDGMENTS

This research was supported by Grant R29 NRO3195, National Institute of Nursing Research, National Institutes of Health, and R29 NRO3195-03S1 Office of Research on Women's Health, Office of the Director, National Institutes of Health.

The authors wish to acknowledge the assistance of DaLynn Clayton, Sharon Rogers, and Ida Miller with data collection.

REFERENCES

Andresen, E., Malmgren, J., Carter, W., & Patrick, D. (1994). Screening for depression in well older adults: Evaluation of a short form of the CES-D. *American Journal of Preventive Medicine, 10*, 77–84.

Anderson, D. W., Ellenberg, J. H., Leventhal, C. M., Reingold, S. C., Rodriquez, M., & Silberberg, D. H. (1992). Revised estimate of the prevalence of multiple sclerosis in the United States. *Annals of Neurology, 31*, 333–336.

Becker, H., Stuifbergen, A., Oh, H., & Hall, S. (1993). The self-rated abilities for health practices scale: A health self-efficacy measure. *Health Values, 17*(5), 42–50.

Becker, H., Stuifbergen, A., & Sands, D. (1991). Development of a scale to measure barriers to health promotion activities among persons with disabilities. *American Journal of Health Promotion, 5*(6), 449–454.

Blair, S. N., Kohl, H., Paffenbarger, R., Clark, D., Cooper, K., & Gibbons, L. (1989). Physical fitness and all-cause mortality. *Journal of the American Medical Association, 262*, 2395–2401.

Brandt, E. N., & Pope, A. M. (Eds.). (1997). *Enabling America: Assessing the role of rehabilitation science and engineering* (Executive Summary). Washington, DC: National Academy Press.

Collins, J. G. (1993). Prevalence of selected chronic conditions, United States, 1986–88. *Vital Health Statistics 10*(182), 1–87.

Ferrans, C., & Powers, M. (1985). Quality of Life Index: Development and psychometric properties. *Advances in Nursing Science, 8*, 15–24.

Freudenheim, E. (1996). *Chronic care in America: A 21st century challenge*. Princeton, NJ: Robert Wood Johnson Foundation.

Joreskog, K. G., & Sorbom, D. (1996). *LISREL 8: User's reference guide*. Chicago: Scientific Software International.

Kurtzke, J. F. (1981). A proposal for a uniform minimal record of disability in multiple sclerosis. *Acta Neurological Scandinavica, 64*(Suppl. 87), 110–129.

Lanig, I., Chase, T. M., Butt, L., Hulse, K., & Johnson, K. (1996). *A practical guide to health promotion after spinal cord injury*. Gaithersburg, MD: Aspen Publications.

Marge, M. (1988). Health promotion for persons with disabilities: Moving beyond rehabilitation. *American Journal of Health Promotion, 2*(4), 29–35.

Minden, S. L., Marder, W. D., Harrold, L. N., & Dor, A. (1993). *Multiple sclerosis: A statistical portrait*. New York: National Multiple Sclerosis Society.

Pender, N. J. (1987). *Health promotion in nursing practice*. Norwalk, CT: Appleton & Lange.

Renwick, R., Brown, I. & Nagler, M. (Eds.). (1996). *Quality of life in health promotion and rehabilitation*. Thousand Oaks, CA: Sage.

Roberts, G., & Stuifbergen, A. (1998). Models of health appraisal in multiple sclerosis. *Social Science and Medicine, 47*(2), 243–254.

Roller, S. (1996). Health promotion for people with chronic neuromuscular disabilities. In D. M. Krotoski, M. A. Nosek, & M. A. Turk (Eds.), *Women with physical disabilities: Achieving and maintaining health and well-being* (pp. 431–440). Baltimore: Paul H. Brookes Publishing Co.

Rosenthal, B. J., & Scheinberg, L. C. (1990). Exercise for multiple sclerosis patients. In J. V. Basmanjian (Ed.), *Therapeutic exercise* (5th ed., pp. 243–244). Baltimore: Williams & Wilkins.

Stuifbergen, A. (1997). Physical activity and perceived health status in persons with multiple sclerosis. *Journal of Neuroscience Nursing, 29*(4), 238–243.

Stuifbergen, A., Gordon, D., & Clark, A. P. (1998). Health promotion: A complementary strategy for stroke rehabilitation. *Topics in Stroke Rehabilitation, 5*(2), 11–18.

Stuifbergen, A., & Roberts, G. (1997). Health promotion practices of women with MS. *Archives of Physical Medicine and Rehabilitation, 78*(Suppl. 5), S3–S9.

Stuifbergen, A., & Rogers, S. (1997). Health promotion: An essential component of rehabilitation for persons with chronic disabling conditions. *Advances in Nursing Science, 19*(4), 1–20.

Stuifbergen, A., Seraphine, A., & Roberts, G. (2000). An explanatory model of health promotion and quality of life in chronic disabling conditions. *Nursing Research, 49*(3), 122–129.

Walker, S. N., & Hill-Polrecky, D. (1996). Psychometric evaluation of the Health-Promoting Lifestyle Profile II. *Proceedings of the 1996 Scientific Session of the American Nurses Association's Council of Nurse Researchers*. Washington, DC.

Walker, S., Sechrist, K., & Pender, N. (1995). *Health Promoting Lifestyle Profile II*. Omaha, NE: Author.

Weinert, C., & Brandt, P. A. (1987). Measuring social support with the Personal Resource Questionnaire. *Western Journal of Nursing Research, 9*(4), 589–602.

U.S. Department of Health and Human Services (USDHHS). (1990). *Healthy people 2000* (DHHS Publication No. PHS 91-50212). Washington, DC: U.S. Government Printing Office.

[18]

Insufficient Access to Elderly Patients' Advance Directives in the Emergency Department

Debbie Travers, Diane Kjervik, and Laurence Katz

Emergency department (ED) clinicians must sometimes balance the need for emergency therapy against a patient's desire to limit treatment, when therapy will only prolong the suffering of patients who have no hope of recovery (Fox & Siegler, 1992; Iserson, 1997). Many elderly persons enact advance directives to limit life-prolonging treatments, in order to protect their right to die and maintain their autonomy (Emanuel, Barry, Stoeckle, Ettelson, & Emanuel, 1991; Hanson, Danis, & Garrett, 1997; Murphy, 1990). Advance directives (AD) include living wills that mandate refraining from life-sustaining treatment under specified circumstances and durable powers of attorney. Do-not-resuscitate (DNR) orders include physicians' written orders to withhold cardiopulmonary resuscitation (CPR), intubation, and/ or resuscitation.

Recent studies suggest that patients' advance directives have little impact on whether or not they receive life-sustaining resuscitative treatments during a hospital visit (Danis et al., 1996; Marco, Bessman, Schoenfeld, & Kelen, 1997; Teno et al., 1994). Communication problems have been identified as one reason for the disparity between these directives and actual treatment (Olsen, Lowenstein, Koziol-McLain, & Summers, 1993; Travers & Mears, 1996).

The emergency arena presents particular challenges in communicating advance directives and DNR orders (Crimmons, 1993). Although chronically ill elderly patients may desire treatment limits and have advance directives and DNR orders, if they present to the ED with life-threatening problems, they may receive unwanted treatments such as CPR, intubation, and defibrillation. These resuscitative efforts often are made because ED personnel do not have information about the patients' treatment preferences at the crucial moment when resuscitation decisions are made (Dull, Graves, Larsen, & Cummins, 1994; Travers & Mears, 1996; Wachter, Luce, Hearst, & Lo, 1989). Also, at the time of the medical emergency, clinicians must verify that written documents or statements from family and friends who accompany the patient to the ED are legally sound evidence of the patient's wishes. In situations in which emergency treatment might be withheld, legally defensible verification of the patient's wishes is a frequently cited concern of emergency physicians, nurses, and paramedics (Marco et al., 1997; Travers & Mears, 1996).

This exploratory, descriptive study explored patient, staff, and family experiences in the ED with the communication of AD/DNR for elderly patients with previously stated wishes for limits on resuscitative treatments. The study explored the factors that contributed to whether resuscitation was initiated in patients with AD/DNR and the resuscitation attempts performed on these elderly patients.

METHODS

The study was part of a larger study of clinicians' access to information about AD/DNR in the ED of a university teaching hospital in the southeastern United States. The study site serves urban and rural clients and has an annual volume of 48,000 ED visits. All ED visits between December 1, 1997, and March 30, 1998, were screened for enrollment in the study. Chronically ill persons age 65 or greater were eligible for the study if they had a life-threatening condition, vital signs were documented on admission to the ED and the patients were likely to need a decision about resuscitation. In addition, inclusion required documented evidence of a prior AD stipulating limits on life-sustaining treatments and/or a prior DNR order. The AD/DNR had to be presented or noted in the online or paper medical record, or documented as a statement regarding the patient's desire for treatment limits from the patient, family, or primary physician. Emergency department visits for major, multiple-system traumatic conditions were excluded.

If a patient visit was considered eligible, a research assistant identified the names of the ED nurse and physician who cared for the patient, the next of kin from the ED record, and the patient, if alive and able to participate in an interview. The nurse, physician, and patient or relative were then contacted and asked to participate in individual interviews at a convenient location. Staff members were asked whether and how they became aware of the patient's resuscitative treatment preference, how sure they were that that preference was honored during the visit, and what suggestions they had for enhancing communication of AD/DNR in the ED. Family members were asked how they conveyed the patient's resuscitative treatment choices during the ED visit. Family and patients were asked how they felt about the specific treatment rendered in light of the patient's wishes, then were asked for suggestions for improving AD/DNR communication in the ED. All interviews were audiotaped and transcribed. No identifying information was retained about informants.

An audit trail was maintained throughout the study with a log of impressions about specific interviews and decisions by the research team. Credibility was established with selected member checks and comparison of emerging themes with previous research (Danis et al., 1996; Dull et al., 1994; Travers & Mears, 1996; Wrenn & Brody, 1992).

Data analysis involved content analysis and identification of themes. Initially, each investigator read the transcripts independently and made notes about emerging themes. The investigators then discussed the analysis and came to consensus on six major themes emerging from the interviews. Next, the investigators met with a qualitative methods consultant and discussed the initial themes derived from the data. They reviewed the transcripts again, carefully examining each line and grouping statements according to commonalities. With this more focused analysis, the investigators concluded that eight themes were evident in the data. Several of these themes were consistent with findings from previous studies, and two clinician investigators who worked in the study ED agreed that the themes were applicable to the ED.

RESULTS

After review of all 2,632 ED visits by patients age 65 and older during the enrollment period, 102 ED visits were identified that potentially met the study inclusion criteria. Of these 102 visits, 32 were excluded because of a lack of previous AD/DNR documented in the patient's medical record, 28 because the patient was not in a life-threatening condition, and 4 because the patient was in cardiac or pulmonary arrest. The final sample comprised 38 ED visits by 32 patients (4 visited twice). All patients had one or more chronic illnesses; the mean was five.

Sixty interviews were conducted by the research team with patients (1), family members (11), nurses (25), resident physicians (12), and attending physicians (11). One family member declined to participate, 16 patients had died, and 15 patients were too ill and/or debilitated to be interviewed. Data saturation was achieved with 60 interviews, so interviews were then discontinued.

Interviews with staff were conducted in an office near the ED. Ten family members and one patient were interviewed by phone, and one family member was interviewed at home. The interviews took place from 1 week to 5 months after the ED visit. The major themes from interviews regarding AD/DNR communication and perceptions of the care rendered in the ED are described below.

ED Clinicians Need Better Access to AD/DNR Information before Resuscitation Decisions

Timing concerns were frequently cited as a barrier to AD/DNR information in the ED. Many ED staff members reported receiving information about the patient's AD/DNR during or after resuscitation treatments. Both staff and family members expressed frustration with situations in which the AD/DNR information was not conveyed before the resuscitative efforts were initiated.

A major source of frustration for nurses and physicians was the multiple locations for AD/DNR evidence. Most staff desired to see documentation of the patient's wishes. But they had to search for a myriad of different source documents, including forms sent to the ED with patients such as photocopies of living wills, powers of attorney, DNR orders, and brightly colored nursing home transfer forms or prehospital DNR order forms. Hospital sources for documented AD/DNR included multiple forms in the paper medical record and many screens in the online record.

Although the ED clinicians expressed a desire to see documentation of patients' AD/DNR, they felt most comfortable honoring patient wishes when the patients were competent and expressed their own wishes. Unfortunately, few situations were reported in which patients were competent to express their wishes. Clinicians reported that family members present at the patient's bedside were the most reliable source of AD/DNR information. As one physician said, family members' confirmation of the patient's wish for limits on resuscitation was "more reassuring than any form in the world."

A frequent topic in both staff and family interviews was poor communication of AD/DNR status for patients sent to the ED from nursing homes. Many patients with life-threatening conditions were transferred to the ED from nursing homes with no information about an AD/DNR. Both nurses and physicians thought that improving communication between nursing homes and the ED would help with AD/DNR communication. Their suggestions included standardized transfer protocols with photocopies of DNR orders, brightly colored transfer forms with DNR status information, an ED/nursing home liaison to facilitate communication, and faxing documents to the ED before patients arrived. Some clinicians suggested that nursing home patients with DNR orders should wear armbands stating their DNR status.

Clinicians also suggested adding prompts on the ED record for AD/DNR status assessment, having automatic computer printouts of previous status on the ED record, and streamlining the online and paper medical records so that AD/DNR status would be located in a uniform place. Staff also suggested that programs promoting greater involvement of family members in communicating AD/DNR (i.e., making sure AD/DNR forms were with patients whenever they went to the clinic or hospital) might improve the communication process.

A Pattern of Physical and/or Mental Deterioration Precedes Readiness for DNR

Although all patients in the study had an AD/DNR and presented to the ED with a life-threatening condition, their acceptance of death varied. Family members of patients who had a DNR order and were not resuscitated in the ED often described a prolonged period of suffering and deterioration prior to the ED visit. One wife described her husband's terminal ED visit: "I told them he was too far gone, he didn't want it. Because he was too old and sick." Staff expressed concern at the futility of resuscitative measures for patients with poor functional status, and felt more comfortable with DNR orders for such severely debilitated patients than for patients with good pre-emergency functional status.

Staff Roles: Treat First versus Proactive Approach to Treatment Status

Two approaches to accessing AD/DNR in the ED emerged from the clinician interviews. Some staff believed that their primary duty was to resuscitate all patients who presented to the ED, and they thought that complex issues like AD/DNR status were better addressed in the inpatient setting. These clinicians believed that the responsibility for conveying patients' wishes for treatment limitations rested with patients, family, nursing home staff, primary care providers, or emergency medical services personnel who brought patients to the ED.

Other nurses and physicians saw themselves as advocates for ED patients desiring treatment limitations. These staff members took a proactive approach to treatment status, seeking out information about patients' preferences. They diligently searched through the myriad of forms in the medical record for evidence of AD/DNR. They also made frequent attempts to phone the patient's family members and/or long-term caregivers about the patient's AD/DNR status. These ED nurses and physicians were most likely to search for AD/DNR information for severely debilitated elderly patients.

The Reversibility of an Emergency Condition Is Important but Difficult to Determine

Advance directives are typically activated when a patient has a terminal illness or incurable condition. The informants in this study described difficulty in determining when a chronically ill patient with a concomitant acute illness had reached the point of being "terminally" or "incurably" ill. Many family members said it was helpful to get prognostic information when faced with a resuscitation decision in the ED. However, many physicians related difficulty in determining the reversibility of a condition in the ED without initiating diagnostic evaluations that might conflict with a patient's AD/DNR.

When the ED clinician conveyed that the patient's life-threatening problem was potentially reversible, patients and/or family members were more likely to override the AD/DNR and choose resuscitation. This was most common for patients with good functional status before the emergency.

People Have Differing Expectations about Advance Directive Specifics

Although those interviewed felt that advance directives and DNR orders were clearly applicable to situations in which patients were in cardiac arrest, staff and family members varied in their views of the applicability of such directives to situations such as potentially reversible life-threatening respiratory compromise, shock, or hemorrhage.

Many staff felt that an AD/DNR needed to give specific instructions, such as whether or not to intubate patients or place them on a ventilator.

One patient's wife said her husband's directive stipulated that he wished to have CPR but not be intubated. However, most of the patients' AD/DNRs were not specific; they merely stated "do not resuscitate."

Some staff felt AD/DNR could not adequately address specific clinical situations. They said no one could anticipate all the possible situations that might be encountered at the end of life, and therefore AD/DNR could not be inclusive of a patient's wishes for every clinical scenario. They preferred to rely on health care proxies to make decisions at the time of the ED visit, rather than try to interpret the intent of a general statement in situations requiring specific decisions. Specific decisions mentioned by staff included whether or not to administer blood products, or perform endoscopy on a patient with a potentially life-threatening gastrointestinal bleed, or perform general surgery on a patient with a bowel obstruction, or consider the insertion of a pacemaker for a life-threatening bradycardia.

Staff Comfort with Helping Patients Die in the ED Varies

Several staff members believed that the ED was not the right place to help patients die, nor did they feel prepared to handle the situation. Some nurses and physicians were also concerned about liability, especially if the patient's wishes were less than clear. In the face of secondhand information from emergency medical personnel about the possible existence of a nursing home DNR order, one staff member said, "I was uncomfortable [enacting the AD/DNR] . . . we had no proof at the time."

However, several nurses described situations in which patients' wishes were clear, and they were comfortable shifting from performing unwanted resuscitation to helping family members cope with their loved one's condition and making the patient as comfortable as possible.

Conflict about Resuscitation Has Repercussions

When family members did not agree with each other or with the patient's desire for limits on resuscitation, the patient was usually resuscitated. Those interviewed all expressed distress in such situations. In one instance, the ED nurse and physician verified a patient's wish for no heroic measures, which was corroborated by the daughter and by documents in the chart. They defended their approach to care and comfort measures to the medical resident and primary physician, who wanted to institute aggressive treatment and admit the patient to the intensive care unit. The medical resident said to the ED nurse: "If I send her to the floor, she'll die." The nurse thought to herself: "Well, that's what the patient wants to do."

Staff, Patient, and Family Have Negative Feelings after Unwanted Resuscitation

Family members expressed anger toward nursing home staff when their relatives with AD/DNR were sent to the ED with life-threatening conditions and received unwanted resuscitation. They attributed these situations to lack of communication of the DNR status. One interviewee's mother had a DNR order at the nursing home but was transferred to the ED without communication of the DNR status. When the daughter arrived at the hospital, she found her mother intubated and in the ICU: "She never wanted to be put on a respirator or anything. She had the living will. They took me in; there she was on the respirator. My mind went blank to see her like that. There's a bill over there that I can't pay right now. With the 10 hours [of care in the hospital], it was over $4,000."

Many staff reported distress at resuscitating patients who they later learned had not wanted heroic efforts. As one staff member put it, "The purpose of the DNR is to let these people die in peace and not to bring them into the ED and have us do all kinds of things to them."

The one patient interviewed for the study was angry with her family for calling 911 when she developed respiratory distress. She was subsequently intubated and hospitalized for several days. During the interview 11 weeks later, she said, "I didn't want it [intubation]. They wanted me to have it. I've got three sons and a daughter, and all of them said we're going to keep you here as long as we can. I said when I die, just let me pass."

DISCUSSION

Elderly patients presenting to the ED with life-threatening conditions are extremely complex patients. Most have multiple chronic medical conditions, and they challenge clinicians to use a range of skills, from adjusting pain management or congestive heart failure treatment regimens to diagnosing acute reversible conditions, to putting acute and chronic problems into the context of the patient's desire for a peaceful death. As in previous studies, the majority of those interviewed in this study recognized that a problem exists with the communication of AD/DNR in the ED (Crimmons, 1993; Dull et al., 1994; Travers & Mears, 1996). Since the ED is not an ideal place for patients who desire end-of-life care and comfort only, it will probably continue to be a place where conflicts about this occur (Iserson, 1997). The family members interviewed here, as well as informants in studies by Balentine, Gaeta, Rao, and Brandon (1996) and Wrenn and Brody (1992), described family members' positive reactions to being asked about their loved one's AD/DNR status during ED visits. The differing expectations about AD/DNR specifics identified in this study are also consistent with previous studies. Singer, Martin, and Kelner (1999) described terminally ill patients' desires for discussions of specific treatments, but challenged clinicians to focus these discussions on treatments likely to alleviate suffering and not provide false hope.

The interviewees here suggested improving the flow and availability of information from nursing homes to the ED, streamlining access to AD/DNR in the ED, creating a climate where staff are proactive in searching for AD/DNR, and advocating more conversations between clinicians, patients, and families regarding prognosis and reversibility. Interviewees felt that these changes would maximize a patient's opportunity to receive care and comfort measures in the ED, while maintaining the right to die with dignity.

The interviewees noted particular problems with the communication of AD/DNR status for nursing home patients, which is consistent with studies by Bradley, Peiris, and Wetle (1998), Hanson and colleagues (1997), and Olsen and associates (1993). Future studies should test educational interventions to improve AD/DNR communication between nursing homes and the ED, especially for elderly, debilitated patients (Balentine et al., 1996). In-service programs for nursing home staff should address both communication of AD/DNR in emergencies and care of the dying patient. The ED physicians and nurses who participated in this study also expressed a need for education in helping patients and families through death and dying experiences in the ED. These findings clearly point to the need for improved family and patient education about communication of AD/DNR status in emergencies, as well as care of the dying.

Hospitals are now using increasingly sophisticated clinical information systems that record, organize, and deliver information to the clinician at the patient's bedside. One solution to the communication and access problems with AD/DNR might be the development of a computer application that streamlines AD/DNR information from multiple clinical entry points and provides it to the ED clinician in a quick online format as well as a printout on the ED record. Murphy and colleagues (1994) and Schonwetter, Walker, Kramer, and Robinson (1993) found that providing patients with information about the poor odds of surviving resuscitation decreased patients' willingness to undergo such usually futile treatments. Effective methods are needed for ED physicians to accurately convey status and prognosis information, without bias, and in light of elderly patients' previous AD/DNR. Primary care and ED providers, researchers, and information technologists must work together to help chronically ill elders and their families communicate AD/DNR across the continuum of care, from outpatient settings to long-term care to the emergency arena.

ACKNOWLEDGMENTS

This study was partially funded by the Center for Research on Chronic Illness at the University of North Carolina at Chapel Hill School of Nursing, grant #P30NR03962, National Institute of Nursing Research, National Institutes of Health. The authors wish to thank research assistant Juliet Stumpf, MSPH, EMT-P, and consultant Sandra Laws, RN, MSN, for their contributions to the study.

REFERENCES

Balentine, J., Gaeta, T., Rao, N., & Brandon, B. (1996). Emergency department do-not-attempt-resuscitation orders: Next-of-kin response to the emergency physician. *Academic Emergency Medicine, 3*(1), 54–57.

Bradley, E. H., Peiris, V., & Wetle, T. (1998). Discussions about end-of-life care in nursing homes. *Journal of the American Geriatric Society, 46,* 1235–1241.

Crimmons, T. J. (1993). Ethical issues in adult resuscitation. *Annals of Emergency Medicine, 22,* 495–501.

Danis, M., Mutran, E., Garrett, J. M., Stearns, S. C., Slifkin, R. T., Hanson, L., Williams, J. F., & Churchill, L. R. (1996). A prospective study of the impact of patient preferences on life-sustaining treatment and hospital cost. *Critical Care Medicine, 24*(11), 1811–1817.

Dull, S. M., Graves, J. R., Larsen, M. P., & Cummins, R. O. (1994). Expected death and unwanted resuscitation in the prehospital setting. *Annals of Emergency Medicine, 23*(5), 997–1001.

Emanuel, L. L., Barry, M. J., Stoeckle, J. D., Ettelson, L. M., & Emanuel, E. J. (1991). Advance directives for medical care—A case for greater use. *New England Journal of Medicine, 324,* 889–895.

Fox, E., & Siegler, M. (1992). Redefining the emergency physician's role in do-not-resuscitate decision-making. *American Journal of Medicine, 92,* 125–128.

Hanson, L. C., Danis, M., & Garrett, J. (1997). What is wrong with end-of-life care? Opinions of bereaved family members. *Journal of the American Geriatrics Society, 45*(11), 1339–1344.

Iserson, K. V. (1997). Sailing life's uncharted seas: Advance directives and emergency medicine patients. *Academic Emergency Medicine, 4,* 933–934.

Marco, C. A., Bessman, E. S., Schoenfeld, C. N., & Kelen, G. D. (1997). Ethical issues of cardiopulmonary resuscitation: Current practice among emergency physicians. *Academic Emergency Medicine, 4*(9), 898–903.

Murphy, D. J. (1990). Improving advance directives for healthy older people. *Journal of the American Geriatric Society, 38,* 1251–1256.

Olsen, E. B., Lowenstein, S. R., Koziol-McLain, J., & Summers, J. G. (1993). Do-not-resuscitate order: What happens after hospital discharge? *Western Journal of Medicine, 158*(5), 484–487.

Schonwetter, R. S., Walker, R. M., Kramer, D. R., & Robinson, B. E. (1993). Resuscitation decision making in the elderly: The value of outcome data. *Journal of General Internal Medicine, 8,* 295–300.

Singer, P. A., Martin, D. D., & Kelner, M. (1999). Quality end-of-life care: Patients' perspectives. *Journal of the American Medical Association, 281*(2), 163–168.

Teno, J. M., Lynn, J., Phillips, R. S., Murphy, D., Youngner, S. J., Bellamy, P., Connors, Jr., A. F., Desbiens, W. F., & Knaus, W. A. (1994). Do formal advance directives affect resuscitation decisions and the use of resources for seriously ill patients? *Journal of Clinical Ethics, 5*(1), 23–30.

Travers, D. A., & Mears, G. D. (1996). Physicians' experiences with prehospital do-not-resuscitate orders in North Carolina. *Prehospital and Disaster Medicine, 11*(2), 91–100.

Wachter, R. M., Luce, J. M., Hearst, N., & Lo, B. (1989). Decisions about resuscitation: Inequities among patients with different diseases but similar prognoses. *Annals of Internal Medicine, 111,* 525–532.

Wrenn, K., & Brody, S. L. (1992). Do-not-resuscitate orders in the emergency department. *American Journal of Medicine, 92,* 129–133.

Part IV

ILLNESS/DISEASE MANAGEMENT

[19]

Effects of Exercise on Fatigue: Aerobic Fitness and Disease Activity in Persons with Rheumatoid Arthritis

Geri B. Neuberger, Allan N. Press, Herbert B. Lindsley, Ruthellyn Hinton, Perri E. Cagle, Katherine Carlson, Stephen Scott, Judy Dahl, and Beth Kramer

Fatigue is a person's response to physiological, psychological, and situational factors (Kellum, 1985). It can occur on a cellular, unconscious level first but, if it persists, will eventually lead to a subjective, generalized response. A major feature of chronic fatigue is self-report of a sustained and significant lack of energy. In persons with rheumatoid arthritis (RA), fatigue is associated with joint pain, and the absence of fatigue is identified as a criterion for remission by the American College of Rheumatology (Schumacher, 1993). Yet despite the fact that fatigue is a common symptom of RA, few investigators have explored the experience of fatigue in persons with RA.

In a small ($N = 20$) descriptive study, Tack (1990) found that 12 of 20 subjects reported fatigue as one of the three most problematic aspects of RA. In a subsequent study, using a self-report instrument to measure the multidimensional aspects of fatigue (severity, distress, consequences), Tack and colleagues found that 40% of their sample of 133 adults with RA reported fatigue every day (Belza [Tack], Henke, Yelin, Epstein, & Gilliss, 1993). Pain, sleep quality, physical activity level, comorbid conditions, functional status, duration of disease, depression, learned helplessness, and social support were all significantly associated with fatigue. Crosby (1991) found that factors identified by subjects as contributing to fatigue included RA disease activity, disturbed sleep, and increased physical effort. Fatigue of subjects experiencing a disease flare was positively correlated with joint pain ($r = .62$), fragmented sleep ($r = .42$), and grip strength of the right and left hands ($r = .52$ and $r = .88$, respectively).

The effects of exercise on fatigue in clients with RA have not been systematically assessed. However, Neuberger, Kasal, Smith, Hassanein, and DeViney (1994) found that 63% of 100 subjects with either RA or osteoarthritis had poor or very poor levels of aerobic fitness. Two exercise intervention studies with RA clients produced reductions in fatigue. However, in one of these studies there was no preexercise measure of fatigue, and fatigue was measured only by a one-item global assessment as worse, same, better, or much better (Harkcom, Lampman, Banwell, & Castor, 1985). In the other study (Perlman et al., 1990), two interventions were tested simultaneously—low-impact aerobic exercise and problem solving—and it was impossible to separate the effects of the two.

The study reported here tested the effects of a low-impact aerobic exercise intervention on fatigue and aerobic fitness. Fatigue was defined as a sensation of general tiredness or lack of energy and was measured by self-report. Participation in the exercise program was expected to decrease fatigue in outpatients with RA and increase the aerobic fitness levels of subjects without increasing disease activity. Because other researchers have found varied levels of participation in exercise interventions (Bradley, 1989; Minor, Hewett, Webel, Anderson, & Kay, 1989; Stenstrom, 1994; Waggoner & LeLieuvre, 1981) and several have raised questions about maintenance of exercise, the study also examined the effects of different degrees of exercise participation on measures of fatigue, aerobic fitness, and disease activity, the extent to which subjects reported continued performance of low-impact aerobic exercise at a 15-week follow-up visit, and the extent to which subjects continued to improve or change at follow-up on measures of fatigue, aerobic fitness, and disease activity.

METHOD

Sample

A convenience sample of persons who had a diagnosis of RA, were mentally competent, able to read and speak English, and able to ambulate, had no history of fibromyalgia or severe COPD, were not presently involved in a regular program of aerobic exercise (defined as 30 minutes of aerobic exercise three times a week or more), and had their rheumatologist's approval were recruited for the study. Letters of invitation were mailed to 64 outpatients with rheumatoid arthritis identified from a university database and were also placed in the offices of several private rheumatologists. Potential subjects were told that the purpose of the study was to examine the signs and symptoms of RA before and after a 12-week program of exercise. They were not told that fatigue was the primary symptom of interest.

Thirty-two subjects began the study, and 25 completed it. Two subjects dropped out before the first assessment period, two subjects dropped out after the first assessment period (one moved, and one's doctor felt she was not ready for this type of exercise), and three subjects dropped out after the second assessment (two due to a change in work schedule and one due to weakness after influenza).

The mean age of the sample was 55, with a range of 30 to 71 years. The mean duration of RA was 9.8 years, with a range of 7 to 30 years. Nineteen subjects were Caucasian, 3 African American, 2 Hispanic, and 1 Asian. There were 14 women and 11 men. Six (24%) of the subjects had attended or graduated from high school, 10 (40%) had some college or equivalent training, and 9 (36%) had a college or master's degree. Eleven subjects were employed full-time, 5 employed part-time, and 9 not employed. Their median yearly income was $41,250. Twenty-two subjects lived with a spouse or significant other. At baseline, 22 subjects were in functional status Class II (able to perform usual self-care and vocational activities, but limited in avocational activities), and 3 were in Class III (able to perform usual self-care activities, but limited in vocational and avocational activities), as defined by the American College of Rheumatology (Schumacher, 1993).

Intervention

The exercise intervention consisted of participation in a low-impact aerobic exercise class for 1 hour three times weekly for 12 weeks, for a total of 36 sessions. The exercise regimen was designed by two physical therapists, an aerobic instructor, and one of the investigators. The class consisted of four phases: warm-up exercises, strengthening exercises, low-impact aerobic exercises, and cool-down exercises. Initially, warm-up and strengthening phases were longer in order to build muscle strength. As aerobic minutes were increased, minutes of warm-up and cool-down were reduced, and this progression of minutes was recorded. The exercise class was held in a room in the exercise facility on the medical center campus. Subjects came to either an early or a late afternoon class. Subjects were encouraged to attend each exercise session, but only one subject attended all 36 sessions.

Measures

Several questionnaires were administered to enable participants to report their symptoms and feelings. These included the Multidimensional Assessment of Fatigue to measure fatigue and the Profile of Mood States—Short Form to measure fatigue, depression, and other moods (anger, tension, etc). The Arthritis Impact Measurement Scales were used to measure pain and the impact of arthritis, along with other disease information. Measures of disease activity were joint count, pain, grip strength, walk time, and sedimentation rate. Aerobic fitness was calculated from a bicycle ergometer test.

Multidimensional Assessment of Fatigue (MAF)

The MAF (Tack, 1991) scale has 16 items that measure four dimensions of fatigue experienced during the previous week: severity (2 items), distress (1 item), timing (2 items), and degree of interference with activities of daily living (11 items). Each item is scored on a scale from 1 (none) to 10 (severe, or a great deal), and items are averaged to create a score for each dimension (Tack, 1990). A Global Fatigue Index, which ranges from 3 (least) to 50 (most fatigue), also can be calculated. Belza and her coauthors (1993) reported concurrent validity of the MAF with the fatigue subscale of the Profile of Mood States as $r = .78$, $p < .001$, and divergent validity with the POMS vigor subscale of $r = -.60$, $p < .001$. For this study, Cronbach's alphas ranged from .83 to .92 across assessment points for global fatigue and from .79 to .92 for the interference with Daily Activities subscale.

Profile of Mood States—Short Form (POMS)

The POMS-Short Form consists of 30 of the original 65 items in the POMS. Validity of the POMS has been supported in numerous clinical studies that showed improvement of symptoms after treatment (McNair, Lorr, & Droppleman, 1992). All mood scales were examined for their relationships to fatigue. In this study, Cronbach's alphas for the fatigue subscale ranged from .83 to .93 across assessment points.

For each of the six subscales (Tension, Anger, Fatigue, Vigor, Confusion, Depression), a mean score of the five items in the subscale was computed.

Item responses ranged from 0 (not at all) to 4 (extremely). One item, "efficient," had to be recoded so that all items were in the same direction prior to the calculation of subscale scores.

Arthritis Impact Measurement Scales (AIMS)

AIMS, a multidimensional measure of health status, was selected because it has a reliable (Cronbach's alpha of .86) and valid subscale for pain (four items) (Meenan, Gertman, Mason, & Dunlaif, 1982). Current medications, duration of arthritis, and arthritis impact are also measured by items on the AIMS. The arthritis impact item asks subjects to mark a visual analog scale that ranges from 0 (very well) to 100 (very poor) in response to this statement: "Considering all the ways your arthritis affects you, mark (X) on the scale for how well you are doing." AIMS subscale scores are converted to a 0 to 10 scale by multiplying the original score by 0.10.

Bicycle Ergometer Testing

The Astrand-Rhyming protocol was used to obtain data for calculating the estimated VO_2 max of each subject (American College of Sports Medicine, 1991). In this protocol, subjects pedal on a stationary bicycle ergometer at the rate of 50 revolutions per minute at a workload (resistance to pedaling) determined by their heart rate, which is monitored every minute during the 6-minute test. The second-minute heart rate must be between 115 and 140, and workload is adjusted up or down accordingly. The fifth- and sixth-minute heart rates must be within five beats; otherwise the subject must pedal an additional 1 or more minutes until a steady state is reached. The American College of Sports Medicine 1991 guidelines were used to determine the safety of performing the test on each subject. Regression equations have been developed for submaximal bicycle ergometer testing for men and women of varying age groups. The correlation between the measured and estimated VO_2 max in one study was .94 (Siconolfi, Cullinane, Carleton, & Thompson, 1982). In the present study, the estimated VO_2 max obtained on each subject was compared to norms to determine the fitness level for each subject at the beginning of the study, after completion of the exercise intervention, and at the 15-week follow-up visit.

Joint Count

Joint count, or the number of painful or swollen joints, was obtained at each assessment by the same trained research assistant, who palpated and/ or moved each joint (total of 81) to determine whether tenderness or swelling was present. The total number of tender and swollen joints was used in the analysis (joint count is high when RA is active and decreases when RA is less active).

Grip Strength

Grip strength was measured in each hand at each assessment by using a rolled-up blood pressure cuff connected to a portable sphygmomanometer with a mercury manometer, which was pumped up to 20 mmHg (the mercury would rise depending on the force of the subject's hand grip). Subjects performed three hand grips for each hand, and the mean for each hand was used in analyses (Hess, 1988).

Walk Time

Walk time, or the number of seconds it took a subject to walk 50 feet, was measured at each assessment (walk time often increases with disease activity). A distance of 50 feet was identified on a flat, straight floor and marked with masking tape. The subject was instructed to start walking 18 feet prior to the marked area so that stride was established before the subject reached the designated starting point. Time used to walk 50 feet was determined using a stopwatch and recorded in seconds.

Sedimentation Rate

Sedimentation rate was assessed with standard laboratory procedures (Corbett, 1992). (The value increases [above 20mm/hr] in inflammatory disorders [Anderson, 1993].)

Procedure

Measures were obtained on all subjects five times: at two baseline assessments (BL), 6 weeks apart; at mid-treatment (MT), after 6 weeks of the exercise intervention; at the end of treatment (ET), after 12 weeks of the exercise intervention; and at follow-up (FU), which occurred 15 weeks after completion of the exercise program. Two baseline assessments were obtained because RA disease activity can vary at short intervals. After the second baseline assessment, subjects began the exercise program. All measures were repeated at each of the five assessment points except for the bicycle ergometer test, which was obtained at BL, ET, and FU only. The time of day of each subject's visit for each of the five assessments was recorded to determine whether diurnal variations occurred in fatigue ratings.

After signing a written consent form at the initial visit, each subject's weight and height were obtained on the same clinic scale, and blood pressure was taken on the same sphygmomanometer by the same research assistant. Subjects then completed the paper-and-pencil instruments. In a private examination room, one research assistant did a joint assessment on each subject and a brief physical examination to rule out gross cardiac and pulmonary abnormalities. Walk time and hand grip measurements also were obtained. Prior to the bicycle ergometer testing, venous blood was obtained for measurement of sedimentation rate. Research assistants who collected data were blinded to previous assessment data and final score calculations.

Data Analysis

To determine the effects of level of participation in the exercise intervention on fatigue and related variables, exercise was treated as a continuous variable (number of classes attended). In order to compare subjects at different ends of the self-selected exercise continuum, participants were separated into high, medium, and low levels of participation. High participants ($n = 8$) attended 31 to 36 of the 36 exercise classes, medium participants ($n = 8$) attended 25 to 30 classes, and low participants ($n = 9$) attended 24 or fewer classes. If subjects attended all three 1-hour sessions of exercise per week during the exercise intervention, they engaged in 180 minutes of exercise weekly. The typical subject who was a high exerciser engaged in 162 minutes weekly ($SD = 1.78$); the corresponding figure for moderate exercisers was 137.5 minutes ($SD = 1.51$) and for low exercisers, 71 minutes ($SD = 9.93$). High-, medium-, and low-exercise participant groups did not differ in level of education, mean age, or gender proportions.

The dependent measures were analyzed in a mixed categorical–continuous analysis of variance (ANOVA) design (Pedhazur, 1982), using the multivariate general linear model routine in the SYSTAT data analysis package. Differences in mean responses on the variables were examined at the three assessment points of baseline (average of the two baseline measures), mid-treatment, and end of treatment. In addition, the analysis determined whether exercise participation (number of classes attended) affected measures of the dependent variables. The results on the main dependent measures are reported first for baseline (BL), mid-treatment

(MT), and end-of-treatment (ET) scores, then for the comparison of changes from end-of-treatment (ET) to follow-up (FU).

RESULTS

Electrolytes, blood chemistries, hematology, and thyroid function were within normal limits for all subjects at all measurement points during the study. Thus, many metabolic processes that might have caused fatigue were normal. There were no significant changes in means on sleep effectiveness, sleep disturbance, or depression across measurement times. From baseline (BL) to end-of-treatment (ET) assessments, medications received for arthritis changed in six subjects, but usually the change was simply to another drug in the same class (e.g., from one nonsteroidal anti-inflammatory drug to another). Medications remained the same for 19 subjects. Therefore, it is unlikely that changes in the variables measured in the study were due to response to medications.

Table 19.1 shows the mean responses for low-, medium-, and high-participation subjects. At baseline all subjects reported at least some fatigue. The average MAF scores were moderately low. There were no significant associations between fatigue ratings and time of day of data collection.

Two of the fatigue measures, the MAF Distress and Severity subscales, changed from baseline to mid-treatment to end of treatment. Contrary to our expectation that exercise would decrease fatigue, the total group means for distress and severity increased from BL to MT, then decreased to their lowest points at ET (see Table 19.1). As Table 19.1 indicates, there were differences in fatigue variables over the three time periods as a function of exercise participation. Global fatigue was not significant at the .05 level for changes over time periods, but when number of exercise classes attended was considered in the analysis (interaction of time period and number of classes attended), global fatigue decreased significantly. A similar pattern occurred for the POMS fatigue scale. The mean fatigue scores for respondents with high-, moderate-, and low-exercise class participation are shown in Table 19.1. Although the low-exercise group initially reported the least fatigue on all measures, their fatigue had increased at ET.

By contrast, improvements in aerobic fitness and disease activity measures were not a function of frequency of exercise. Aerobic fitness was not measured at mid-treatment, but it improved significantly from BL to ET (see Table 19.2). Four of the disease measures, left and right hand grip strength, walk time, and pain ratings, significantly improved over time (pain rating showed significant improvement from BL to ET only, $F(1,23) = 5.95$, $p = .05$). Another disease activity measure, impact of arthritis, also improved

TABLE 19.1 Mean Scores and *F* Values for Time Period and Interaction of Time Period with Number of Exercise Classes on Fatigue Scales for Low, Moderate, and High Exercisers for Three Time Periods

Dependent Measure	Time Period[a]	Exercise Participation			Total Group Mean	Time *F*	ANOVA Time-by-# Classes *F*
		Low Mean	Moderate Mean	High Mean			
MAF Distress[b]	BL	2.11	2.69	3.25	2.66	3.87*	6.05**
	MT	3.89	2.75	3.50	3.40		
	ET	2.89	2.13	2.63	2.56		
MAF Severity[b]	BL	3.78	3.78	4.03	3.86	3.25*	4.34*
	MT	5.39	3.75	3.94	4.40		
	ET	4.22	2.69	3.38	3.46		
MAF Global[b]	BL	17.50	18.50	19.90	18.59	2.87#	3.58*
	MT	23.40	16.80	20.30	20.31		
	ET	19.40	13.70	17.10	16.75		
POMS Fatigue Scale[c]	BL	1.13	1.39	1.23	1.24	0.60	3.38*
	MT	1.49	0.73	1.36	1.20		
	ET	1.36	0.83	1.05	1.05		

# $p < .10$ * $p < .05$ ** $p < .01$
[a] BL = Baseline; MT = Mid-treatment; ET = End-of-treatment
[b] MAF = Multidimensional Assessment of Fatigue; possible ranges are 1–10 for the Distress and Severity subscales and 3–50 for the global scale
[c] POMS = Fatigue Subscale of Profile of Mood States; possible range = 0–4

TABLE 19.2   Mean Scores and *F* Values for Aerobic Fitness and Disease Activity Measures for Three Time Periods (BL, MT, ET)

Measures	BL	MT	ET	F
		Time Period[a]		
Aerobic fitness	22.71	na	30.78	20.86**
Left grip strength	127.00	138.00	150.00	18.54**
Right grip strength	121.00	129.00	139.00	10.11**
Impact of arthritis	3.27	2.92	2.51	2.53#
Pain	5.09	4.64	4.50	2.31
Walk time	10.41	9.86	9.44	3.74*
Sedimentation rate	30.70	29.60	30.00	.045
Joint count	31.50	28.00	30.10	.925

#$p < .10$ *$p < .05$ **$p < 0.001$
[a]BL = Baseline; MT = Mid-treatment; ET = End-of-treatment; F = F values for ANOVAs comparing the three time points.

over time, but the change was not significant. As expected, sedimentation rate and total joint count showed little or no change.

Eighty percent, or 20 of the 25 subjects, reported continued performance of some type of low-impact exercise at the 15-week follow-up visit. Seventeen reported walking, while three reported joining a formal low-impact exercise class. The mean number of minutes of exercise per week reported at follow-up (FU) was 81 minutes. High exercisers reported an average of 124 minutes (SD = 65.0) weekly; middle exercisers, 71 minutes (SD = 67.3); and low exercisers, 51 minutes (SD = 66.8). There were no significant changes in fatigue scores from end of treatment to follow-up.

There was a significant decrease in mean sedimentation rates from ET (M = 30.0) to FU (M = 16.2). There were also a continued increase in right grip strength and continued decreases in total joint count. Aerobic fitness levels did not change from ET to FU. However, aerobic fitness both at ET and FU varied significantly depending on the self-selected amount of exercise. The mean aerobic fitness levels at FU were 29.3 for low-, 31.9 for medium-, and 32.3 high-exercise groups.

DISCUSSION

Although fatigue was reported by all subjects at baseline, the ratings of fatigue severity were lower than anticipated. One possible explanation is that subjects who volunteer for exercise studies may be more active and less fatigued than those not volunteering. However, it also is possible that following an initial adjustment period after diagnosis of RA, these persons readjust their expectations of their energy level to a lower norm. If the latter is true, persons with RA who report higher levels of fatigue may not have adjusted to their reduced energy level or may have more severe disease symptoms. There are no controlled studies available to shed light on either of these possibilities.

Those subjects who were low exercisers showed increased fatigue from BL to ET; however, the more frequent exercisers showed a significant decrease in fatigue. This suggests that the positive effects of exercise on fatigue are dose-related. However, any increase in aerobic exercise can have positive effects and persons with RA need to be encouraged to exercise to their individual tolerance. As found in this study, persons with RA may experience increased fatigue as they increase the minutes of aerobic exercise performed; but if they continue to exercise over a period of weeks, that exercise-induced fatigue will decrease.

In contrast to the findings about fatigue, in which changes across time periods varied by level of exercise participation, disease activity remained stable and aerobic fitness improved for exercise groups from BL to MT and ET. These results are consistent with earlier findings of increased aerobic fitness after an exercise intervention for persons with RA (Ekblom, Lovgren, Alderin, Fridstrom, & Satterstrom, 1975; Ekdahl, Anderson, Moritz, & Svensson, 1990; Harkcom et al., 1985; Karper & Evans, 1986; Lyngberg, Danneskiold-Samsoe, & Halskov, 1988; Minor et al., 1989). Although impact of arthritis scores improved over measurement times, the improvement was not significant. However, such a global, one-item measure may not be sensitive to the small or moderate improvements in functioning experienced by subjects during and at the end of the intervention.

There was no significant change in aerobic fitness levels from ET to FU. The mean number of minutes of exercise per week dropped from ET to FU, so it is not surprising that mean aerobic fitness levels did not increase. However, aerobic fitness did not decrease significantly from ET to FU, indicating that subjects did not lose all that they had gained from the exercise classes. The decreased pain found after the exercise intervention is similar to findings of other researchers who have studied exercise for persons with RA (Harkcom et al., 1985; Minor et al., 1989; Nordemar, Ekblom, Zachrisson, & Lundqvist, 1981; Perlman et al., 1990; Stenstrom, 1994). The finding of no increase in mean sedimentation rate as a function of exercise is also consistent with the findings of other investigators (Ekdahl et al., 1990; Lyngberg, Harreby, Bentzen, Frost, & Danneskiold-Samsoe, 1994), as is the decrease in the time needed to walk 50 feet following the intervention (Minor et al., 1989; Perlman et al., 1990). This finding indicates that increased fitness can improve a daily function such as walking.

In this study, exercise decreased fatigue for those respondents who chose to exercise to a moderate or high degree. All subjects showed improvement in aerobic fitness levels and improvement, or at least no worsening, on a number of measures of disease activity. This is particularly important clinically, because it indicates that the exercise intervention did not worsen arthritis disease activity. Hesitancy to engage in or recommend exercise is often due to fear that such activity will worsen the RA. Our findings provide strong evidence to alleviate such fears.

Nurses in clinical practice should encourage persons with RA to consult their health care provider about participating in appropriate regular exercise. Exercises such as walking, aquatic, or aerobic exercise programs sponsored by local Arthritis Foundation chapters are appropriate for most persons with RA. Participation in exercise may assist these persons to control symptoms such as fatigue and pain and improve their endurance for carrying out daily activities.

ACKNOWLEDGMENTS

This study was supported by the Center for Biobehavioral Studies of Fatigue Management under a grant from the National Institute of Nursing Research NIH (P20 NR03270), Lauren S. Aaronson, RN, PhD, principal investigator/center director. Additional support was obtained from Delta Chapter, Sigma Theta Tau and the Research Office of the University of Kansas School of Nursing. The authors acknowledge the assistance of Nancy Potter, RN, BSN, MA, and Barbara Adkins, RN, MS, as research assistants. For help with recruitment of subjects, the authors thank rheumatologists Drs. Daniel Stechschulte and Kathryn Welch and nurse clinicians Nadine Colbert, Tracey Castleman, and Glenda Virtue. This chapter is adapted from Neuberger, G. B., Press, A. N., Linsley, H. B., Hinton, R., Cagle, P. E., Carlson, K., Scott, S., Dahl, J., & Kramer, B. (1997). Effects of exercise on fatigue, aerobic fitness, and disease activity measures in persons with rheumatoid arthritis. *Research in Nursing and Health, 20,* 195–204. Copyright 1997 by John Wiley & Sons, Inc. Printed with permission.

REFERENCES

American College of Sports Medicine. (1991). *Guidelines for exercise testing and prescription.* Philadelphia: Lea & Febiger.

Anderson, R. J. (1993). Rheumatoid arthritis: Clinical features and laboratory. In H. E. Schumacher (Ed.), *Primer on rheumatic diseases* (pp. 90–95). Atlanta: Arthritis Foundation.

Belza, B., Henke, C. J., Yelin, E. H., Epstein, W. V., & Gilliss, C. L. (1993). Correlates of fatigue in older adults with rheumatoid arthritis. *Nursing Research, 42*, 93–99.

Bradley, L. A. (1989). Adherence with treatment regimens among adult rheumatoid arthritis patients: Current status and future directions. *Arthritis Care and Research, 2*, S33–S39.

Corbett, J. V. (1992). *Laboratory tests and diagnostic procedures with nursing diagnoses.* Norwalk, CT: Appleton & Lange.

Crosby, L. A. (1991). Factors which contribute to fatigue associated with rheumatoid arthritis. *Journal of Advanced Nursing, 16*, 974–981.

Ekblom, B., Lovgren, O., Alderin, M., Fridstrom, M., & Satterstrom, G. (1975). Effect of short-term physical training on patients with rheumatoid arthritis I. *Scandinavian Journal of Rheumatology, 4*, 80–86.

Ekdahl, C., Andersson, S. I., Moritz, U., & Svensson, B. (1990). Dynamic versus static training in patients with rheumatoid arthritis. *Scandinavian Journal of Rheumatology, 19*, 17–26.

Harkcom, T., Lampman, R., Banwell, R., & Castor, C. (1985). Therapeutic value of graded aerobic exercise training in rheumatoid arthritis. *Arthritis and Rheumatism, 28*, 32–39.

Hess, E. V. (1988). Rheumatoid arthritis: Treatment. In H. R. Schumacher (Ed.), *Primer on the rheumatic diseases* (pp. 93–96). Atlanta: Arthritis Foundation.

Karper, W. B., & Evans, B. W. (1986). Cycling programme effects on one rheumatoid arthritic. *American Journal of Physical Medicine, 65*, 167–172.

Kellum, M. D. (1985). Fatigue. In M. M. Jacobs & W. Geels (Eds.), *Signs and symptoms in nursing* (pp. 103–118). Philadelphia: Lippincott.

Lyngberg, K., Danneskiold-Samsoe, B., & Halskov, O. (1988). The effect of physical training on patients with rheumatoid arthritis: Changes in disease activity, muscle strength and aerobic capacity. A clinically controlled minimized crossover study. *Clinical Experimental Rheumatology, 6*, 253–260.

Lyngberg, K. K., Harreby, M., Bentzen, H., Frost, B., & Danneskiold-Samsoe, B. (1994). Elderly rheumatoid arthritis patients on steroid treatment tolerate physical training without an increase in disease activity. *Archives of Physical Medicine and Rehabilitation, 75*, 1189–1195.

McNair, D., Lorr, M., & Droppleman, L. F. (1992). *EdITS manual for the profile of mood states (POMS).* San Diego, CA: Educational and Industrial Testing Services.

Meenan, R. F., Gertman, P. M., Mason, J. H., & Dunaif, R. (1982). The Arthritis Impact Measurement Scales: Further investigation of a health status measure. *Arthritis and Rheumatism, 25*, 1048–1053.

Minor, M., Hewett, J. E., Webel, R. R., Anderson, S. K., & Kay, D. R. (1989). Efficacy of physical conditioning exercises in patients with rheumatoid arthritis and osteoarthritis. *Arthritis and Rheumatism, 32*, 1396–1405.

Neuberger, G., Kasal, S., Smith, K., Hassanein, R., & DeViney, S. (1994). Determinants of exercise and aerobic fitness in outpatients with arthritis. *Nursing Research, 43*, 11–17.

Nordemar, R., Ekblom, B., Zachrisson, L., & Lundqvist, K. (1981). Physical training in rheumatoid arthritis: A controlled long-term study, I. *Scandinavian Journal of Rheumatology, 10*, 17–23.

Pedhazur, E. J. (1982). *Multiple regression in behavioral research.* Chicago: Holt, Rinehart & Winston.

Perlman, S. G., Connell, K. J., Clark, A., Robinson, M. S., Conlon, P., Gecht, M., Caldron, P., & Sinacore, J. M. (1990). Dance-based aerobic exercise for rheumatoid arthritis. *Arthritis Care and Research, 3*, 29–35.

Schumacher, H. E. (Ed.) (1993). *Primer on the rheumatic diseases.* Atlanta: Arthritis Foundation.

Siconolfi, S. F., Cullinane, E. M., Carleton, R. A., & Thompson, P. D. (1982). Assessing VO_{2max} in epidemiologic studies: Modification of the Astrand-Rhyming test. *Medicine and Science in Sports and Exercise, 14*, 335–338.

Stenstrom, C. H. (1994). Home exercise in rheumatoid arthritis functional class II: Goal setting versus pain attention. *Journal of Rheumatology, 21*, 627–634.

Tack, B. B. (1990). Fatigue in rheumatoid arthritis: Conditions, strategies and consequences. *Arthritis Care and Research, 3*, 65–70.

Tack, B. B. (1991). *Dimensions and correlates of fatigue in older adults with rheumatoid arthritis.* Unpublished doctoral dissertation, University of California, San Francisco.

Waggoner, C., & Le Lieuvre, R. (1981). A method to increase compliance to exercise regimen in rheumatoid arthritis patients. *Journal of Behavioral Medicine, 4*, 191–201.

[20]

Helping Patients with Localized Prostate Cancer: Managing after Treatment

Merle H. Mishel, Barbara B. Germino, Michael Belyea, Lorna Harris, Janet Stewart, Donald E. Bailey, Jr., James Mohler, and Cary Robertson

Psychoeducational interventions have been studied for over 15 years, and a number of these have been found effective in improving quality of life for cancer patients (Andersen, 1992). However, they have focused primarily on breast cancer patients and, secondarily, on lung and melanoma cancer patients (Fawzy, Fawzy, Arndt, & Pasnau, 1995). Even though lung and melanoma cancer populations include men, less attention has been given to men with cancer and far less to men with prostate cancer. Yet prostate cancer is the second most common form of malignant disease in men in the United States, and the incidence is increasing, particularly among African-American men (Catalona, Smith, Ratliff, & Basler, 1993).

Since the advent of prostate cancer screening that includes PSA testing, more men have been diagnosed with localized prostate cancer and treated by radical prostatectomy or external beam radiation therapy. For men with localized prostate cancer (which is usually stages 2,a,b,c, and 3a), the most common treatment is radical prostatectomy, which leaves the men with urine leakage and compromised erectile function (Scher, 1999). These side effects of treatment have great influence on quality of life. Erectile dysfunction and incontinence generate uncertainties about masculine roles and create changes in relationships that the patient may not know how to manage. For men who receive radiation as their treatment for localized prostate cancer, fatigue, urinary frequency, erectile dysfunction, and bowel problems are side effects that peak several weeks into treatment (Shipley et al., 1999). Furthermore, the uncertainty about treatment benefit and the possibility of recurrence of the cancer are common concerns.

Because of the side effects from surgery and radiation, along with the potential for disease reoccurrence, interventions to help men manage treatment side effects, handle the uncertainty of the cancer diagnosis and treatment, and improve their quality of life are needed. The purpose of this study, therefore, was to test the effectiveness of an uncertainty management intervention delivered by a nurse via telephone using two different structures for delivery—directly to the patient (treatment direct, TD), or directly to the patient with supplementation through a family care provider (treatment supplemented, TS)—to reduce uncertainty, manage uncertainty, manage treatment-related side effects, increase self-care behaviors, and improving quality of life among Caucasian and African-American men receiving treatment for localized prostate cancer.

METHODS

The design for the study was a 3×2 randomized block, repeated measures design with three levels of the intervention factor: (1) the uncertainty management intervention (UMI) delivered directly (TD), (2) UMI delivered directly plus supplementation (TS), and (3) the control condition, crossed with two levels on the ethnicity factor (Caucasian and African American).

Subjects

Both Caucasian and African-American men with localized prostate cancer (stages 2,a, b, c, and 3a) who had had their catheter removed following prostatectomy or were in their third week of radiation treatment, had a family member living with them willing to participate in the study, had access to a telephone, and planned to remain in their current locale for 12 months were eligible to participate in the study. The sample included men and their family members from each ethnic group, who were blocked on race, then randomly assigned to intervention and control groups, resulting in a total of six groups, three Caucasian and three African-American. The final sample included 134 Caucasian and 105 African-American subjects, with 85 subjects in the treatment direct group, 66 in the treatment supplemented group, and 88 in the control group. The groups were approximately the same age (63 to 65 on average) and had similar levels of education (13 to 14 years). The majority of the subjects (70% to 90% of each group) were married. The numbers of African-American and Caucasian subjects in the treatment direct and control groups were similar, but there were fewer African-American subjects than Caucasian subjects in the treatment supplemented group because study entrance criteria required that the family member live with the subject. Many African-American men did not meet that criterion, and we were able to enroll only 20 subjects in the African-American treatment supplemented cell.

Approximately 69% of the subjects had stage 2 prostate cancer, which is cancer confined to the prostate, followed by approximately 30% in early stage 3, which is cancer in the capsule. The majority of the subjects (80%) had received surgery, primarily prostatectomy. Only a small percentage had received a nerve-sparing prostatectomy. Twenty percent had received external beam radiation.

Measures

Outcomes measured included uncertainty, uncertainty management, symptom management, self-care behaviors, and quality of life. Uncertainty was measured by a shortened version of the Uncertainty in Illness Scale (UIS). The UIS (Mishel & Braden, 1987) was modified to a shortened version of 26 items in order to reduce respondent burden. Items were deleted when they were judged by the investigators and a clinical specialist as not highly relevant for prostate cancer patients. The reliability of the shorter version was an alpha of .86 for the total sample, an alpha of .88 for Caucasian men, and an alpha of .82 for African-American men. Validity of the shortened version was supported by the relationship between this version of the uncertainty scale and emotional distress in African-American men (Mishel et al., 1999).

Uncertainty management was conceptualized to occur through four components: problem solving, cognitive reframing, cancer knowledge, and patient-provider communication. Problem solving and cognitive reframing were measured by two subscales on the Self-Control Scale (Rosenbaum, 1983). Problem solving was defined as the ability to identify and define concerns and generate solutions. The internal consistency of the 11-item problem-solving subscale with this sample was an alpha of .90; alphas were

.90 for Caucasian men and .86 for African-American men. Cognitive reframing was defined as the ability to view concerns as manageable. The 10-item cognitive reframing scale had an alpha of .90 with this sample and identical alphas of .89 for Caucasian and African-American men. Validity of both subscales was supported by their correlation with uncertainty in the predicted direction (Braden, Mishel, & Longman, 1998). Patient-provider communication, a third component of uncertainty management, was measured by five investigator-developed items that asked about communication between the patient and health care providers during a typical visit. Two items looked at how much information was given to the patient by either the nurse or the doctor, two items tapped into how much information the patient gave to either the nurse or the doctor, and one item asked how much the patient helped with planning treatment. The reliability of the total scale was an alpha of .71 for the sample. Each item was addressed individually in the analysis. An investigator-developed prostate cancer knowledge scale, the fourth measure of uncertainty management, had an alpha of .67 for the total sample.

Symptom management was measured by one dimension from the Southwest Oncology Group Quality of Life Questionnaire (SWOG-QOL) (Moinpour, Hayden, Thompson, Feigl, & Metch, 1990). This dimension is comprised of the Symptom Distress Scale plus 15 items specific to prostate cancer added by SWOG investigators. The symptom component of the SWOG-QOL has been refined in four clinical trials with cancer patients (Moinpour et al., 1990). Reliability of the symptom portion of the SWOG-QOL in this sample was an alpha of .70.

Self-care was measured by the Self-Care Inventory—Wellness Promotion Scale (Pardine, Napoli, & Dytell, 1983). This 14-item scale with a Likert response format measures nutrition, relaxation, activity, and safety areas of self-care. Reliability of the scale was a coefficient alpha of .79 for the total scale (.75 for Caucasian men and .82 for African-American men).

Quality of life was measured by six subscales on the Psychosocial Adjustment to Illness Scale (PAIS) (Morrow, Chiarello, & Derogatis, 1978). Each subscale taps into a different area of quality of life: The Vocational Environment subscale refers to participation in work or home activities, the Domestic Environment subscale deals with current relationship with family, the Sexual Relationship subscale explores current interest and participation in sexual activity, the Extended Family Environment subscale covers contact with family residing outside of the home, the Social Environment subscale refers to participation in the social activities that one was involved in prior to illness, and the Emotional State subscale indexes current emotional status including anger, depression, and guilt. The PAIS is a semi-structured interview to assess the quality of a patient's adjustment to current medical illness or its residual effects. The reliability of the total PAIS with this sample was an alpha of .90; subscale alphas ranged from .65 to .83. The Sexual Relationship subscale had the lowest alpha coefficient, and findings from that scale are open to question. Validity of the subscales has been reported for Caucasian subjects (Mishel, Hostetter, King, & Graham, 1984) and is supported for African-American men by a significant relationship between uncertainty and the psychological distress factor of the PAIS (Mishel et al., 1999).

Procedure

Men were recruited from major medical centers and private oncology practices in central and eastern North Carolina. Recruiters approached all men who met the study criteria, explained the study, and left brochures with those who conveyed interest. These men were then sent a recruitment video, followed with a call from the study office to determine willingness to participate. Of those who entered the study, we had an attrition rate of 6% for Caucasian subjects and 11% for African-American subjects. These are low attrition rates for a longitudinal study over 7 months.

At entry into the study, time 1 (T1), or baseline, data were collected from the men and from their family member; time 2 (T2) data collection for subject and family member occurred 4 months from baseline, with time 3 (T3) three months later. All subjects and family members were in the study for 7 months. A data collector matched to the subject by race collected all data in the subject's home.

The intervention was given to subjects in the treatment groups for 8 weeks following time 1 data collection. For these subjects, there were 2 months between completion of the intervention and time 2 data collection.

Intervention

The purpose of the intervention was to teach the patient or family member how to manage uncertainty from diagnosis and treatment. The intervention was telephone delivered through eight weekly phone calls by a nurse matched to the subject, or subject and family member, by race and gender. Intervention components were tailored to the subject's concerns using a computer-generated protocol.

The intervention was derived from Mishel's theory of uncertainty in illness (Mishel, 1988) and delivered through a semi-structured interview in which the nurse assessed the subject's problems or concerns, categorized each problem according to type of uncertainty, and evaluated the degree of distress or threat attributed to the problem by the subject using established criteria. Interventions based on this assessment included reinforcing the subject's plan of action to handle the problem, providing information on the problem or on managing the problem, problem solving possible solutions to the problem with the subject, providing access to resources, teaching problem management methods, and promoting patient advocacy by teaching assertive behaviors. Many of the interventions involved providing information or explanations, depending on the nature of the uncertainty. Often the subject was informed about resources that he could activate, or the nurse would structure expectations by laying out, to the degree possible, the trajectory of the problem or concern. The trajectory was personalized by finding markers or timelines that were meaningful for the individual. A number of strategies were provided to help the person manage the problem, such as Kegel exercises to gain urine control, potency enhancement methods for impotence, and information on other approaches to express intimacy. Problem solving with the subject was used to generate options, look at alternatives, and consider resources. Also, the subject was taught how to monitor himself concerning a symptom or side effect so that he could find a pattern to the problem. The subject's ability to manage his uncertainties was strengthened by teaching him how to use resources, problem solve, and be an advocate in his own treatment. These interventions were applied to concerns about diagnosis, treatment, response to treatment, living with cancer, caring for self, and lifestyle issues. The range of interventions was contained in the protocol, but the application of interventions was targeted to the specific concerns and needs of each patient at each phone call.

The intervention protocol was delivered similarly to both the subject and the family member in the treatment-supplemented cell. In delivery of the intervention to the family member, the focus was on the prostate cancer patient's concerns and how the family member could assist in modifying these concerns.

Data Analysis

A repeated measures MANOVA was conducted for each outcome variable looking at treatment group, ethnic group, and the interactive effects of treatment and ethnic group. To look at patterns of change over time, planned contrasts between T1 and T2 and T2 and T3 were tested for all major outcome variables. Contrasts for these time differences were also tested within ethnic groups to see if differences existed for only one ethnic group. Subject randomization was checked by comparing the treatment and control groups on baseline data. The only significant difference was preexisting health problems. Therefore, this variable was included in all analyses as a covariate.

RESULTS

Uncertainty

There were no significant effects from the intervention in reducing uncertainty. Uncertainty levels significantly decreased over time for subjects in all groups as they became more familiar with their illness and treatment.

Uncertainty Management

Of the four uncertainty management methods, a significant treatment effect was found for cognitive reframing, which refers to the ability to reframe events as manageable, and for problem solving, which refers to generating alternative approaches to manage problems.

For cognitive reframing, there was a significant difference between subjects in the treatment direct group, the treatment supplemented group, and the control group in the change from baseline (T1) to 4 months postbaseline (T2), $F(4,456) = 3.81$, $p < .01$ (see Figure 20.1). The effect

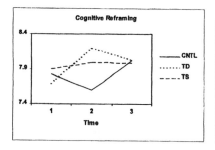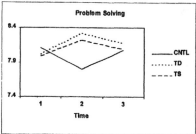

FIGURE 20.1   Changes in managing uncertainty by treatment groups (cognitive reframing and problem solving).

did not hold over time, however, and subjects were at the same level of cognitive reframing by T3, 7 months from baseline.

Similarly, for problem solving, from baseline to T2, subjects who received the intervention either directly or with supplementation improved more than the control subjects in their ability to problem solve, $F(4,456) = 2.40$, $p < .05$. However, there was no difference between the groups by T3.

Symptom Management

Lack of control over urine flow was the major side effect from prostate cancer surgery. Using the items from the Symptom Distress Scale referring to control over urine flow, subjects in both the treatment direct and treatment supplemented groups showed significantly better control over urine flow than did control subjects from baseline to T2, 4 months postbaseline, $F(2,212) = 3.71$, $p < .03$ (see Figure 20.2). From T2 to T3 (7 months after baseline), subjects in the treatment supplemented group, in which both the subject and the family member received the intervention, continued to improve in control over urine flow, whereas those in the treatment direct and control groups leveled off. However, these differences were not significant.

Using items from the Symptom Distress Scale, the change in number of symptoms was calculated over time. All groups decreased in the number of symptoms over time; however, among Caucasian men, the decrease in the treatment supplemented group from baseline (T1) to 4 months postbaseline (T2) was significantly greater than for the Caucasian control

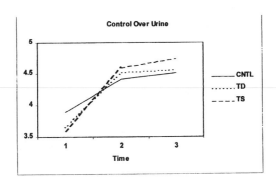

FIGURE 20.2   Changes in control over urine flow by treatment groups.

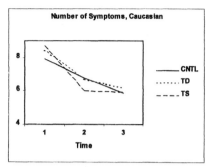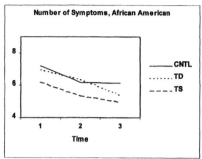

FIGURE 20.3   Changes in the number of symptoms by ethnicity and treatment groups.

group, $F(2,228) = 3.07$, $p < .05$ (see Figure 20.3). From T2 to T3, all of the Caucasian groups leveled out. However, among African-American men, those in the treatment direct group had a greater decrease in number of symptoms from T2 to T3 than the African-American control group, $F(1,229) = 3.96$, $p < .05$.

Self-Care

Subjects in all groups declined in their ability to implement self-care behaviors for managing treatment side effects from T1 to T2; however, Caucasian subjects in the treatment direct group showed less decline from baseline to 4 months postbaseline than did those in the treatment supplemented and control groups, $F(1,229) = 4.95$, $p < .03$ (see Figure 20.4). From T2 to T3, those in the control group stayed about level, whereas Caucasians in the treatment supplemented group improved in self-care abilities, with a gain that distinguished them from the treatment direct group, $F(1,229) = 4.72$, $p < .03$.

Quality of Life

Two areas of psychosocial adjustment were significantly affected by the intervention. From baseline to 4 months postbaseline, Caucasian men who received the intervention, both those in the treatment direct group and those in the treatment supplemented group, showed significant improve-

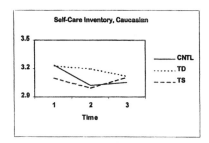
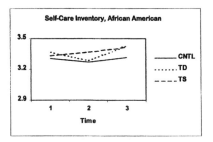

FIGURE 20.4   Changes in self care by ethnicity and treatment groups.

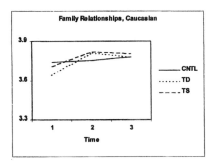
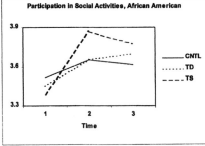

FIGURE 20.5   Changes in quality of life by ethnicity and treatment groups.

ments in their family relationships, $F(2,229) = 4.80$, $p < .03$ (see Figure 20.5). They maintained this improvement over time but did not improve further from T2 to T3. For African-American men, those in the treatment supplemented group improved more in their social relationships from baseline to 4 months postbaseline than did the control group, $F(1,229) = 4.54$, $p < .03$.

CONCLUSIONS

The Uncertainty Management Intervention provided a personal and supportive structure for men to explore their issues and concerns about prostate cancer. With this supportive interaction between nurse and patient, patients were able to reevaluate the cancer experience and cognitively restructure their expectations. Patients also improved in problem-solving skills when they were shown how to use their experience and knowledge to identify resources and management strategies.

As noted by Lepore and Helgeson (1998), sharing perceptions with knowledgeable and supportive others facilitates integration of the cancer experience into the patient's life. In this study, validating the thoughts and feelings of men with prostate cancer, reinforcing the appropriateness of their concerns for the circumstances, and providing them with information and management strategies helped them reframe the cancer experience into something that was manageable.

The strategies used in the intervention did not differ greatly from those currently used in practice. However, instead of being applied indiscriminately, they were used only when they specifically addressed a subject's concern. This individualized tailored approach delivered through the convenient medium of the telephone appeared to lessen social constraints about talking about sensitive topics and promoted open communication about concerns.

With a mean length of phone time of 23 minutes, subjects were able to learn cognitive skills that were applicable beyond their immediate concerns. The management strategies taught to subjects appear to have been applied to manage urine flow and reduce the number of treatment side effects. Similarly, these strategies seemed to stave off the decline in self-care strategies that tends to follow prostate cancer treatment. Once treatment side effects could be managed, then other areas of social functioning could improve, as shown in the areas of family and social relationships.

It is important to note that the primary benefits from this intervention came in the first 4 months after treatment. As time extended, learning occurred in all patients and the control subjects improved over time. Yet it is in the first 4 months when side effects are most adverse and the impact of the cancer experience is greatest. Thus, this is the period when it is most important to intervene. Nurses have more contact with patients during the early period after treatment, and it is important for them to recognize that this is the time when the intervention will be most effective for men with localized prostate cancer.

ACKNOWLEDGMENTS

This work was supported in part by grant # R01 NR03782 from the National Institute of Nursing Research at the National Institutes of Health.

REFERENCES

Andersen, B. L. (1992). Psychological interventions for cancer patients to enhance the quality of life. *Journal of Consulting and Clinical Psychology, 60,* 552–568.

Braden, C. J., Mishel, M. H., & Longman, A. J. (1998). Self-help intervention project: Women receiving breast cancer treatment. *Cancer Practice, 6,* 87–98.

Catalona, W. J., Smith, D. S., Ratliff, T. L., & Basler, J. W. (1993). Detection of organ-confined prostate cancer is increased through prostate-specific antigen-based screening. *Journal of the American Medical Association, 270,* 948–954.

Fawzy, F. I., Fawzy, N. W., Arndt, L. A., & Pasnau, R. O. (1995). Critical review of psychosocial interventions in cancer care. *Archives of General Psychiatry, 52,* 100–113.

Lepore, S. J., & Helgeson, V. S. (1998). Social constraints, intrusive thoughts, and mental health after prostate cancer. *Journal of Social and Clinical Psychology, 17,* 89–106.

Mishel, M. H. (1988). Uncertainty in illness. *Image: Journal of Nursing Scholarship, 20,* 225–231.

Mishel, M. H., Belyea, M., Hamilton-Spruill, J., Germino, B., Bohlig, M., Braden, C. J., & Harris, L. (1999). *Predictors of emotional distress in African-American cancer patients.* Manuscript in review.

Mishel, M. H., & Braden, C. J. (1987). Uncertainty: A mediator between support and adjustment. *Western Journal of Nursing Research, 9*(1), 43–57.

Mishel, M. H., Hostetter, T., King, B., & Graham, V. (1984). Predictors of psychosocial adjustment in patients newly diagnosed with gynecological cancer. *Cancer Nursing, 7,* 291–299.

Moinpour, C. M., Hayden, K. A., Thompson, I. M., Feigl, P., & Metch, B. (1990). Quality of life assessment in Southwest Oncology Group trials. *Oncology, 4,* 79–89, 227–230.

Morrow, Y., Chiarello, R., & Derogatis, L. (1978). A new scale for assessing patients' psychosocial adjustment to medical illness. *Medicine, 8,* 605–610.

Pardine, P., Napoli, A., & Dytell, R. (1983, August). *Health-behavior change mediating the stress-illness relationship.* Paper presented at the 91st annual convention of the American Psychological Association, Anaheim, CA.

Rosenbaum, M. (1983). Learned resourcefulness as a behavioral repertoire for the self-regulation of internal events: Issues and speculations. In M. Rosenbaum, C. M. Franks, & Y. Jaffe (Eds.), *Perspectives on behavior therapy in the eighties* (pp. 54–73). New York: Springer.

Scher, H. I. (1999). Management of prostate cancer after prostatectomy: Treating the patient, not the PSA. *Journal of the American Medical Association, 281,* 1642–1645.

Shipley, W. U., Thames, H. D., Sandler, H. M., Hanks, G. E., Zietman, A. L., Perez, C. A., Kuban, D. A., Hancock, S. L., & Smith, C. D. (1999). Radiation therapy for clinically localized prostate cancer. *Journal of the American Medical Association, 281,* 1598–1604.

[21]

Management of Problematic Behavioral Symptoms Associated with Dementia: A Cognitive Developmental Approach

Mary Ann Matteson, Adrianne D. Linton,
Brenda L. Cleary, Susan J. Barnes, and
Michael J. Lichtenstein

Dementia associated with Alzheimer's disease and related disorders (ADRD) involves both memory impairment and one or more of the following cognitive disturbances: aphasia, apraxia, agnosia, and disturbance in executive functioning. These cognitive deficits cause significant impairments in social and occupational functioning and lead to significant declines from previous levels of functioning (American Psychiatric Association, 1994).

Behaviors such as wandering, screaming, verbal abuse, pacing, and resisting care are common and troublesome symptoms of ADRD. Behavioral interventions have been used to decrease agitated and wandering behaviors and catastrophic reactions (Beck, Heacock, Mercer, & Walton, 1991; Hall, 1994; Hellner & Norberg, 1994; Jorm, 1994; Maas, 1988; Rapp, Flint, Herrmann, & Proulx, 1992; Ryden & Feldt, 1992; Steward, 1995; Syme, 1995), but, unfortunately, these interventions have yielded inconsistent results.

The inadequate management of problematic behavioral symptoms of dementia has resulted in the high use of psychotropic medications in spite of 1987 Omnibus Reconciliation Act (OBRA) regulations; indeed, 20% to 50% of nursing home residents are taking these medications (Ray et al., 1993). Psychotropic medications may alleviate behavioral symptoms associated with ADRD; however, the drugs have frequent and dangerous side effects, including movement disorders, tardive dyskinesia, anticholinergic toxicity, postural hypotension, and excessive sedation, and thus they increase the risk of falls and hip fractures in aged individuals. Furthermore, because the drugs interfere with neurotransmitter function, they may actually increase the cognitive impairment associated with dementia, decrease function, and produce more problem behaviors (Pollock & Mulsant, 1995; Ray, 1992; Schneider, Pollock, & Lyness, 1990; Thapa, Gideon, Fought, & Ray, 1995). Clearly, a different approach is needed to alleviate these behaviors.

Reisberg (1984) has identified several stages of decline in ADRD:

1. Normal forgetfulness—no impairment but subjective concern about memory loss
2. Early and late confusion (borderline to mild Alzheimer's disease)—decreased ability to perform in demanding employment and social interactions, deficit in memory and ability to concentrate
3. Early dementia (moderate Alzheimer's disease)—unable to recall phone number; little assistance required with eating or toileting; difficulty choosing proper clothing; coaxing required for bathing
4. Middle dementia (moderately severe Alzheimer's disease)—unable to recall own name; disturbed diurnal rhythm; generally unaware of surroundings; personal hygiene dysfunction; urinary and fecal incontinence; agitation and wandering; obsessive symptoms
5. Late dementia—speech and motor dysfunction; inability to walk; inability to eat.

The similarities between the common regressive pattern of behaviors associated with ADRD (Almkvist, Basun, Wahlund, & Lannfelt, 1995; Crockett, Tuokko, Koch, & Parks, 1989; Hughes, Berg, & Danzinger, 1982; O'Carroll et al., 1995; Reisberg, Ferris, & Franssen, 1985) and Jean Piaget's (1952) progressive stages of cognitive development hold promise for developing a consistent approach to these behaviors. According to Piaget, human beings progress through four stages of cognitive development: (1) sensorimotor (0 to 24 months), (2) preoperational (24 months to 7 years), (3) concrete operations (7 to 12 years), and (4) formal operations (12 years onward). The progression occurs in a systematic manner; however, the rate of progression varies among individuals. Several studies of both cognition and behavior in ADRD have noted the similarities between Piaget stages and Reisberg's stages of ADRD (Emery, 1985; Emery & Breslau, 1987; Jacobs et al., 1995; Matteson, Linton, & Barnes, 1996; Matteson, Linton, Barnes, Cleary, & Lichtenstein, 1996; Mitrushina, Uchiyama, & Satz, 1995; Thornbury, 1993). The study reported here tested the efficacy of behavioral and environmental interventions based on Piaget's cognitive developmental stages, for persons at all stages of ADRD in nursing home and special care units. Psychotropic drugs for behavioral management were withdrawn as interventions were implemented. It was expected that the behavioral and environmental interventions would decrease problem behaviors that seem to occur because of ADRD patients' misunderstanding, misinterpretation or fear of behavioral and/or environmental cues, or caregivers' inappropriate expectations of patients.

METHOD

Design

The study used a quasi-experimental design to determine the efficacy of cognitive developmental care to reduce problematic behavioral symptoms, with concurrent withdrawal of psychotropic drugs.

Setting and Sample

Two nursing home facilities with dementia special care units (SCUs) were used for the study; both had dementia patients on regular units and in SCUs. A Veterans' Affairs Medical Center in southern Texas was used for the treatment group, and a privately owned, Medicaid-supported nursing home in the same area served as the control.

A total of 93 residents who were in all stages of dementia, taking psychotropic medications according to chart records, and demonstrating at least one problem behavior were randomly selected to participate in the study. Patients' records were reviewed by a research assistant to determine eligibility for the study, and information on demographics, medications, and medical diagnoses was obtained. The diagnosis of dementia was based on demonstrated decline in memory and other cognitive functions in comparison with the person's previous level of function (McKhann et al.,1984). Two nondemented subjects (Folstein Mini-Mental State Exam [MMSE] scores >24) who were not taking psychotropic medications or demonstrating behavior problems also were included in the sample to examine the relationships among higher Piaget levels and MMSE scores over time. Consent was obtained from subjects if they were able and from family members or guardians if subjects were deemed incompetent to give consent. The initial sample consisted of 63 subjects in the treatment group and 30 in the control group. There were 64 males and 29 females, with a mean age of 77. Twenty-nine of the subjects resided in special care units (20 in the treatment group, and 9 in the control group). Baseline testing was carried out to determine ADRD stages and Piaget levels as well as behavior problems and psychotropic drug use.

The staff members in the VA nursing home were more highly trained, and the control group residents were more impaired in activities of daily living, but these differences were not significant. No differences in mean age, ADRD stages based on mental status scores, Piaget levels, medical diagnoses, number and types of medications, percent of persons taking psychotropic medications, or number of problem behaviors were found at baseline between the two groups. However, the VA group included significantly more Caucasians, $t(193) = 5.06$, $p < .0005$, and men, $t(158) = 10.82$, $p <. 0005$, than the private nursing home group.

Instruments

The Folstein Mini-Mental State Exam (MMSE)

The MMSE was used to establish ADRD levels at baseline and following the intervention. The MMSE is a screening instrument with established psychometric properties, including adequate evidence of reliability and validity, which separates patients with cognitive disturbances from those without such disturbances. The instrument assesses orientation, registration, attention and calculation, recall, and language. There is a total possible score of 30; a score of less than 24 indicates some degree of cognitive impairment (Folstein, Folstein, & McHugh, 1975).

The Linton-Piaget Test

The Linton-Piaget Test was developed for this study to determine Piaget levels in older subjects with dementia. The instrument uses a set of 14 simple tasks representing each cognitive level, and completion of certain tasks is used to classify subjects as follows: (1) formal operations—correctly performs one or two tests of formal operations, (2) concrete operations—correctly performs at least three (50%) concrete tasks but no formal tasks, (3) preoperational—correctly performs at least one (34%) preoperational task but no concrete or formal tasks, (4) sensorimotor substages 2–6—correctly performs at least one sensorimotor task but no higher level tasks, and (5) sensorimotor substage 1—does not perform any task or respond as expected. The instrument was tested for validity and reliability, and found to be acceptable for use with this population (Matteson, Linton, Barnes, et al., 1996).

The Nursing Home Behavior Problem Scale (NHBPS)

The NHBPS is a 29-item scale developed to measure behaviors that are disruptive or stressful enough in a nursing home to warrant the use of antipsychotic medications or physical restraints. The instrument is designed to be completed quickly and easily by nurses and nursing assistants with minimal education and training. There are six subscales: (1) Uncooperative or Aggressive Behavior, (2) Irrational or Restless Behavior, (3) Sleep Problems, (4) Annoying Behavior, (5) Inappropriate Behavior, and (6) Dangerous Behavior. The rater is asked to report the frequency of each behavior in the past 3 days using a 5-point scale (0 = never to 4 = always). The instrument has shown high convergent validity in a nursing home population, with Pearson correlations of .75 with the widely used NOSIE and .91 with the Cohen-Mansfield Agitation Index (CMAI). Interrater correlations were .83 and .75 (Ray, Taylor, Lichtenstein, & Meador, 1992).

Behavioral and Cognitive Status of Sample

The most frequent individual behavior problems noted on the NHBPS were (1) talks/mumbles to self, (2) resists care, (3) upsets easily, (4) fidgets, and (5) awakens during night. The NHBPS behavior problem subscales on which high scores most commonly were observed were Irrational or Restless Behavior, Sleep Problems, and Uncooperative or Aggressive Behavior. The most frequently taken psychotropic medications were hydroxyzine (34%), haloperidol (21%), tricyclic antidepressants (8%), thioridazine (5%), and lorazepam (4%).

The ranges of MMSE scores viewed as ADRD stages and Piaget levels were as follows: Normal Forgetfulness (formal operations) = 24–30; Early and Late Confusion (concrete operations) = 22–23; Moderate Alzheimer's Disease (preoperational) = 7–20; Moderately Severe Alzheimer's Disease

(Sensorimotor I—substages 3/4/5/6) = 2–6; and Late Dementia (Sensori-motor II—substages 1/2) = 0–1.

Behavioral and Environmental Interventions

Specific behavioral interventions were prescribed for all subjects based on their Piaget levels. Care plans included interventions for carrying out activities of daily living and for alleviating specific behavioral symptoms (see Table 21.1). For example, if a subject at the preoperational level resisted dressing, strategies were implemented that would be appropriate for an individual at that cognitive developmental level. A person with preoperational abilities was expected to be able to dress with most independence and least resistance when clothes were laid out in order of use and verbal coaching was employed.

Modifications in the environment were also made based on Piagetian concepts. For example, from the late sensorimotor stage on up, individuals are able to recognize many symbols, including letters, short words, pictures, and signs. Thus, for subjects in these stages, symbols were used to provide cues to various locations and activities. In addition, music was used as a behavioral and environmental intervention to provide comfort and stimulate memories and give cues to locations and activities.

Psychotropic Drug Withdrawal Protocol

Drug withdrawal was carried out by the physician's assistant and medical director of the nursing home, with oversight by the physician coinvestigator. Drug withdrawal followed close assessment of behavior. The dose was initially decreased by 50%. Drugs prescribed to treat side effects of antipsychotics also were stopped. When the subject remained stable for 7 days, the dose was again decreased by 50%. The process was repeated until the calculated decreased dose was less than the minimum standard dose. If a drug had to be initiated or reinstituted because of behavioral problems, subjects were evaluated to identify possible contraindications and establish baseline behaviors. A drug was selected, and subjects were started on a very low dose and observed for positive and negative effects. If there was no significant improvement, a standard protocol permitted the physician's assistant in consultation with the physician to gradually increase the dose in specified steps until a maximum dose was reached. Subjects were assessed daily while the dose was being adjusted.

TABLE 21.1   Examples of Care Plans Based on Piaget Levels

Activities	Piaget Levels/ADRD Stages		
	Preoperational Moderate ADRD	*Sensorimotor I* *(3/4/5/6)* Moderately Severe ADRD	*Sensorimotor II* *(1/2)* Late ADRD
Eating/ nutrition	Assist with cutting foods. Give verbal encouragement.	Use finger foods for meals and snacks. Demonstrate hand-to-mouth motion.	Feed patient. Talk to patient in a warm, accepting voice. Avoid rushing patient.
Dressing	Lay clothes out in order. Provide verbal coaching.	Have patient imitate caregiver with step-by-step demonstration.	Dress patient.
Sleep/rest	Follow previous sleep patterns and routines. Check for pain, hunger, or other physical discomfort.	Maintain bedtime routine. Provide music or read when patient has difficulty falling asleep or awakens during night.	Give cues for sleeping (music, dim lights). Provide comfort measures (rocking, stuffed animal).
Bathing	Explain shower care in simple terms; break tasks into steps. Use verbal prompting as needed. Assist patient as needed.	Give cues to bath time; gather bath supplies, etc. Use simple, one-step commands. Give patient comfort item to hold. Use distraction and redirection in the form of singing or having patient "help" hold something. Use handheld showerhead if patient is afraid of overhead shower.	Approach patient slowly and calmly. Match verbal and visual cues. Use sponge bath rather than shower or tub if patient is fearful. Give patient comfort item to hold.

Intervention Procedure

In the treatment group, individualized care plans based on Piaget levels were used for behavioral interventions while concurrently subjects were systematically withdrawn from psychotropic medications. Care plans were laminated and color coded according to Piaget levels to address problem behaviors related to functions such as bathing, dressing, sleeping, and eating, and were readily available for quick reference. Colored "dots" corresponding to the color codes for Piaget levels were placed on patients' arm bands, name plates on the doors to their rooms, and Kardex cards to alert the staff to their cognitive developmental level. Before the interventions began, all staff associated with the treatment group, including all nursing and medical staff, allied health, housekeeping, and dietary personnel, were required to participate in an educational program for environmental and behavior management. The care plans were updated as necessary when changes were noted in the yearly Piaget tests. In the control group, subjects received usual care.

Data Collection

Subjects were tested three times at yearly intervals (year 1—baseline; year 2 and year 3) for Piaget levels of cognitive development and for cognitive impairment using the Folstein Mini-Mental State Exam (MMSE). Piaget testing was conducted by one research assistant and the MMSE by a second. Neither communicated findings to the other.

Observations of disruptive behaviors and records of psychotropic drug use were obtained at baseline and 3, 12, and 18 months posttreatment. Treatment began immediately after baseline data collection. The initial posttest data were collected 3 months after the treatment began to allow time for withdrawal of the psychotropic medications and for the behavioral interventions to take effect. The primary research assistant collected data on problem behaviors from the nursing staff who were primary caregivers of the subjects. The raters noted whether the staff had observed a problem behavior on their shifts during the past 3 days. The rating sheets were then filled out once a week for 4 weeks at each data collection period. Data on psychotropic drug use for the previous month, including date, time, circumstances, and frequency of use, were obtained from subjects' charts.

RESULTS

A total of 57 subjects (43 in the treatment group and 14 in the control group) completed the study. Seventeen resided in the special care units, with 12 in the treatment group and 5 in the control group. Forty-six were male and 11 were female, with a mean age of 76. There were 53 Caucasians, 2 non-Hispanic Caucasians, and 2 African Americans. The number of these subjects at each Piaget level at baseline was formal operations, $n = 1$; concrete operations, $n = 22$; preoperational, $n = 13$; sensorimotor II, $n = 7$; and sensorimotor I, $n = 14$. At baseline, subjects' mean Folstein MMSE score was 12.5 ($SD = 11.4$). Mean scores on the MMSE decreased slightly over the 2 years (year 2 = 11.3, and year 3 = 9.4), and MMSE scores were significantly correlated with Piaget levels at baseline (year 1) ($r = .84$, $p < .0005$), year 2 ($r = .85$, $p < .0005$), and year 3 ($r = .80$, $p < .0005$). MMSE scores of the two subjects who did not demonstrate behavioral symptoms and were not taking psychotropic medications decreased slightly, and one went down one Piaget level (formal to concrete operations), whereas the other stayed in the concrete operations level. Neither developed behavioral symptoms or began taking psychotropic medications during the course of the study.

Behavior Problems

Among the 55 subjects with problem behaviors, the treatment group's overall NHBPS scores did not change significantly between baseline and 3 months; however, there were significant decreases at 12 months, $t(12) = -2.39$, $p = .034$, and 18 months, $t(11) = -2.65$, $p = .023$. The control group's overall NHBPS scores decreased significantly at 3 months, $t(12) = -2.38$, $p = .037$, and 12 months, $t(11) = 2.26$, $p = .023$, but scores at 18 months increased to pretest levels (see Table 21.2). Repeated measures ANOVA comparisons of overall scores showed a significant difference between groups over time, $F(1,51) = 5.8$, $p = .02$.

TABLE 21.2 Mean NHBPS Scores and Psychotropic Drug Use in Mean Equivalent Doses in Milligrams

	Treatment Group ($n = 43$)				Control Group ($n = 14$)			
	Baseline	3m	12m	18m	Baseline	3m	12m	18m
NHBPS scores	2.9	2.5	2.1	2.1	4.3	2.9	2.3	4.0
Neuroleptics	5.2	3.0	2.4	0.9	4.6	4.5	5.3	4.4
Anxiolytics	44.0	15.0	6.0	9.7	70.0	29.0	70.0	79.0
Antidepressants	7.5	8.6	3.5	1.3	10.5	10.2	13.7	2.5

Psychotropic Medications

The types of psychotropic drugs administered fell into three categories: (1) anxiolytic, (2) neuroleptic, and (3) antidepressant medications. Dose equivalents were computed using a standard comparison drug for each category. The largest amounts given were anxiolytic agents, followed by antidepressants and neuroleptics. Paired t-tests comparing pretest amounts taken in each category with amounts at 3, 12, and 18 months showed significant decreases over 18 months in the experimental group in anxiolytics (pretest to 3 months: $t(42) = -3.16$, $p = .003$; pretest to 12 months: $t(42) = -4.1$, $p < .0005$; pretest to 18 months: $t(42) = -.3.56$, $p = .001$) and neuroleptic medications (pretest to 18 months: $t(42) = -2.7$, $p = .01$), but no difference in antidepressants. In the control group, there were no significant changes in any of the categories at any point (refer to Table 21.2).

Repeated measures analysis of variance of amounts of medication by category revealed no significant differences between the groups for neuroleptics and antidepressants; however, there were significant differences over time in the amounts of anxiolytic medications. The treatment group had a significantly greater decrease than the control group, $F(3,165) = 3.02$, $p = .031$, in the amount of anxiolytic medications given over time.

DISCUSSION

The results of this study suggest that using behavioral and environmental interventions based on Piaget levels of cognitive development may be effective in managing problem behaviors and decreasing the use of psychotropic medications in institutionalized ADRD patients. The sequence of losses in ADRD has been described by others (Reisberg, 1984; Reisberg et al., 1985; Thornbury, 1993; Turkington, 1985); however, we have taken this a step further by applying that information in a practical way to develop an acceptable, useful program of care for participants.

At baseline, behavior problems occurred most frequently in the Irrational/Restless Behavior subscale, followed by Uncooperative/Aggressive and Inappropriate Behaviors. Overall scores decreased in the treatment group; however, 3-month posttest scores did not decrease significantly. Indeed, we observed that some behavior problems increased during the first 3 months, most probably because of the weaning from psychotropic medications. As staff comfort levels with the program increased and behavioral interventions based on the protocol continued, behavior problems began to decrease significantly. It is not clear why in the control group overall scores decreased on the NHBPS at 3 and 12 months but increased at 18 months.

In the treatment group, we were most successful in decreasing behaviors in the Irrational/Restless and Inappropriate Behavior categories, which include behaviors related to wandering, pacing, restlessness, and agitation. In a previous study (Matteson & Linton, 1996; Matteson, Linton, & Byers, 1992), we found a positive correlation between the amount of wandering and pacing and the use of psychotropic medications: restlessness and agitation were as frequent in persons receiving psychotropic medications as in those who were not. These data and the findings of the present study suggest that reducing psychotropic medications may be effective in reducing these behaviors.

There were few untoward reactions when psychotropic medications were decreased. During the first 3 months of the intervention, four subjects showed increases in aggressive behavior. Daily progress notes were kept on each of these subjects for 2 months. One resumed his medications, and the others settled down with no need for medication. Some subjects were more active and agitated in the evening; others improved in self-care and were more alert.

Progress notes were kept on 20 subjects in the treatment group who were not completely removed from medications. Some of these subjects were changed from one category or type of psychotropic medication to another; others decreased the dosages of the medications they were taking. The behavior problems most often demonstrated by these subjects were found in the NHBPS Uncooperative/Aggressive Behavior subscale (i.e., uncooperative, aggressive, and refuses or resists care).

An impact of the project on staff for the treatment group was observed in terms of their approach to care and their attitudes toward residents. When behavioral interventions rather than psychotropic medications were used for behavior problems, the staff began to look at problem behaviors from the perspective of patients' cognitive developmental levels and intervened in creative, appropriate ways. In addition, in spite of misgivings about a "childlike" approach to care of dementia patients, caregivers did not patronize or infantalize subjects. Rather, they treated subjects with dignity and understanding of the consequences of the disease process. This appeared to be due to the formal education required of all study staff, which emphasized an adult approach using methods that would be most comfortable for patients at various cognitive levels.

ACKNOWLEDGMENTS

This chapter is adapted from Matteson, M. A., Linton, A. D., Cleary, B. L., Barnes, S. J., & Lichtenstein, M. J. (1997). Management of problematic behavioral symptoms associated with dementia: A cognitive developmental approach. *Aging: Clinical and Experimental Research, 9*(5), 342–355. Copyright 1997 by Editrice Kurtis S.r.l. Printed with permission. The research reported in this chapter was funded by a grant from the National Institute of Nursing Research and the National Institute on Aging (R01 NR02998).

REFERENCES

Almkvist, O., Basun, H., Wahlund, L., & Lannfelt, L. (1995). Cognitive functions of family members with and without the $APP_{670/671}$ mutation. In K. Iqbal, J. Mortimer, B. Winblad, & H. Wisniewski (Eds.), *Research advances in Alzheimer's disease and related disorders* (pp. 251–259). New York: Wiley.

American Psychiatric Association. (1994). *Diagnostic and statistical manual of mental disorders* (4th ed.). Washington, DC: Author.

Beck, C., Heacock, P., Mercer, S., & Walton, C. (1991). Decreasing demented older adults' need for assistance with dressing: Third National Conference on Research for Clinical Practice. In *Key aspects of elder care: Managing falls, incontinence and cognitive impairment* (pp. 309–319). Chapel Hill, NC: University of North Carolina.

Crockett, D., Tuokko, H., Koch, W., & Parks, R. (1989). The assessment of everyday functioning using the Present Functioning Questionnaire and the Functional Rating Scale in elderly samples. *Clinical Gerontology, 3*–25.

Emery, O. B. (1985). Language and aging. *Experimental Aging and Research, 11*, 3–60.

Emery, O. B., & Breslau, L. (1987). The acceleration process in Alzheimer's disease: Thought dissolution in Alzheimer's disease early onset and senile dementia Alzheimer's type. *American Journal of Alzheimer's Care and Related Disorders and Research, 9/10*, 24–30.

Folstein, M., Folstein, S., & McHugh, P. (1975). "Mini-mental state": A practical method for grading the cognitive state of patients for the clinician. *Journal of Psychiatric Research, 12*, 189.

Hall, G. R. (1994). Chronic dementia: Challenges in feeding a patient. *Journal of Gerontological Nursing, 20*, 21–30.

Hellner, B. M., & Norberg, A. (1994). Intuition: Two caregivers' descriptions of how they provide severely demented patients with loving care. *International Journal of Aging and Human Development, 38*, 327–338.

Hughes, C. P., Berg, L., & Danzinger, W. L. (1982). A new clinical scale for the staging of dementia. *British Journal of Psychiatry, 140*, 566–572.

Jacobs, D. M., Sano, M., Dooneief, G., Marder, K., Bell, K. L., & Stern, Y. (1995). Neuropsychological detection and characterization of preclinical Alzheimer's disease. *Neurology, 45*, 956–962.

Jorm, A. F. (1994). Disability in dementia: Assessment, prevention, and rehabilitation. *Disability and Rehabilitation, 16*, 98–109.

Maas, M. (1988). Management of patients with Alzheimer's disease in long-term care facilities. *Nursing Clinics in North America, 23*, 57–64.

Matteson, M. A., & Linton, A. D. (1996). Wandering behaviors in institutionalized persons with dementia. *Journal of Gerontological Nursing, 22,* 39–46.

Matteson, M. A., Linton, A. D., & Barnes, S. J. (1996). The cognitive developmental approach to dementia. *Image: Journal of Nursing Scholarship, 28,* 233–240.

Matteson, M. A., Linton, A. D., Barnes, S., Cleary, B. L., & Lichtenstein, M. J. (1996). The relationship between Piaget and cognitive levels in persons with Alzheimer's disease and related disorders. *Aging: Clinical and Experimental Research, 8,* 61–69.

Matteson, M. A., Linton, A. D., & Byers, V. (1992). Wandering behavior in institutionalized Alzheimer's patients. *The Gerontologist, 32,* 202.

McKhann, G., Drachman, D., Folstein, M., Katzman, T., Price, D., & Stallan, E. M. (1984). Clinical diagnosis of Alzheimer's disease: Report of the NINCDS-ADRDA work group under the auspices of the Department of Health and Human Services task force on Alzheimer's disease. *Neurology, 34,* 939–944.

Mitrushina, M., Uchiyama, C., & Satz, P. (1995). Heterogeneity of cognitive profiles in normal aging: Implications for early manifestations of Alzheimer's disease. *Journal of Clinical and Experimental Neuropsychology, 17,* 374–382.

O'Carroll, R. E., Prentice, N., Murray, C., vanBeck, M., Ebmeier, K. P., & Goodwin, G. M. (1995). Further evidence that reading ability is not preserved in Alzheimer's disease. *British Journal of Psychiatry, 167,* 659–662.

Piaget, J. (1952). *The origins of intelligence in children* (M. Cook, trans.). New York: International Universities Press.

Pollock, B. G., & Mulsant, B. H. (1995). Antipsychotics in older patients: A safety perspective. *Drugs and Aging, 6,* 312–323.

Rapp, M. S., Flint, A. J., Herrmann, N., & Proulx, G. B. (1992). Behavioural disturbances in the demented elderly: Phenomenology, pharmacotherapy and behavioural management. *Canadian Journal of Psychiatry, 37,* 651–657.

Ray, W. A. (1992). Psychotropic drugs and injuries among the elderly: A review. *Journal of Clinical Psychopharmacology, 12,* 386–396.

Ray, W., Taylor, J. A., Lichtenstein, M. J., & Meador, K. G. (1992). The nursing home behavior problem scale. *The Journals of Gerontology: Medical Sciences, 47,* M9–16.

Ray, W. A., Taylor, J. A., Meador, K. G., Lichtenstein, M. J., Griffin, M. R., Gought, R., Adams, M. L., & Blazer, D. G. (1993). Reducing antipsychotic drug use in nursing homes: A controlled trial of provider education. *Archives of Internal Medicine, 153,* 713–721.

Reisberg, B. (1984). Stages of cognitive decline. *American Journal of Nursing, 84,* 225–228.

Reisberg, B., Ferris, S. H., & Franssen, E. (1985). An ordinal functional assessment tool for Alzheimer's-type dementia. *Hospital and Community Psychiatry, 36,* 593–595.

Ryden, M. B., & Feldt, K. S. (1992). Goal-directed care: Caring for aggressive nursing home residents with dementia. *Journal of Gerontological Nursing, 18,* 35–42.

Schneider, L. S., Pollock, V. E., & Lyness, S. A. (1990). A metaanalysis of controlled trials of neuroleptic treatment in dementia. *Journal of the American Geriatric Society, 38,* 553–563.

Steward, J. T. (1995). Management of behavior problems in the demented patient. *American Family Physician, 52,* 2311–2317, 2321–2322.

Syme, S. (1995). Independence through finger food. *Contemporary Nurse, 4,* 80–81.

Thapa, P. B., Gideon, P., Fought, R. L., & Ray, W. A. (1995). Psychotropic drugs and the risk of recurrent falls. *American Journal of Epidemiology, 142,* 202–211.

Thornbury, J. M. (1993). The use of Piaget's theory in Alzheimer's disease. *American Journal of Alzheimer's Care and Related Disorders and Research, 7/8,* 16–21.

Turkington, C. (1985). Alzheimer's losses reverse child's gains. *American Psychological Association Monitor, 11,* 17.

[22]

Patient Knowledge and Self-Efficacy for Diabetes Management: Impact of Home Care Nurse Interventions

Cynthia Fryhling Corbett

Diabetes mellitus (DM) is the third most common ICD-9 category of home health care (HHC) admissions (National Association for Home Care, 1996). However, although it is a common diagnosis among HHC clients, DM is rarely the primary reason for HHC services (Milone-Nuzzo, 1993). Clients with DM, especially those over 60 years of age, frequently have a myriad of other acute and chronic health problems. Because DM affects nearly every body system and self-care of DM requires a multitude of daily activities, DM management and/or educational interventions are frequently performed by HHC nurses regardless of the primary reason for home care. The goal of the nurse "is to increase patients' and caregivers' knowledge of diabetes and help develop the technical skills necessary to manage their diabetes, resulting in positive physical and mental health outcomes" (Caffrey, 1996, p. 759).

Improving patients' abilities to self-manage diabetes requires both patient education and development of confidence in self-management. The process begins with teaching basic DM knowledge and skills. Unfortunately, many patients with diabetes, including the majority of older patients with

261

type 2 diabetes, have never attended DM education classes (Coonrod, Betschart, & Harris, 1994; Hendricks & Hendricks, 1998). Therefore, patients with diabetes who are admitted for HHC services may have limited knowledge of DM and DM management even if they have had diabetes for months or years.

Bolstering patients' confidence in their ability to successfully manage the illness is the next crucial step (Ellison & Rayman, 1998; Paterson, Thorne, & Dewis, 1998). Patients' perceptions of their competence to perform certain behaviors is termed self-efficacy (Bandura, 1986). Patients with diabetes who show more self-efficacy have been found to use better care practices and to have better outcomes (Crabtree, 1986; Glasgow et al., 1992; Hockmeyer, 1990; Hurley, 1988; Kavanagh, Godey, & Wilson, 1993; Kingery & Glasgow, 1989; Ludlow & Gein, 1995; Padgett, 1991; Skelly, Marshall, Haughey, Davis, & Dunford, 1995). Thus, nursing actions to enhance patients' confidence should lead to improved outcomes.

Self-efficacy varies across persons, situations, and time and is amenable to change. There are four primary methods of enhancing self-efficacy or perceived confidence: enactive attainment, vicarious experience, verbal persuasion, and physiological state (Bandura, 1977, 1986). All methods are routinely used by home health care nurses. Enactive attainment is actual performance of the behavior, which leads to mastery; this mastery is most effective in increasing self-efficacy (Bandura, 1977). Enactive attainment occurs, for example, when patients practice until they demonstrate mastery of the skills of glucose monitoring, insulin preparation, and dose adjustment.

Vicarious experience, or observing others perform, is another method of developing self-efficacy. When patients see that someone else can perform a certain behavior, they assume that perhaps they too can accomplish that behavior. Home care nurses use this technique when they show the patient how to perform a skill. Verbal persuasion is incorporated into care when nurses coax and provide reinforcement for new behaviors such as meal planning, insulin preparation, and daily exercise.

A final method of increasing self-efficacy is learning to interpret physiological state or internal feedback from the body. For example, patients who are able to recognize low blood glucose based on physiologic signs and symptoms before hypoglycemia becomes critical are likely to have greater confidence that they can prevent reactions than patients who recognize low blood glucose only when it is severe. This method of boosting confidence is used when nurses instruct patients to monitor blood glucose whenever they suspect symptoms of hypoglycemia or hyperglycemia.

The study reported here assessed diabetes knowledge and self-efficacy in patients before and after knowledge and efficacy-enhancing home-based nursing interventions. Additionally, the type and frequency of nursing interventions delivered to patients with high baseline knowledge and self-efficacy were compared to the nursing interventions provided to patients with low baseline knowledge and self-efficacy.

METHODS

Sample and Setting

A pre-post design was used for the study. Insulin-requiring adult home care patients with diabetes were interviewed regarding DM knowledge and self-efficacy prior to their first nursing visit (T1) and after HHC nursing services (T2). The T2 interview occurred after the patient was discharged from HHC or after the patient had received 60 days of HHC nursing service, whichever came first. All interviews were conducted by the primary investigator.

The study intervention was routine diabetes-related education and efficacy-enhancing activities provided by nurses. No special training was provided to the nurses for the research. Nurses were notified that their patients were involved with the study, but nurses were not aware of the specific knowledge and self-efficacy questions that were asked of patients. Chart reviews were done at least 1 month after the T2 interview to allow time for all documentation to be filed in the medical record. Records were analyzed to determine the type and number of diabetes knowledge and efficacy-enhancing interventions provided to patients.

Study participants (N = 115) received HHC nursing services from a hospital-based HHC agency and a free-standing visiting nurse agency in the northwestern United States. Both HHC agencies served approximately the same geographic region, and both were Medicare certified. Each agency made roughly 85,000 skilled nursing visits during the 2 years of data collection. The educational levels of the nurses were diploma (10%), associate degree (17%), baccalaureate degree (58%), and master's degree (15%). Patients included in the study were primarily responsible for their own DM management, able to speak and read English, and recipients of at least two nursing visits. The average number of visits per patient was 11 (range: 2 to 62). Patients had had a diagnosis of diabetes for an average of 16 years (range: 2 months to 62 years) and had been insulin-dependent for an average of 8.7 years. Most (70%) had cardiac problems. In addition, participants had a wide range of other health problems. Most (76%) were on Medicare or Medicaid. Their mean age was 65 (SD = 13.8). Most were

Caucasian (64%) and female (69%). About a third lived alone, while the remaining mostly lived with a spouse or other family members.

Measures

Diabetes knowledge was measured using the Diabetes Knowledge Test (DKN) (Dunn et al., 1984). The DKN has 15 multiple choice items that cover the spectrum of basic diabetes knowledge needed by insulin-requiring persons with diabetes (diet, exercise, insulin, signs and symptoms of reaction). Each test item is followed by four possible answers, and the tool is scored from 0 to 15, with each correct response worth 1 point. Thus, higher scores indicate more knowledge. Adequate content validity and reliability have been established for this tool (see Dunn et al., 1984), and acceptable reliability was also achieved in this study (Kuder Richardson-20 reliability of .76 for both T1 and T2).

Self-efficacy was measured using the Insulin Management Diabetes Self-Efficacy Scale (IMDSES), which assesses patients' "beliefs in their capability to plan, carry out, monitor, and adjust their diabetes activities of daily living" (Hurley, 1990, p. 3). The IMDSES has 28 items that reflect the full range of DM self-care activities. Each item is worded so that patients rate perceived confidence in their ability to perform a specific DM routine. Items are measured on a Likert scale ranging from 1 (strongly disagree) to 6 (strongly agree). A "not applicable" response is also an option. Scores are computed as a percentage based on the number of items each patient believes apply to himself or herself. Potential scores range from 0 (all responses "not applicable") to 100% (all responses "strongly agree"). Content and construct validity, as well as reliability, have been established and are reported elsewhere (Hockmeyer, 1990; Hurley, 1988, 1990). Internal consistency reliability for the IMDSES in this study was also acceptable (Cronbach's alpha of .77 for T1 and .78 for T2).

Nursing Interventions

The Nursing Intervention Classification (McCloskey & Bulechek, 1996) was used to categorize the type and frequency of knowledge and efficacy-enhancing interventions delivered by nurses. The Nursing Intervention Classification is a taxonomy that identifies 433 nursing interventions, their definitions, and the activities usually performed with each intervention. The taxonomy is a reliable and valid method of organizing nursing interventions (McCloskey & Bulechek, 1996). Nursing interventions are defined as "any treatment, based upon clinical judgment and knowledge, that a nurse performs to enhance patient/client outcomes" (McCloskey & Bulechek, 1996, p. xvii). Nursing activities are defined as "the specific behaviors or actions that nurses do to implement an intervention and which assist patients/clients to move toward a desired outcome. Nursing activities are at the concrete level of action. A series of activities is necessary to implement an intervention" (McCloskey & Bulechek, 1996, p. xvii).

All nursing activities associated with diabetes management were recorded based on the medical record of each participant. Activities were then matched with nursing interventions in the taxonomy. This procedure resulted in a list of nursing interventions and activities received by patients as well as information about the proportion of clients who received each activity. For example, many patients received knowledge and efficacy-enhancing information for hypo/hyperglycemia management. Specifically, 43% of patients were instructed on recognition of signs and symptoms of hypo/hyperglycemia, 39% were instructed to keep a log of blood glucose and insulin administration, 31% were taught self-care for hypo- and hyperglycemia, 19% were informed of when the physician should be notified, 17% were instructed about appropriate blood glucose levels, 17% were told about factors that affect blood glucose, and 12% were given other specific information to help them prevent hypo- and hyperglycemic episodes. Qualitative chart review data were used to determine if interventions to enhance DM knowledge and self-efficacy were provided to patients, and if changes in knowledge and self-efficacy reflected the frequency of activities and interventions that patients received.

RESULTS

Diabetes Knowledge

Overall, DM knowledge improved significantly after HHC, $F(1,114) = 6.04$, $p < .05$. The participants were able to answer one more question correctly at T2 (after HHC; $M = 11.0$) than at T1 (before HHC admission, $M = 10.0$). It was hypothesized that patients who had high DM knowledge at T1 might not improve much at T2 (ceiling effect). To test this hypothesis, the sample was divided into three approximately equal-size groups based on T1 knowledge: low (DKN score ≤ 8), moderate (DKN score ≥ 9 or ≤ 11), high (DKN score ≥ 12). Those who had the least baseline understanding had the greatest improvement at T2 (see Figure 22.1). Clinically, this is the desired outcome: improved knowledge in those with lower levels and maintenance of information in those demonstrating adequate knowledge. The group with the highest initial scores improved significantly on only 8 of the 15 questions, whereas the low and moderate groups improved on all of the 15 questions ($p < .05$). Unfortunately, the participants in the lower groups still had serious knowledge deficits even after HHC. The low and moderate groups were significantly different from the high knowledge group in all analyses related to degree of knowledge and type and frequency of interventions. Therefore, these two groups (low and moderate) were combined into one low group ($n = 71$) for ease of comparison with the high group.

More educational interventions to improve understanding of diabetes principles were performed for the 71 participants in the lower group than for those in the higher knowledge group (see Table 22.1). However, even after these interventions, more than 40% of the lower knowledge participants still could not identify that (1) poor control can result in a greater chance of complications, (2) rice is a carbohydrate, (3) the presence of ketones in the urine is bad, (4) all persons with diabetes should use diet as a form of glycemic control, (5) a hypoglycemic reaction may be caused

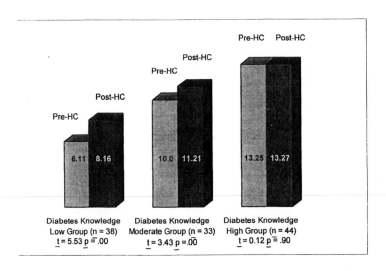

FIGURE 22.1 Improvement in diabetes knowledge in patients with low, moderate, and high knowledge before home care.

TABLE 22.1 Educational Interventions Provided to High Knowledge and Low Knowledge Groups

Specific Documented Educational Interventions Related to Diabetes Knowledge Test Questions	% High Knowledge Group Who Received Intervention	% Low Knowledge Group Who Received Intervention
Effect of exercise on blood glucose*	2.3	9.1
Prevention of hypo/hyperglycemia	0.0	7.0
Treatment of hypo/hyperglycemia	29.5	36.6
Interpret blood glucose results	11.4	19.7
Appropriate blood glucose range*	9.1	22.5
Factors other than diet that affect blood glucose*	2.3	18.3
Ketone testing*	4.5	1.4
Possible adverse effects of medications	36.4	31.0
Use of sliding scale insulin	15.9	15.5
Sick day care*	6.8	14.1
Allowed versus restricted	6.2	67.6
Reinforce dietary compliance	43.2	50.7
Possible drug/food interactions	31.8	35.2
Recognize signs and symptoms of hypo/ hyperglycemia	25.0	49.2
Referral to dietitian	2.3	1.4
Possible diabetes-related complications*	31.8	35.2
Measures to prevent or minimize diabetes-related complications	9.1	15.5

*Statistically significant difference between frequency of intervention provided to high knowledge group versus low knowledge group ($p < .05$).

by too much insulin, and (6) weight control is one reason exercise is important. The latter two questions were also incorrectly answered by 34% of the high knowledge group after HHC. There were no significant differences in the average number of nurse visits provided to patients with low, moderate, or high knowledge. Each group received approximately 11 visits (10.6 low knowledge group, 11.5 moderate, and 10.8 high group).

Diabetes Self-Efficacy

Self-efficacy for diabetes management improved significantly after home care (T1 $M = 77.6$, T2 $M = 81.1$; $F(1,114) = 5.15$, $p = .01$). Again, it was expected that a ceiling effect might occur. To test this hypothesis, patients were divided into three groups based on their self-efficacy before the home care intervention. Those with low and moderate confidence showed significant improvements ($p < .05$ for both), whereas the group with the highest self-efficacy improved only slightly. The average numbers of nurse visits for each group were as follows: 11.3 for the high self-efficacy group, 10.0 for the moderate self-efficacy group, and 12.4 for the low self-efficacy group. The differences in number of visits were not significant. Thus, for ease of comparison with the group that had high self-efficacy, the low and moderate self-efficacy groups were combined into one low group ($n = 78$). The same pattern of differences between groups was observed when pre– and post–home care diabetes self-efficacy was analyzed by individual items on the questionnaire. Patients with lower self-efficacy scores prior to home care improved their self-efficacy on 5 of the 28 items, whereas patients in the high group ($n = 37$) improved on only 2 of the 28 items. Confidence in dietary management improved in both groups, and the group with low self-efficacy also gained confidence in recognizing low blood sugar and felt more competent in diabetes management in general.

Efficacy-enhancing Interventions

As with DM knowledge, patients with lower preintervention confidence received more efficacy-enhancing interventions than patients with high pre–home care confidence. The intervention was routine home care nursing services, so the findings suggest that nurses assess the need for and provide more interventions to patients who have the poorest knowledge and the least confidence. Table 22.2 displays the percent of patients who received each documented efficacy-enhancing intervention in the high baseline efficacy group and in the low group. Demonstration and feedback focusing on use of the glucose meter, insulin preparation and administration, and self-care on sick days were documented significantly more often for patients with low confidence than for patients with high confidence. In contrast, prevention of hypo- and hyperglycemia and insulin self-adjustment were documented significantly more frequently for patients with high baseline self-efficacy than for patients with low feelings of competence at baseline. Thus, basic skills were emphasized for patients with low self-efficacy whereas advanced management activities were taught to those who had more confidence prior to home care.

Post–home care self-efficacy ratings specific to complex diabetes management (e.g., adjusting insulin, preventing hypoglycemia) reflected the percentage of patients who received teaching in these areas. Patients in the

TABLE 22.2 Documented Efficacy-Enhancing Nursing Interventions for High Self-Efficacy and Low Self-Efficacy Groups

Specific Documented Educational Interventions Related to Insulin Management Diabetes Self-Efficacy Scale	% High Self-efficacy Group Who Received Intervention	% Low Self-Efficacy Group Who Received Intervention
Recognize signs and symptoms of hypo/hyperglycemia	35.1	46.2
Keep log of blood glucose and insulin	35.1	41.0
Treatment of hypo/hyperglycemia	27.0	33.3
Interpretation of blood glucose levels	18.9	15.4
Appropriate blood glucose range	21.6	15.4
Factors other than diet that affect blood glucose	10.8	12.8
Prevention of hypo/hyperglycemia*	8.1	2.6
Check urine sugar/ketones	2.7	2.6
Actions of each medication	51.4	59.0
Possible side effects of each medication	35.1	32.1
Use of sliding scale insulin*	24.3	11.5
Foot care	32.4	25.6
Sick day care*	5.4	14.1
Allowed vs. restricted foods	59.5	71.8
Reinforce dietary compliance	51.4	60.3
Possible drug/food interactions	32.4	39.7
Demonstrate use of glucose meter*	8.1	17.9
Step-by-step instruction about use of glucose meter	24.3	39.7
Give feedback re return demo of glucose meter use*	27.0	42.3
Demonstrate insulin administration	0.0	2.7
Step-by-step instruction about administering insulin*	10.8	29.5
Give feedback re return demo of insulin administration	32.4	33.3
Demonstrate insulin preparation	21.6	19.2
Step-by-step instruction about insulin preparation*	10.8	25.6
Effects of exercise on blood glucose	2.7	6.4

*Statistically significant difference between frequency of intervention provided to high knowledge group versus low knowledge group ($p < .05$).

low group ($n = 78$) reported lack of confidence (< 4 on the self-efficacy scale) for the following diabetes care behaviors: exercising despite not feeling like exercising, adjusting insulin based on blood glucose, determining insulin dosage changes based on altered daily routines, preventing low blood glucose when exercising, and adjusting DM self-care when ill. In contrast, all patients in the high self-efficacy group ($n = 37$) were moderately confident (scores of 5 or greater) in their ability to implement all but two diabetes care behaviors. They were slightly confident (score of between 4 and 5) about exercising despite not feeling like exercising and determining insulin dose when changes occurred in daily routines.

DISCUSSION

The major purpose of this research was to determine whether knowledge of DM and self-efficacy for DM management improved after knowledge and efficacy-enhancing home care nursing interventions. Patients with diabetes did increase their understanding of diabetes management after HHC. However, after home care nearly one third of the participants continued to have poor knowledge of almost every facet of diabetes and DM management. Prior research suggests that adequate baseline knowledge is necessary to engage in active DM self-management (deWeerdt, Visser, Kok, & Van der Veen, 1990; Ellison & Rayman, 1998; Paterson et al., 1998) and improve glucose control (Lockington, Farrant, Meadows, Dowlatshahi, & Wise, 1988; Peyrot & Rubin, 1994). Therefore, a primary implication for HHC nurses is to conduct a detailed baseline assessment of diabetes-related knowledge and tailor subsequent nursing interventions to patient needs. For example, despite the fact that dietary topics were some of the most frequently documented educational interventions, over 40% of patients in the lower knowledge group did not know after HHC that rice was a carbohydrate/starch. A patient who cannot accurately identify foods that fit into each food group will not understand much dietary teaching or be able to implement suggestions for improved dietary management. Thus, in addition to providing education, nurses must evaluate patients' understanding of and ability to implement suggested modifications.

Overall, patient confidence about diabetes care increased significantly after home health services. The finding of higher self-efficacy after the interventions is similar to results in other settings. Rubin, Peyrot, and Saudek (1989), for example, found that patients' confidence in diabetes care improved significantly immediately following and 6 months after an intensive 5-day outpatient diabetes education and behavioral management program. Glasgow and colleagues (1992), who targeted interventions to enhance diet and exercise, found that patient confidence increased 3 months after baseline, although the gain was not statistically significant, largely because over half of the patients in their study rated self-efficacy in the 90th percentile at baseline, leaving little room for improvement. Glasgow and colleagues' results are similar to the pattern found in this study: Patients who had high initial confidence improved only slightly after home care.

It is not known what level of self-efficacy is associated with the best diabetes management. However, greater confidence has been consistently linked with better diabetes self-care (Crabtree, 1986; Glasgow et al., 1992; Hockmeyer, 1990; Hurley, 1988; Kavanagh et al., 1993; Kingery & Glasgow, 1989; Ludlow & Gein, 1995; Padgett, 1991; Skelly et al., 1995). In addition, Rubin and associates (1989) and Ludlow and Gein (1995) reported that lower glycosylated hemoglobin was correlated with higher self-efficacy.

In this study, patients with lower diabetes self-efficacy scores at baseline received more interventions to enhance confidence, although they did not receive more visits than other patients. They also received more interventions to develop basic DM management skills. Patients with greater confidence received more instruction on two advanced self-care activities— prevention of hypo and hyperglycemia and adjustment of insulin—than did patients with less self-efficacy. Clearly, patients with less perceived ability also need instruction and efficacy-enhancing interventions in these complex areas of self-management. The fact that patients with lower self-efficacy received less instruction on advanced self-care, but the same number of visits as those with higher baseline self-efficacy suggests that patients with lower self-efficacy require more visits and many more interventions. If patients remain homebound, continue to improve self-care capabilities, and are willing to further expand their management skills, home services should be provided until patients are competent to independently perform even the most complex management behaviors.

Active self-care is considered the cornerstone of diabetes management. Unfortunately, many patients in this home care study reported low confidence in the skills that involved active self-management. Thus, all home care nurses should strive to improve self-efficacy in their patients. Offering patients opportunities to repeatedly demonstrate self-care behavior is the most effective way to increase self-efficacy. In addition, patients should be encouraged to self-critique their techniques and management decisions between nursing visits. On subsequent visits the nurse can discuss patient actions and provide feedback to further boost confidence. If patients are able to understand the principles of insulin adjustment, the nurse should collaborate with the physician to initiate teaching on this, since previous research has shown self-adjustment of insulin to be one of the most effective methods of improving glycemic control (Peyrot & Rubin, 1994). Also, many patients with type 2 diabetes may benefit from newer classes of oral antidiabetic medications such as thiazlidinediones and biguanides (e.g., Glucophage), and these options should be discussed with the physician. Ideally, nursing care will guide patients to increasingly use their own judgment to incorporate diabetes self-care into their daily life.

Home care nurses can improve care by requesting access to clinical specialists and assisting in the development of nursing care plans or clinical paths that reflect current care standards and delineate patient outcomes (Adams & Biggerstaff, 1995; Adams & Cook, 1994; Corbett & Androwich, 1994). Care paths should address the entire scope of outcomes suggested by the American Diabetes Association (1998). Although blood glucose monitoring, insulin preparation and administration, and ability to recognize hypoglycemia are "survival skills," prophylactic foot care, managing sick days, and avoiding hypoglycemia when daily activities change are equally important for health maintenance and prevention of complications. Care guidelines can serve as prompts for quality home care and assist agency personnel to advocate for the appropriate numbers of visits.

ACKNOWLEDGMENTS

The author gratefully acknowledges financial support of this study from the American Nurses Foundation, Alpha Beta Chapter of Sigma Theta Tau International, and Delta Chi Chapter at Large of Sigma Theta Tau International. This chapter is adapted from Corbett, C. F. (1999). Research-based practice implications for patients with diabetes: Parts I & II. *Home Health Care Nurse, 17*(8, 9). Copyright 1999 by Lippincott, Williams & Wilkins. Printed with permission.

REFERENCES

Adams, C., & Biggerstaff, N. (1995). Reduced resource utilization through standardized outcome-focused care plans. *Journal of Nursing Administration, 25*(10), 43–50.

Adams, C., & Cook, D. (1994). The impact of a diabetes nurse educator on nurses' knowledge of diabetes and nursing interventions in a home care setting. *Diabetes Educator, 20*, 49–53.

American Diabetes Association. (1998). Clinical practice recommendations 1998. *Diabetes Care, 21*(Suppl. 1).

Bandura, A. (1977). Self-efficacy: Toward a unifying theory of behavioral change. *Psychological Review, 84*, 191–215.

Bandura, A. (1986). *Social foundations of thought and action.* Englewood Cliffs, NJ: Prentice-Hall.

Caffrey, R. (1996). Diabetes update and implications for care. *Home Healthcare Nurse, 14,* 756–776.

Coonrod, B., Betschart, J., & Harris, M. (1994). Frequency and determinants of diabetes patient education among adults in the U.S. population. *Diabetes Care, 17,* 852–858.

Corbett, C., & Androwich, I. (1994). Critical paths: Implications for improving practice. *Home Healthcare Nurse, 12*(6), 27–34.

Crabtree, K. (1986). *Self-efficacy and social support as predictors of diabetic self-care.* Unpublished doctoral dissertation, University of California, San Francisco.

de Weerdt, I., Visser, A. P., Kok, G., & Van der Veen, E. A. (1990). Determinants of active self-care behavior of insulin treated patients with diabetes: Implications for diabetes education. *Social Science and Medicine, 30,* 605–615.

Dunn, S., Bryson, J., Hoskins, P., Alford, J., Handelman, M., & Turtle, J. (1984). Development of the Diabetes Knowledge (DKN) Scales: Forms DKNA, DKNB, and DKNC. *Diabetes Care, 7,* 36–41.

Ellison, G., & Rayman, K. (1998). Exemplars' experience of self-managing Type 2 diabetes. *Diabetes Educator, 24,* 325–329.

Glasgow, R., Toobert, D., Riddle, M., Donnelly, J., Michell, D., & Calder, D. (1992). Diabetes-specific social learning variables and self-care behaviors among persons with Type II diabetes: The "Sixty Something . . . " study. *Patient Education and Counseling, 19,* 61–74.

Hendricks, L., & Hendricks, R. (1998). Greatest fears of Type 1 and Type 2 patients about having diabetes: Implications for diabetes educators. *Diabetes Educator, 24,* 168–173.

Hockmeyer, M. (1990). *The influence of self-efficacy and health beliefs, considering treatment mode, on self-care behaviors of adults diagnosed within 3 years with non-insulin dependent diabetes.* Unpublished doctoral dissertation, University of Maryland, Baltimore.

Hurley, A. (1988). *Diabetes health beliefs and self care of individuals who require insulin.* Unpublished doctoral dissertation, Boston University, Boston.

Hurley, A. (1990). Measuring self-care ability in patients with diabetes: The Insulin Management Self-Efficacy Scale. In O. Stricklan & C. Waltz (Eds.), *Measurement of nursing outcomes: Measuring client self-care and coping skills* (Vol. 4, pp. 28–44). New York: Springer.

Kavanagh, D., Godey, S., & Wilson, P. (1993). Prediction of adherence and control in diabetes. *Journal of Behavioral Medicine, 16,* 509–522.

Kingery, P., & Glasgow, R. (1989). Self-efficacy and outcome expectations in the self-regulation of non-insulin dependent diabetes mellitus. *Health Education, 20,* 13–19.

Lockington, T., Farrant, S., Meadows, K., Dowlatshahi, & Wise, P. (1988). Knowledge profile and control in diabetic patients. *Diabetic Medicine, 5,* 381–386.

Ludlow, A., & Gein, L. (1995). Relationship among self-care, self-efficacy and HbA1c levels in individuals with non-insulin dependent diabetes mellitus (NIDDM). *Canadian Journal of Diabetes Care, 19*(1), 10–15.

McCloskey, J., & Bulechek, G. (1996). *Iowa Intervention Project: Nursing intervention classification.* St. Louis: Mosby.

Milone-Nuzzo, P. (1993). Third-party reimbursement for home care of clients with diabetes. *Diabetes Educator, 19,* 513–516.

National Association for Home Care. (1996). *Statistics about home care 1996.* Washington, DC: Author.

Padgett, D. (1991). Correlates of self-efficacy beliefs among patients with non-insulin dependent diabetes mellitus in Zagreb, Yugoslavia. *Patient Education and Counseling, 18,* 139–147.

Paterson, B., Thorne, S., & Dewis, M. (1998). Adapting to and managing diabetes. *Image, 30,* 57–62.

Peyrot, M., & Rubin, R. (1994). Modeling the effect of diabetes education on glycemic control. *Diabetes Educator, 20,* 143–148.

Rubin, R. R., Peyrot, M., & Saudek, C. (1989). Effect of diabetes education on self-care, metabolic control, and emotional well-being. *Diabetes Care, 12,* 673–679.

Skelly, A., Marshall, J., Haughey, B., Davis, P., & Dunford, R. (1995). Self-efficacy and confidence in outcomes as determinants of self-care practices in inner-city African American women with non-insulin dependent diabetes. *Diabetes Educator, 21,* 38–46.

[23]

HIV Self-Care Management by African-American Mothers

Margaret S. Miles, Diane Holditch-Davis,
and Beth Black

In the United States, infection with the human immunodeficiency virus (HIV) poses a growing threat to women in the childbearing years (Centers for Disease Control and Prevention [CDC], 1996, 1998; Fowler, Melnick, & Mathieson, 1997), especially poor African-American women (Wortley, Chu, & Berkelman, 1997). HIV affects cell-mediated and antibody-mediated immunity, causing a progressive, severe depression of the immune system (Kahn & Walker, 1998). Thus, HIV involves a variety of related health problems and symptoms that unfold over time and that, if untreated, can cause serious life-threatening complications (Farizo et al., 1992).

Early diagnosis and advances in the treatment of HIV have prolonged the life expectancy of individuals with the virus, and HIV is now viewed as a chronic albeit still fatal disease (Feinberg, 1996). The course of the disease is more rapid in women than in men. Ongoing, regular health care is vital to the successful management of HIV. Women with HIV, however, are less likely than men to use health services, more likely to present at clinical facilities with advanced disease, and less likely to use antiretroviral therapy (Butz et al., 1993; CDC, 1996; Cohn, 1993; Hankins & Handley, 1992; Hellinger, 1993; Hogan, Solomon, Bouknight, & Solomon, 1991; Misener & Sowell, 1998; "Women and AIDS," 1995). Thus, women's prognosis and survival may be affected by their differential access to and follow-through with preventive care and treatment (Williams, Shahryarinejad, Andrews, & Alcabes, 1997).

Women's self-care and health care seeking may be affected by their emotional responses to their diagnosis, including fear, anxiety, sadness, and depression (Jaccard, Wilson, & Radecki, 1995; Kaplan, Marks, & Mertens, 1997; Miles, Burchinal, Holditch-Davis, Wasilewski, & Christian, 1997; Stevens & Doerr, 1997), as well as feelings of shame and stigma (Bunting, 1996; Lawless, Kippax, & Crawford, 1996). As a result, women may cope with their diagnosis through avoidance or denial (Jaccard et al., 1995; Stevens & Doerr, 1997).

The more rapid course of HIV in women may also be related to their lack of knowledge about HIV and its manifestations during the early stages of the disease. HIV symptoms in low-income women are the result of complex interrelationships between their life circumstances, lifestyle, previous health problems, and the HIV infection (Butz et al., 1993; Lyons & DeHovitz, 1995). Women may not attribute symptoms they are experiencing to HIV and may ignore them. Yet when the symptoms are left untreated, the infection may further compromise their immune status, leading to more rapid progression of the infection (Clark, 1997; Landesman & Holman, 1995).

Low-income African-American women with HIV face particular challenges that may affect self-care as well as treatment seeking. These include lack of available or adequate health care resources, lack of insurance, child care and family responsibilities, inadequate support, and lack of transportation (Butz et al., 1993; Williams et al., 1997). Health care seeking by HIV-infected women is also affected by their focus on their children rather than themselves (Andrews, Williams, & Neil, 1993; Butz et al., 1993; Regan-Kubinski & Sharts-Hopko, 1995).

To date, little attention has been focused on self-care issues for women with HIV. Nurses working with HIV-positive women need a clearer understanding of the symptoms and health problems these women experience early in the course of the disease in order to help women understand and cope with their HIV diagnosis, and prevent and manage symptoms and related health problems. This chapter, therefore, describes the physical health problems, depressive symptoms, perceptions of stigma, perceptions of having HIV, and barriers to care reported by African-American mothers with HIV. Data for the chapter were derived from a longitudinal study, *Parental Caregiving of Infants Seropositive for HIV* (Miles, 1997). Based on these data and relevant literature about HIV, we present an HIV self-care management model to guide nursing interventions for women with HIV.

METHODS

Subjects and Setting

Caregivers of infants born to HIV-positive mothers (foster mothers, kin, and biological mothers) were recruited from two university-based pediatric infectious disease clinics where the infants were being followed to determine their HIV status. They were recruited after the infant's first clinic visit to avoid a time of distress for the caregivers. Caregivers were told about the purpose of the study and signed an informed consent form.

Eighty-seven caregivers were enrolled in the study. Sixty-seven caregivers were the biological mothers of the infants. All of the biological mothers were HIV positive, and most (88%) were African-American. The mean age of the biological mothers was 26 years (SD = 5.9). Their mean educational level was 11 years, with a range from 7 to 16 years; most (54%) had at least a high school diploma. A majority of the mothers were single (58%), unemployed (76%), and on public assistance (78%). The mean household income was $10,130. The mothers had an average of three children.

Data Collection Methods

Three self-report questionnaires were used to assess physical health, depressive symptoms, and stigma at four data collection points—at enrollment when the infant was 3 to 4 months of age and when the infant was 6, 12, and 18 months; a subset of cases was followed to 24 months. In addition, semi-structured interviews were conducted at every contact. Some data collection occurred in the clinic and some in the home setting.

Physical Health

The mother's health was evaluated at every contact using the Short Health Survey adapted from the Medical Outcomes Study health survey (Ware & Sherbourne, 1992). This scale includes three subscales: Perception of Health, Activity Limitations, and Physical Symptoms. On the Perception of Health scale, respondents rate four statements—"My health is excellent," "I am somewhat ill," "I am as healthy as anyone I know," and "I have been feeling bad lately"—using a 4-point rating scale, ranging from 1 (definitely true) to 4 (definitely false), with a 3 indicating "not sure." Scores for negative items on this scale are reversed so that a higher score indicates poorer health. In this study, Cronbach's alphas for the Perception of Health scale ranged from .68 to .83 over time.

On the Activity Limitations scale, respondents rate the degree to which their health limits them in carrying out seven activities. These activities include activities of daily living and various types of physical activities such as walking, lifting, running, and moving objects. The items are rated on a 3-point descriptive scale; the descriptors are "not limited," "limited for less than 3 months," and "limited for more than 3 months." A higher score indicates more limitations. Cronbach's alphas for this scale ranged from .76 to .91 in this study.

A Physical Symptoms list was developed for the study reported here in order to assess HIV-related symptoms and health problems. The list was based on several health questionnaires and on literature related to health problems experienced in early HIV. Respondents rate the prevalence of 13 physical symptoms (e.g., difficulty eating, unwanted weight loss, infections, low energy, and problems thinking and remembering). A 3-point rating scale is used with 1 indicating that the symptom is "never experienced," 2 indicating it is "sometimes experienced," and 3 indicating that it is "often experienced." A higher score indicates more symptoms. Cronbach's alphas ranged from .79 to .84 in this study.

Depressive Symptoms

The Center for Epidemiological Studies Depression Scale (CES-D) was used to assess depressive symptoms at every contact. The 20-item CES-D assesses the frequency of self-reported blues, loneliness, difficulty concentrating, sleeping, and eating problems. Higher scores indicate more depressive symptoms; a score of 16 or higher is considered to indicate risk for depression (Radloff, 1977; Roberts & Vernon, 1983). Cronbach's alphas in our study ranged from .89 to .92.

Stigma

Feelings related to the stigma of having HIV were assessed using the Demi Stigma Scale (Demi, 1995) at 6, 12, 18, and 24 months. On this tool, respondents indicate how often they have experienced feelings such as feeling blamed, fearing loss of a job or friend, and thinking the illness is a punishment. The 13 items are rated on a 4-point frequency rating scale ranging from "not at all" to "often." A higher score indicates more stigma. Cronbach's alphas in our study ranged from .77 to .84 over time.

Interviews

The semi-structured interviews focused both on the mother and her concerns, symptoms, and health problems, and on the mother's experiences and perceptions of caring for her child. Interviews were tape-recorded and transcribed verbatim. At each data collection contact, research assistants recorded extensive field notes about their observations and conversations that were not recorded.

RESULTS

Data on physical health, depressive symptoms and stigma are presented here for 34 biological mothers who were followed to the 24-month data collection point.

Physical Health

On the Perceptions of Health scale, means ranged from 2.2 to 2.5 over time (see Table 23.1). The women rated statements between "mostly true" (moderately positive) and "not sure."

On the Activity Limitations scale, responses indicating any limitations were combined and scored as a limitation. The percentages of women

TABLE 23.1 Means and Standard Deviations for Perception of Health, Stigma, and Depressive Symptoms of 34 Women

	Times				
	3 months	6 months	12 months	18 months	24 months
Variables	M (SD)	M (SD)	M (SD)	M (SD)	M (SD)
Perception of Health[a]	2.5 (.93)	2.5 (.91)	2.5 (.95)	2.2 (.93)	2.3 (.99)
CES-D	16.1 (11.7)	15.8 (12.0)	13.6 (10.2)	12.5 (10.5)	13.2 (11.3)
Demi Stigma Scale	(na)[b]	1.7 (.51)	1.8 (.54)	1.8 (.62)	1.8 (.57)

[a]A higher score indicates a poorer perception of health.
[b]Not administered.

reporting activity limitations were low to moderate, ranging from 3% to 26% (see Table 23.2). Few women had problems with activities of daily living (6% to 10% over time), walking a block (6% to 23%) or work-related activities (8% to 16%). More women reported difficulty with vigorous physical activities (17% to 24%) or moderate physical activities (15% to 21%), with walking uphill or climbing (12% to 26%), and with bending, lifting, and stooping (15% to 21%).

On the Physical Symptoms scale, responses noted as "sometimes" and "often" were combined to reflect the presence of the symptom. The percentages of women reporting specific physical symptoms varied, ranging from

TABLE 23.2 Frequencies on Selected Items Measuring Activity Limitations and Physical Symptoms of 34 Women

	Times				
Items	3 months n (%)	6 months n (%)	12 months n (%)	18 months n (%)	24 months n (%)
Activity limitations					
Walking uphill/ climbing	6 (19)	8 (26)	7 (21)	4 (12)	7 (21)
Bending, lifting, stooping	6 (19)	5 (16)	7 (21)	6 (18)	5 (15)
Vigorous activities	5 (17)	7 (23)	8 (24)	6 (18)	8 (24)
Moderate activities	5 (16)	6 (19)	5 (15)	5 (15)	7 (21)
Work	5 (16)	5 (16)	4 (12)	4 (12)	3 (08)
Walking one block	4 (12)	7 (23)	5 (15)	2 (06)	4 (12)
Activities of daily living	2 (06)	3 (10)	2 (06)	1 (03)	1 (03)
Physical symptoms					
Infections/MD visit	13 (41)	11 (36)	11 (33)	9 (27)	6 (18)
Problems thinking	13 (41)	12 (39)	14 (42)	10 (30)	7 (21)
Low energy levels	13 (41)	15 (48)	16 (59)	21 (64)	16 (47)
Female problems	13 (41)	11 (36)	12 (36)	7 (21)	8 (24)
Difficulty eating	9 (28)	7 (23)	6 (18)	8 (24)	4 (12)
Difficulty eating	9 (28)	7 (23)	6 (18)	8 (24)	4 (12)
Difficulty moving	6 (19)	5 (16)	6 (18)	5 (15)	6 (18)
Problems breathing	5 (16)	10 (32)	11 (33)	5 (15)	9 (27)
Fevers	5 (16)	7 (23)	7 (21)	4 (12)	3 (09)
Weight loss	4 (13)	6 (19)	15 (46)	8 (24)	12 (35)
Difficulty using hands	3 (9)	6 (19)	5 (15)	4 (12)	5 (15)
Problems hearing	3 (9)	4 (13)	4 (12)	3 (9)	4 (12)

9% to 64% (see Table 23.2). Symptoms most often reported were infections requiring a health visit (18% to 41%), problems thinking and remembering (21% to 42%), low energy levels (41% to 64%), and female problems (21% to 41%). The percentage reporting problems in breathing and fevers varied greatly over time (9% to 33%). The percentage reporting weight loss ranged from 13% to 46%; this percentage increased over time, probably reflecting the women's postpartum status. Also, at some points, almost a quarter of the women reported problems with eating (12% to 28%). At least seven women experienced a hospitalization, and two women died in the course of the study. One mother who revealed in the interviews that she was not seeking health care because she was avoiding dealing with her diagnosis died of a sudden overwhelming infection. The other mother was murdered in a drug-related incident.

The interviews and field notes from a sample of 10 mothers who had data available at all five data collection points were content analyzed to identify symptoms and health problems reported by the mothers. The most commonly reported symptoms were fatigue, nausea, shortness of breath, depression, low self-esteem, and anxiety. Although these symptoms may be related to HIV, the mothers were also bothered by symptoms unrelated to HIV such as backache, elevated blood sugar, high blood pressure, and poor vision due to myopia.

Depressive Symptoms

As a group, the mothers exhibited a high level of depression. Mean depression scores ranged from 12.5 to 16.1 across time (see Table 23.1). The percent of mothers with CES-D scores above the cut-off of 16, which indicates risk for depression, ranged from 30% to 45% at various time periods. In addition, 25% of all the biological mothers were categorized as "chronically depressed" because their CES-D scores were over 16 at most data contact points.

Stigma

The mean total scores on the Demi Stigma Scale ranged from 1.7 to 1.8 over the four contact points when this scale was used (6, 12, 18, and 24 months) (see Table 23.1). Three items had the highest mean scores: "I felt ashamed," "I thought the illness was a punishment," and "I feared I would lose my friends." Consistent with the stigma scale scores, interviews with mothers indicated intense fear of stigma. This fear affected their disclosure to others, even family members and health care professionals.

Responses to HIV Diagnosis

The 12-month interview asked about the woman's response to HIV and related problems. This was a time when the mothers had gained enough trust in the research team to be honest and spontaneous in their interviews. Field notes and interviews from the 24 mothers who completed this data collection point were content analyzed, and the analysis indicated that the mothers showed avoidance of their HIV status, with many stating that they did not worry about HIV. A number of mothers said they lacked knowledge of HIV and did not understand test results or know the name of medicines, and they mentioned not being regular about obtaining health care or taking medications for HIV.

Barriers to Health Care Seeking

The interviews also identified several barriers to health care seeking and preventive health care, including financial constraints, lack of support, caregiving responsibilities for both children and other adults in the household, and fear of disclosure should the women attend the clinic too often. Many women, especially those from small towns and rural areas, revealed a distrust of local clinics and physicians and fear of public disclosure of their infection. The distance to tertiary care centers was often long, and transportation was limited. Another barrier to mothers seeking health care was worries about their child's HIV status. They made repeated trips to the pediatric infectious disease clinics to assess the child's health status, and often focused on the child's needs to the exclusion of their own.

DISCUSSION

These African-American mothers with HIV reported changes in their physical health as well as depressive symptoms and feelings of stigma. They also reported avoiding thinking about their HIV because of their intense feelings about the diagnosis. Many lacked understanding of the HIV infection and its manifestations. Their worry about their child's HIV status, lack of resources such as child care and transportation, and fear of disclosure and stigma in local health care settings affected their health care–seeking patterns. Inconsistent health care–seeking patterns and lack of attention to prevention can result in potentially serious health problems, such as infections, which can cause premature death. Escalating health problems can also decrease the mother's ability to work, function in her family, and provide adequate care to her children.

HIV Self-Care Management Intervention Model

Based on the data from this study, we have developed an HIV Self-Care Management Intervention model aimed at helping African-American mothers cope with their illness and begin to prevent, recognize, and manage HIV-related symptoms. The University of California-San Francisco Symptom Management Model (1994) provided a basis for the development of the model, but the specifics came from the information we gained from mothers. Figure 23.1 depicts the model.

The core of the model is helping mothers face their HIV diagnosis by allowing them opportunities to tell how they got HIV and share their responses to having the infection. Facing their feelings about having HIV is important in helping women to become more comfortable in talking about HIV and more open to informational support. The informational support component of the intervention model has two interrelated goals: (1) increasing the woman's knowledge of HIV and related treatments in

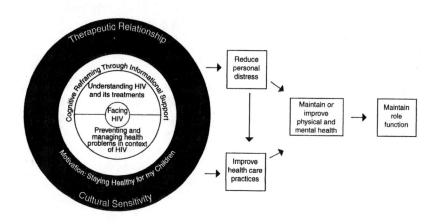

FIGURE 23.1   HIV self-care management intervention model.

order to reframe her view of HIV to a chronic (albeit still fatal) illness over which she can have some control and (2) increasing the woman's knowledge about healthy living, preventive health practices, and recognition and early treatment of health problems within the context of HIV.

The informational modules developed for our intervention offer a structure for assessing women and providing information to them about their disease. The information is based on our research and on the literature about early symptoms of HIV that may be particularly important for African-American women. The emphasis is on preventing, managing, and treating symptoms and health problems that are salient to women with HIV, such as respiratory and gastrointestinal infections, gynecologic problems, skin problems, and problems with fatigue and sleep (Landesman & Holman, 1995; Lyons & DeHovitz, 1995; Minkoff & DeHovitz, 1991). There are also modules on dealing with depression and the blues, and coping with memory loss and disorganization (Kaplan et al., 1997; Miles et al., 1997; Wilkie et al., 1998). The modules focus on how and why these problems are important to women and give information about prevention and management strategies that fit with the unique needs and circumstances of the women. Keeping regular HIV care appointments and complying with medications are also emphasized. The modules are attractively packaged with accurate drawings of African-American women and children, they include African-American quotes and inspirational messages, and they are written in an easy-to-read question-and-answer format. All modules have some focus on the mother's maternal role or on the needs of her children.

An important aspect of the intervention is motivating the mother to focus on her own health care needs in order to "stay healthy to be there for her children." Because African-American mothers with HIV regard their maternal role as very important to their self-identity and worry about whether they will be able to care for their children, this can be a potent motivator for focusing on their own needs (Regan-Kubinski & Sharts-Hopko, 1995).

The informational intervention is embedded in a semi-structured clinical interview informed by sensitivity to the African-American culture of the mothers. This includes paying attention to the establishment of trust, understanding time and timing issues for the mothers, listening to the mothers' own agenda and needs, encouraging storytelling, and giving unconditional regard and acceptance to the mothers no matter what they discuss or how they behave.

IMPLICATIONS FOR PRACTICE

The HIV Self-Care Management Intervention is a tertiary prevention model in that it involves prevention within the context of an already existing chronic illness. The intervention has potential as a case management or clinical intervention model for use by public health nurses visiting the home and nurses who work with HIV-infected women in primary care or specialty clinics.

Intervening with African-American women with HIV must begin with concern about and interest in the women themselves. We have found that going into women's homes and focusing on their needs and concerns is very effective in getting them to pay attention to their HIV diagnosis and overall health. It is important to allow women to tell their stories about how they found out about their diagnosis and share their feelings about the diagnosis. Additionally, it is important to be sensitive to the cultural and social issues of the women and to be nonjudgmental and caring in interactions with them.

Teaching an African-American woman with HIV should begin with an assessment of the woman's knowledge of and views about HIV and related treatments, the relationship between HIV and general health, and specific aspects of prevention and management of health problems in the context of HIV. Teaching should then focus on areas where the woman needs and wants help. It is important to provide information about prevention and management of health problems, and about the importance of keeping regular HIV clinic appointments and taking medications correctly.

While the HIV Self-Care Management Intervention was developed for African-American mothers with HIV infection, this intervention also might be used with mothers with other chronic conditions such as hypertension and diabetes. Low-income mothers with these seemingly mild but potentially serious health problems also tend to focus their attention on their family and parenting roles and often do not seek or follow through with health care for themselves. And like HIV, these conditions have symptoms that are easy to avoid or ignore until they cause serious complications. Thus, the HIV Self-Care Management Intervention has potential as a model for intervention programs for women with HIV and other chronic conditions.

ACKNOWLEDGMENTS

The authors wish to acknowledge primary support for this chapter from the National Institute of Mental Health (MH R0151019). We also acknowledge partial support from the National Institute of Allergies and Infectious Diseases (2V01A127535), the UNC General Clinical Research Center (RR00046), the Center for Research on Chronic Illness (P30 NR03965), and the Center for Aids Research (P30 HD27360). The authors also wish to acknowledge the research team including Joann Haggerty, Tanya Kewson, Shiela Santacroce, and Yvonne Wasilewski.

REFERENCES

Andrews, S., Williams, A. B., & Neil, K. (1993). The mother-child relationship in the HIV-1 positive family. *Image, 25,* 193–198.

Bunting, S. (1996). Sources of stigma associated with women with HIV. *Advances in Nursing Science, 19,* 64–73.

Butz, A. M., Hutton, N., Joyner, M., Vogelhut, J., Greenberg-Friedman, D., Schreibeis, D., & Anderson, J. R. (1993). HIV-infected women and infants: Social and health factors impeding utilization of care. *Journal of Nurse-Midwifery, 38*(2), 10–109.

Centers for Disease Control (CDC). (1996). HIV testing among women aged 18–44 years—United States, 1991 and 1993. *Morbidity and Mortality Weekly Report, 45,* 733–737.

Centers for Disease Control (CDC). (1998). Diagnosis and reporting of HIV and AIDS in states with integrated HIV and AIDS surveillance—United States, January 1994–June, 1997. *Morbidity and Mortality Weekly Report, 47,* 1–6.

Clark, R. (1997). Clinical manifestations and the natural history of HIV in women. In D. Cotton & D. H. Watts (Eds.), *The medical management of AIDS in women* (pp. 115–124). New York: Wiley-Liss.

Cohn, J. A. (1993). Human immunodeficiency virus and AIDS: 1993 update. *Journal of Nurse-Midwifery, 38,* 65–85.

Demi, A. S. (1995). *Psychometric evaluation of the Demi HIV Stigma Scale.* Unpublished manuscript, Georgia State University, Atlanta.

Farizo, K. M., Buehler, J. W., Chamberland, M. E., Whyte, B. M., Froelicher, E., Hopkins, S. G., Reed, C. M., Mokotoff, E., Cohn, D. L., & Troxler, S. (1992). Spectrum of disease in persons with human immunodeficiency virus infection in the United States. *Journal of the American Medical Association, 267*(13), 1798–1805.

Feinberg, M. B. (1996). Changing the natural history of HIV disease. *The Lancet, 348*(9022), 239–246.

Fowler, M. G., Melnick, S. L., & Mathieson, B. J. (1997). Women and HIV: Epidemiology and global overview. *Obstetrics and Gynecology Clinics of North America, 24,* 705–729.

Hankins, C. A., & Handley, M. A. (1992). HIV disease and AIDS in women: Current knowledge and a research agenda. *Journal of Acquired Immune Deficiency Syndrome, 5,* 957–971.

Hellinger, F. J. (1993). The use of health services by women with HIV infection. *Health Services Research, 28,* 543–561.

Hogan, A., Solomon, D., Bouknight, R., & Solomon, S. (1991). Underutilization of medical care services by HIV-infected women? Some preliminary results from the Michigan Medicaid Program. *AIDS, 5,* 338–339.

Jaccard, J. J., Wilson, T. E., & Radecki, C. M. (1995). Psychological issues in the treatment of HIV-infected women. In H. Minkoff, J. A. DeHovitz, & A. Duerr (Eds.), *HIV infection in women* (pp. 87–106). New York: Raven Press.

Jewett, J. F., & Hecht, F. M. (1993). Preventive health care for adults with HIV infection. *Journal of the American Medical Association, 269*(9), 1144–1153.

Kahn, J. O., & Walker, B. D. (1998). Acute human immunodeficiency virus type 1 infection. *New England Journal of Medicine, 339*(1), 33–39.

Kaplan, M. S., Marks, G., & Mertens, S. B. (1997). Distress and coping among women with HIV infection: Preliminary findings from a multiethnic sample. *American Journal of Orthopsychiatry, 67*, 80–91.

Landesman, S. H., & Holman, S. (1995). Epidemiology and natural history of HIV infection in women. In P. Kelly, S. Holman, R. Rothenberg, & S. P. Holzemer (Eds.), *Primary care of women and children with HIV infection* (pp. 19–35). Boston: Jones and Bartlett.

Lawless, S., Kippax, S., & Crawford, J. (1996). Dirty, diseased and undeserving: The positioning of HIV positive women. *Social Science and Medicine, 43*, 1371–1377.

Lyons, & DeHovitz, J. A. (1995). Care of women with HIV disease. In P. Kelly, S. Holman, R. Rothenberg, & S. P. Holzemer (Eds.), *Primary care of women and children with HIV infection* (pp. 37–58). Boston: Jones and Bartlett.

Miles, M. S. (1997). *Parental caregiving of infants sero-positive for HIV.* Unpublished final report for Grant No. MH 51019.

Miles, M. S., Burchinal, P., Holditch-Davis, D., Wasilewski, Y., & Christian, B. (1997). Personal, family, and health-related correlates of depressive symptoms in mothers with HIV. *Journal of Family Psychology, 11*, 23–34.

Minkoff, H. L., & DeHovitz, J. A. (1991). Care of women infected with the human immunodeficiency virus. *Journal of the America Medical Association, 266*, 2253–2258.

Misener, T. R., & Sowell, R. L. (1998). HIV-infected women's decisions to take antiretrovirals. *Western Journal of Nursing Research, 20*, 431–447.

Radloff, L. (1977). The CES-D scale: A self report depression scale for research in the general population. *Applied Psychological Measurement, 1*, 385–401.

Regan-Kubinski, M. J., & Sharts-Hopko, N. (1995). Illness cognition of HIV-infected mothers. *Issues in Mental Health Nursing, 16*, 327–344.

Roberts, R. E., & Vernon, S. W. (1983). The Center for Epidemiologic Studies Depression Scale: Its use in a community sample. *American Journal of Psychiatry, 140*, 41–46.

Stevens, P. E., & Doerr, B. T. (1997). Trauma of discovery: Women's narratives of being informed they are HIV-infected. *Aids Care, 9*(5), 523–538.

University of California-San Francisco School of Nursing Symptom Management Faculty Group. (1994). A model for symptom management. *Image: Journal of Nursing Scholarship, 26*, 272–276.

Ware, J. E., & Sherbourne, C. D. (1992). The MOS 36-item Short-Form Health Survey: I. Conceptual framework and item selection. *Medical Care, 30*, 473–483.

Wilkie, F. L., Goodkin, K., Eisdorfer, C., Faster, D., Morgan, R., Fletcher, M. A., Blaney, N., Baum, M., & Szapocznik, J. (1998). Mild cognitive impairment and risk of mortality in HIV-1 infection. *Journal of Neuropsychiatry and Clinical Neurosciences, 10*, 125–132.

Williams, A. B., Shahryarinejad, A., Andrews, W., & Alcabes, P. (1997). Social support for HIV-infected mothers: Relation to HIV care seeking. *Journal of the Association of Nurses in AIDS Care, 8,* 91–98.

Women and AIDS—Unexplained higher risk of death. (1995). *AIDS Treatment News, 214,* 2–3.

Wortley, P. M., Chu, S. Y., & Berkelman, R. L. (1997). Epidemiology of HIV/AIDS in women and the impact of the expanded 1993 CDC surveillance definition of AIDS. In D. Cotton & D. H. Watts (Eds.), *The medical management of AIDS in women* (pp. 3–14). New York: Wiley-Liss.

[24]

A Survey of Leading Chronic Disease Management Programs

Edward H. Wagner, Connie Davis, Judith Schaefer, Michael Von Korff, and Brian Austin

The past several years have seen an explosion of "disease management" efforts directed at major chronic illnesses. The movement has been fueled by the struggle to find how to best care for patients with chronic illness in an era of cost constraints and performance expectations imposed by purchasers. Recent surveys have documented the intensity of the efforts (National Managed Health Care Congress, 1996) without, however, providing much evidence as to the characteristics and quality of the programs or the effects on patients.

We recently surveyed the chronic disease management activities of 72 programs noted by experts in the field of chronic illness care as particularly innovative and effective. Our survey was guided by the Model for Effective Chronic Illness Care, derived from the literature and expert review. The model attempts to identify specific practice and system changes employed in published, successful programmatic efforts to improve the care of patients with chronic illness (see Figure 24.1).

According to the model, effective chronic illness management requires an appropriately organized health care system linked with necessary policies and resources in the broader community. These policies and resources may provide access to critical supportive or educational services otherwise unavailable in health care systems. The model also points out characteristics

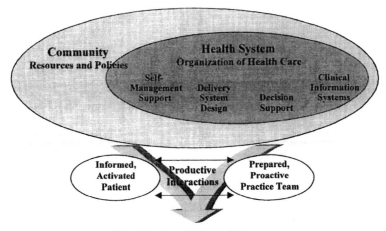

Functional and Clinical Outcomes

FIGURE 24.1   A model for effective chronic illness care.

of the larger health care system without which care improvement is unlikely. These include a coherent approach to system improvement, leadership committed to improving clinical outcomes, and incentives to providers and patients to improve care and adhere to guidelines. The aim is to support the development of informed, activated patients and prepared, proactive professional practice teams. Providers must have the necessary expertise, information, time, and resources to assure effective clinical management. Patients must also have the information and confidence to make the best use of their involvement with their practice team. Productive interactions between providers and patients ensure the delivery of services that achieve desired outcomes, measured by clinical care, health status, satisfaction, health care utilization, and cost.

   Productive interactions include creation of a patient-centered, collaborative care plan based on regular assessment tailored to the needs of the individual patient and targeted to chronic illness. Treatment plans must be responsive to psychological, social, and biological needs, and include the systematic application of proven therapies. The care plan describes mechanisms for sustained follow-up to ensure early detection of complications and patient concerns and to support adherence to the plan.

   The model includes enhancements to practice that contribute to productive interactions between providers and patients. Effective *self-management support* helps patients and families cope with the challenges of living with and treating chronic illness (Von Korff, Gruman, Schaefer, Curry, & Wagner, 1997). Successful self-management is based on a collaborative process between patients and providers to define problems, set priorities, establish goals, create treatment plans, and solve problems along the way. Effective educational resources, skills training, and avenues for psychosocial support provide a self-management support structure.

Effective chronic illness management requires more than simply adding interventions to a system focused on acute care; attention must also be paid to *delivery system design*. Practice team members need clear, complementary roles. Many management functions will require the delegation of care from the physician to nurse case managers and health educators who have the knowledge and time to carry out the range of tasks required to manage complex chronic conditions (Payne et al., 1995). These professionals also need time to assess patients and interact with them, prompts to ensure proper management, and protocols for regular, planned follow-up. To achieve these, innovations may be required in the scheduling and organization of visits such as planned or group visits (Beck et al., 1997; McCulloch, Price, Nindmarsh, & Wagner, 1998) or telephone care (Aubert et al., 1998; Kirkman et al., 1994; Wasson et al., 1992; Weinberger et al., 1995).

Effective chronic illness management programs ensure that providers have decision support (i.e., access to the expertise necessary to care for patients). Most use evidence-based practice guidelines or protocols. These are especially useful for primary care providers, who may be less familiar than specialists with the latest techniques for treating specific conditions. In addition to guidelines, practice teams benefit from appropriate input from relevant medical specialties (Katon et al., 1996; McCulloch et al., 1998).

Timely, useful data about individual patients and populations of patients with chronic conditions is a critical feature of effective programs, especially those that employ population-based approaches (Grenlick, 1992; Wagner, 1995). The first step in establishing a clinical information system is to set up a disease registry for individual practices that includes information about the performance and results of important elements of care. Health care teams with access to a registry can call patients with specific needs, deliver planned care, receive feedback on their performance, and implement reminder systems.

METHODS

To assess the state of the art of chronic illness management, we identified programs for patients with chronic illness considered particularly innovative and/or successful, then surveyed representatives of those programs by telephone to collect information about program design, experience, and effects. On the basis of these interviews, we conducted site visits with a smaller number of particularly interesting programs.

Program Selection and Contact

An advisory committee recommended exemplary programs in chronic illness care. Ninety-one chronic disease management programs throughout the United States and in Western Europe were named. Three interviewers then attempted to contact each nominated program. We failed to contact a relevant person at six organizations (7%), and four others (4%), all proprietary, refused to participate. Nine additional nominated programs (10%) were eliminated because they had not yet begun providing services or were not involved directly with the care of patients. Interviewers then identified program staff most likely to have comprehensive knowledge of the design and implementation of the program and conducted telephone interviews with representatives of the remaining 72 (79%) programs. Program coordinators, directors, or physician champions for the programs were most frequently interviewed.

Survey Instruments

The advisory committee and the authors drafted the questionnaire for interviewing program directors. The questionnaire was organized according to the elements of the model and included a combination of yes-no questions and open-ended questions with specific probes. For example, to assess efforts at improving decision support, we asked: Does the program make specific efforts to educate providers? If the answer was yes, the interviewer probed for the use of any of the following modalities: conventional continuing medical education, computer decision support, local experts, academic detailing, guidelines, or other. The interview instrument also allowed interviewees to describe their experiences with the design and implementation of the interventions.

RESULTS

Tables 24.1 and 24.2 summarize key characteristics of the 72 programs surveyed, which were based in 69 different organizations. Most were located

TABLE 24.1 Characteristics of Interviewed Programs and Health Systems (N = 72)

Characteristic	# of Responses	% of Programs
Organization type		
HMO	35	49%
Other health care organization	14	19%
Government agency	6	8%
Business	6	8%
Mixed	11	15%
Coverage in plan		
Covered benefit	56	78%
Out of pocket	1	1%
Mixed	7	10%
No response	8	11%
Status of organization		
Not-for-profit	35	49%
For profit	20	28%
Mixed	5	7%
No response	12	17%
Relationship to primary care		
Integral part of care	25	35%
Linked to care	38	53%
Not linked	8	11%
Missing	1	1%
Patient population		
Limited to those with ADL deficit	22	31%
Children only	5	7%
Adults	18	25%
Elderly only	22	31%
Mixed ages	27	38%
Diabetes	11	15%
Asthma	4	6%
Congestive heart failure	3	4%
Heart disease	3	4%
Geriatrics	7	10%
Terminally ill	2	3%
Multiple conditions	34	47%
Others specific conditions	8	11%

(continued)

TABLE 24.1   *(continued)*

Characteristic	# of Responses	% of Programs
Entrance to the program*		
Specific criteria	52	72%
Provider referral	46	64%
Self-referral	33	46%
Actively identified	42	58%
Provider incentives		
None	31	43%
Financial	11	15%
Assistance with difficult patients	12	17%
Other	5	7%
Mixed	2	3%
No response	11	15%
Patient incentives		
None	33	46%
Financial	4	6%
Personal relationship with provider	10	14%
Other	7	10%
Mixed	6	8%
No response	12	17%
Financial support for program*		
Internal budget	54	75%
Special fund	21	29%
Outside support	24	33%
Evaluation type		
None	11	15%
Random controlled trials	15	21%
Outcomes	14	19%
Satisfaction	4	6%
Mixed	27	38%
Missing	1	1%

*Multiple responses accepted.

within a health care organization, and approximately half were located in health maintenance organizations. Programs were equally likely to be based on expert opinion, literature review, or other successful programs. Most programs were provided as a covered benefit or required small copayments. Three quarters were funded by internal budgets, and the remainder were dependent on special funds or external sources. By assuming risk under

TABLE 24.2   Implementation of Chronic Care Model Elements in Interviewed Programs

	# of Responses	% of Programs
Patient education		
None	2	3%
Moderate	15	21%
Extensive	53	74%
Missing	3	5%
Self-management support		
None	14	19%
Moderate	43	60%
Extensive	13	17%
Missing	3	5%
Provider education*		
Included as part of program	59	82%
Through CME	45	63%
Computerized decision support	11	15%
Local experts	34	47%
Academic detailing	20	28%
Guideline use		
None	18	25%
Moderate	21	29%
Extensive	27	38%
Missing	5	7%
Information systems*		
Updated system for program	33	46%
Registry	23	32%
Reminder system	25	35%
Care plan	19	26%
Feedback	22	31%
Data input by frontline staff	26	36%
Delivery system design changes*		
Appointments restructured	34	47%
Patient flow	23	32%
Follow-up	34	47%
Care planning	40	56%
Patient education	37	51%
Personnel types*		
Medical specialists	24	33%
Nurse specialists	36	50%
Case managers	23	32%

*Multiple responses accepted.

capitation, a few programs were able to increase their funding to support a broader array of interventions. The Program for All-inclusive Care of the Elderly (PACE) (Eng, Pedulla, Eleazer, McCann, & Fox, 1997) and Community Medical Alliance in Boston (Master et al., 1996) are examples of programs that combined Medicare and Medicaid funding to provide services in the home not covered by Medicare or Medicaid guidelines.

Nearly half of the programs addressed multiple chronic conditions, and another 10% focused on the needs of older adults, especially those with long-term care needs. Most of the remainder targeted a particular condition; diabetes was the most common (15% of all programs). Nearly three quarters of the programs had specific entry criteria for patients, and 58% actively identified and recruited patients. However, physician referral and self-referral continued to be important patient sources.

The relationship of the program to the patient's source of primary care was an important consideration. Primary care was an integral component of only one third of these largely health system–based programs; another 53% were linked to primary care, but often the linkage depended on written communications. We asked program representatives if they used special providers, such as medical specialists, nurse specialists, or case managers, to provide primary care for specific patient groups. Nurse specialists (50% of programs), medical specialists (33%), and nurse or social worker case managers (32%) were used most frequently.

Prevalence of Model Elements

Nearly half of the programs had developed linkages with community-based resources such as patient education programs, counseling services, or long-term care providers. Because many community services were either provided at minimal cost or covered by existing benefit packages, these linkages appeared to be a cost-effective way of providing a broader array of services.

Incentives for providers to improve care of chronic illness were infrequent. Less than 20% of programs offered financial incentives to providers, and the equally infrequent nonfinancial incentives were generally confined to offers of help with tough patients. New patient incentives were also uncommon. Enthusiastic organizational leadership was repeatedly mentioned in interviews as an important element in program success, and its absence was a major obstacle. Although most of the organizations surveyed had endorsed total quality management, we obtained little evidence that organized quality improvement approaches were being used to improve chronic illness care.

While essentially all organizations provided patient education to assist patients with self-management, most depended on traditional, information-oriented resources (see Table 24.2). Only 18% of the programs offered self-management support that employed approaches found to be effective in recent research (Von Korff et al., 1997), and these programs tended to focus on self-management support using techniques that emphasized patient activation or empowerment, collaborative goal setting, and problem-solving skills. All programs reported the availability of psychosocial support for patients or families in need, but few offered it routinely.

Most programs surveyed had made some efforts to reorganize care to meet the needs of patients with chronic illness; most commonly, this included greater involvement of nonphysicians in the care of patients as members of a practice team, changes to the appointment schedule to accommodate chronically ill patients, and more aggressive follow-up. About half of the programs described themselves as delivering team care, although the formality of team operation and role delegation varied widely.

Most of the programs (82%) used some form of case management. In some programs, case management was integrated with primary care provision; in others, case management operated as a carve-out, with minimal or no feedback to primary care. Some used a risk stratification tool to provide case management only for those at the highest risk. Programs typically developed a care plan involving some patient or self-management education, proactive follow-up by the case manager, and referral to other resources as needed. Programs frequently attempted to expedite care across settings, or to provide access to needed social service interventions that might affect medical conditions. Case managers were most frequently registered nurses or social workers, although some programs used nurse practitioners. Some case management programs had well designed clinical protocols, whereas others were clearly more interested in utilization management and moving patients to less expensive clinical venues. Case management programs were still struggling to find optimal ways to relate to primary care to ensure care coordination and appropriate referrals. Changes to appointment systems usually took the form of greater flexibility in visit lengths. However, a few programs were experimenting with different forms of group visits.

Sixty percent of the programs used explicit practice guidelines, and most supported them with provider training of some sort. Computerized decision support was infrequent. About half of the programs attempted to increase access to specialized expertise either through identifying and training local experts or by providing greater opportunities for collaboration and information exchange between generalists and specialists.

Forty-six percent of the programs said that they had updated computer systems as part of the program. Information systems enhanced programs through the use of registries for active identification of patients (32%), automatic flagging systems or reminders (35%), feedback to providers (26%), data capture from front-line workers (37%), and assistance in care planning (26%).

Of the 72 programs surveyed, only 1 had undertaken efforts in all six areas of the Model for Effective Chronic Illness Care, although 5 had made efforts in all areas except links to the community. Some programs addressed only one aspect of care, such as self-management support.

We also asked respondents to describe their experience in program development. Resistance to changing practice patterns was the most frequently cited barrier to program implementation. It was difficult for providers to find the time, patience, or resources to develop treatment plans, encourage self-management, and work toward incremental improvements. They also found it difficult to meet the preventive and psychosocial needs of chronically ill patients and respond to their symptoms during the same brief visits.

Respondents stated that active support and commitment from top leadership in the administration, such as a medical director or chief executive officer, were important to program growth. Leaders reinforce the acute care orientation of established systems by measuring and rewarding productivity as number of visits. New programs often require changes in the culture of an organization; thus, supporting a philosophical match between the administrative leadership, program innovators, and the provider team(s) is essential.

Flux in the organizational structure and culture of health care systems was repeatedly cited as a barrier to program implementation. Program staff noted difficulty in implementing amidst tremendous instability, and administrators found it challenging to coordinate a large organization while making basic changes. Problems included significant decreases or turnover in staff. Many program staff felt their programs were underresourced and had difficulty finding funding. Still others reported tensions between projects competing for funding within the organization.

The results of our survey indicate that many systems have implemented efforts to improve chronic illness care, but their effectiveness is often limited by lack of a comprehensive approach to chronic illness care.

EXAMPLES OF EFFECTIVE CHRONIC ILLNESS PROGRAMS

We selected programs for site visiting that appeared to have particularly innovative or effective elements of the model and collectively covered a range of chronic conditions and geographic locations. We site visited programs using a semi-structured interview schedule similar to that used in the larger survey. Four programs that illustrate the application of the model to practice are described here. These successful programs provide a picture of how innovative organizations have used various model elements to respond to the needs of patients with chronic illnesses, and how these applications differ in kind or intensity from more conventional disease management programs.

Congestive Heart Failure

Rich and colleagues (1993, 1995) developed a multidisciplinary team to reduce rehospitalizations among elderly patients with congestive heart failure (CHF) at Washington University Medical Center. Using hospitalization for CHF as the basis of a CHF registry, patients were randomized to receive the multidisciplinary team intervention or usual care. Nurse case managers developed care plans for intervention group patients based on practice guidelines and interactions with geriatric cardiologists. Dietitians and social workers were involved as needed. Patients received one-on-one instruction and a comprehensive booklet to describe their role in the management of CHF. Their transition to the community was eased by a care plan shared by the hospital and home care. Outcomes included decreased costs of care and improved quality of life for intervention group patients. This comprehensive approach to improving chronic illness care used elements of the model, and improved outcomes resulted.

Diabetes Roadmap

Group Health Cooperative of Puget Sound (GHC) has implemented a population-based model for delivery of care, called Roadmaps, for three chronic diseases: diabetes, heart disease, and depression (Wagner, 1995). The Diabetes Roadmap addresses five model components: guidelines for diabetes care, patient education, and self-management support; primary care practice redesign; access to expert support; a diabetes registry; and organizational leadership (McCulloch et al., 1998). The program encourages proactive routine care by the primary care team. Guidelines for the care of patients with diabetes are available on the intranet. Through an automated diabetes registry, providers have access to guideline-driven information on their diabetic patients such as pertinent lab values and dates of the last foot examination and retinal screening. Patients who do not meet guideline criteria are flagged. The provider team can then organize care to meet the needs of a specific panel of patients. An expert team consisting of a diabetologist and nurse specialist travel to primary care clinics to provide support to front-line providers through educational offerings, guideline revision, and joint patient-expert-provider meetings. A patient self-management book that is consistent with the guidelines is provided to patients and used for patient teaching.

The Diabetes Roadmap serves approximately 16,000 people with diabetes, all of whom have received some of the available services. Published results indicate increased adherence to guidelines (McCulloch et al., 1998). Implementation of the program, however, is in part dependent on the readiness of primary care providers to adopt new practice methods.

Cooperative Health Care Clinics

Kaiser-Permanente in Colorado has made systematic efforts to improve patient care and provider satisfaction in caring for chronically ill, high-utilizing elderly patients by redesigning the structure of a typical office visit (Beck et al., 1997). Providers reasoned that the chronically ill elderly had similar needs and that these might be met by providing care in a structured group interaction. The Cooperative Health Care Clinic (CHCC) in Denver, Colorado, brings together about 25 patients with their primary care provider and registered nurse. Visits consist of supportive sharing, information exchange such as a presentation on medication safety by the clinic pharmacist, and individual assessments and triage of patients for individual appointments. Providers and patients plan the session topics together, and patients maintain records of their care in notebooks that they bring to each monthly group session. During a 1-year randomized trial, CHCC visits were found to increase adherence to preventive services, increase satisfaction of patients and providers, and reduce the cost of care for CHCC participants. Alignment of incentives by providers has been made possible by agreement about the appropriate formula for assigning productivity credits for the time devoted to the clinics by providers (Beck et al., 1997). This creative program emphasizes the practice redesign and self-management elements of the model, the components requiring the most substantial changes to traditional clinical practice.

Nurse Case Management for Diabetes

A recently reported randomized trial of nurse case management, conducted at the Jacksonville Health Care Group clinics in Florida, compared to usual care is another example of a systematic effort to improve diabetes care (Aubert et al., 1998). The nurse manager uses behavioral techniques to assist patient self-management efforts, including access to high-quality educational offerings. She follows explicit guidelines for diabetes management and discusses patients regularly with clinical experts and the primary care provider. The case manager follows patients intensively through the use of nurse-initiated telephone calls. Patients are identified from a diabetes registry, and data available from the project are used to support population-based care, such as reminders and feedback to the primary care team. This systematic effort to manage diabetes has resulted in significantly improved HbA1C levels and improved patient health status.

DISCUSSION

We believe the Model for Effective Chronic Illness Care captures the key elements of successful chronic illness programs. Programs with positive results have generally involved comprehensive system changes consistent with the model. Systems contemplating new programs would do well to consider using the model as a checklist to ensure that all critical areas are being addressed.

Most of the "best practice" programs surveyed proved to be limited in their reach and effectiveness. For example, about half of the programs could not identify the size of the population they were to serve or its individual members, and relied on referrals. Of those that could identify their potential patients, nearly half reported that they were serving a minority of the population. Few programs involved large-scale change or redesign of a delivery system, and most were limited to pilot sites. The lack of an effective organizational strategy for implementation and weak linkages to primary care limited the ability of promising pilot programs to expand beyond specialty clinics or pilot sites. Incentives to providers to involve their patients or to patients to become involved were uncommon, which may partially explain the low enrollment in many programs.

Programs that showed improved outcomes in rigorous evaluations ensured the delivery of effective treatments through careful adherence to guidelines. Most used guidelines moderately or extensively and supported guideline implementation by a variety of means: reminder systems, case managers, or specialty involvement in care. In these programs follow-up tended to be more intense than usual care and relied more on telephone calls than on face-to-face visits, which led to earlier identification of patients needing more intensive or more specialized treatment. Finally, successful programs used modern self-management approaches, rather than the more traditional patient education.

Despite the recent flurry of activity around improving chronic illness care in organized health systems, our review of the "best practices" identified relatively few organizations that have made the comprehensive system changes associated with demonstrably better patient and system outcomes. The Model for Effective Chronic Illness Care may provide a road map for organizations wanting to change their systems to better meet the needs of patients with chronic problems.

ACKNOWLEDGMENTS

Adapted with permission from Wagner, E. H., Davis, C., Schaefer, J., Von Korff, M., & Austin, B. (1999). A survey of leading chronic disease management programs: Are they consistent with the literature? *Managed Care Quarterly, 7*(3), 56–66. ©1999, Aspen Publishers, Inc.

REFERENCES

Aubert, R. E., Herman, W. H., Waters, J., Moore, W., Sutton, D., Peterson, B. L., Bailey, C. M., & Koplan, J. P. (1998). Nurse case management to improve glycemic control in diabetic patients in a health maintenance organization: A randomized, controlled trial. *Annals of Internal Medicine, 129*(8), 605–612.

Beck, A., Scott, J., Williams, P., Robertson, B., Jackson, D., Gade, G., & Cowan, P. (1997). A randomized trial of group outpatient visits for chronically ill older HMO members: The Cooperative Health Care Clinic. *Journal of the American Geriatrics Society, 45*(5), 543–549.

Eng, C., Pedulla, J., Eleazer, G. P., McCann, R., & Fox, N. (1997). Program of All-inclusive Care for the Elderly (PACE): An innovative model of integrated geriatric care and financing. *Journal of the American Geriatrics Society, 45*(2), 223–232.

Greenlick, M. R. (1992). Educating physicians for population-based clinical practice. *Journal of the American Medical Association, 267*(12), 1645–1648.

Katon, W., Robinson, P., Von Korff, M., Lin, E., Bush, T., Ludman, E., Simon, G., & Walker, E. (1996). A multifaceted intervention to improve treatment of depression in primary care. *Archives of General Psychiatry, 53*(10), 924–932.

Kirkman, M. S., Weinberger, M., Landsman, P. B., Samsa, G. P., Shortliffe, E. A., Simel, D. L., & Feussner, J. R. (1994). A telephone-delivered intervention for patients with NIDDM: Effect on coronary risk factors. *Diabetes Care, 17*(8), 840–846.

Master, R., Dreyfus, T., Connors, S., Tobias, C., Zhou, Z., & Kronick, R. (1996). The community medical alliance: An integrated system of care in greater Boston for people with severe disability and AIDS. *Managed Care Quarterly, 4*(2), 26–37.

McCulloch, D. K., Price M. J., Nindmarsh, M., & Wagner, E. H. (1998). A population-based approach to diabetes management in a primary care setting: Early results and lessons learned. *Effective Clinical Practice, 1*, 12–22.

Payne, T. N., Galvin, M., Taplin, S. H., Austin, B., Savarino, J., & Wagner, E. H. (1995). Preaching population-based care in an HMO: Evaluation after 18 months. *HMO Practice, 9*, 101–106.

Rich, M. W., Beckham, V., Wittenberg, C., Leven, C. L., Freedland, K. E., & Carney, R. M. (1995). A multidisciplinary intervention to prevent the readmission of elderly patients with congestive heart failure. *New England Journal of Medicine, 333*(18), 1190–1195.

Rich, M. W., Vinson, J. M., Sperry, J. C., Shah, A. S., Spinner, L. R., Chung, M. K., & Davila-Roman, V. (1993). Prevention of readmission in elderly patients with congestive heart failure: Results of a prospective, randomized pilot study. *Journal of General Internal Medicine, 8*(11), 585–590.

Von Korff, M., Gruman, J., Schaefer, J., Curry, S. J., & Wagner E. H. (1997). Collaborative management of chronic illness. *Annals of Internal Medicine, 127*(12), 1097–1102.

Wagner, E. H. (1995). The current status of HMO research. *HMO Practice, 9*(3), 97–98.

Wasson, J., Gaudette, C., Whaley, F., Sauvigne, A., Baribeau, P., & Welch, H. G. (1992). Telephone care as a substitute for routine clinic follow-up. *Journal of the American Medical Association, 267*(13), 1788–1793.

Weinberger, M., Kirkman, M. S., Samsa, G. P., Shortliffe, E. A., Landsman, P. B., Cowper, P. A., Simel, D. L., & Feussner, J. R. (1995). A nurse-coordinated intervention for primary care patients with non-insulin-dependent diabetes mellitus: Impact on glycemic control and health-related quality of life. *Journal of General Internal Medicine, 10*(2), 59–66.

Part V

CAREGIVING

[25]

Coping with Chronic Illness: Lessons from AIDS Caregivers

Susan Folkman

This chapter focuses on coping during the final stages of long-term illness from the perspective of the primary informal caregiver of the person who is dying. In traditional family caregiving situations, informal caregivers are usually spouses or adult children. In the study that formed the basis of this discussion, the primary informal caregivers were gay men whose partners had AIDS. The men were in committed relationships—the average length of relationship was over 6 years, which may not sound like much until one knows that their average age was about 39. The concerns of the men and their responses to their partners' sickness and death are comparable to those of family caregivers. Thus, we can all learn from their experiences and the ways they coped with them.

Let me place this discussion in the context of my own work. Throughout the course of my career I have been intrigued by the question of how people remain sane in the midst of severe and prolonged stress. The question is very different from the question that is traditionally asked about stress, namely: What are its pathological effects? The two questions are two sides of the same coin, but they lead to very different kinds of observations.

STUDY BACKGROUND

In the study reported here, we followed 253 caregiving partners of men with AIDS for up to 5 years. We interviewed them every 2 months for 2

307

years, then every 6 months for 3 additional years. Interviews included a stress and coping battery, measures of mood, and clinical assessments of mental and physical health, among other measures. Nearly two thirds of the caregivers became bereaved during their first 2 years of participation in the research, and of the 145 participants who completed all 5 years of the study, 125 (86%) were bereaved. In short, this was a prospective study of both caregiving and bereavement.

One expected finding was that caregivers reported very high levels of depressive symptoms throughout caregiving. Most had symptoms at levels that meant they were at risk for clinical depression—one to two standard deviations above the mean in the general population (Folkman, 1997). The pattern was comparable to that reported in studies of family caregivers of people with other diseases and by bereaved spouses.

However, despite the very high levels of depressive symptomatology, the incidence of diagnosable major depressive disorder rarely exceeded 5%, which is about what we find in the general population. Further, there were no significant adverse effects on CD4 cells in HIV-infected caregivers as a result of caregiving. Their CD4 cells declined at the same rate as in a comparison group of HIV-positive men in relationships with healthy individuals. Nor were there any significant increases in illness symptoms associated with caregiving in either the HIV-negative or HIV-positive caregivers. Finally, except during the weeks immediately preceding their partner's death, most caregivers reported experiencing positive affect at a frequency comparable to the frequency of negative affect (Folkman, 1997). This finding that caregivers maintained a positive affect in the presence of intense distress is key to understanding how these caregivers managed to remain sane and possibly resistant to adverse physical health effects, throughout caregiving.

During the study, we collected over two thousand accounts of stressful events related to caregiving. No two caregiving events were the same in the details of what happened, but there were three clear underlying themes: coping with uncertainty, the unexpected, and the time of death.

UNCERTAINTY

Dealing with uncertainty is one of the major challenges of caregiving in any disease (Mishel, 1995). Although AIDS is now a chronic albeit eventually fatal disease, until recently AIDS presented one opportunistic infection after another and people never knew what was going to happen next or when, or what the event would be, or whether it could be managed, or what the sequelae would be. Uncertainty was something people had to live with day in and day out, often for years.

Caregivers described a number of different ways of coping with the uncertainty of their partner's disease. Some caregivers used task-oriented or problem-focused coping to deal with the uncertainty. They read up on the disease, took courses on caregiving that were offered by community organizations, and went with their partner to the clinic and tried to learn as much as possible there (Wrubel & Folkman, 1997). (Today these same people would be making wide use of the Internet.) Acquisition of information and skills helped caregivers feel prepared for whatever might happen. It gave them a sense of control, even if such control was illusory, and in this way it bolstered their well-being (Moskowitz, Folkman, Collette, & Vittinghoff, 1996).

This type of preparation was good for caregivers who liked to think into the future and plan. Not every caregiver wanted to do this. Some caregivers dealt with uncertainty by not thinking too far in advance and taking each day as it came. This strategy was useful for regulating distress, but it did little to bolster positive well-being. Still others engaged in denial-like coping to avoid thoughts about the future. This form of coping not only did not bolster well-being, it also increased distress (Moskowitz et al., 1996).

One aspect of coping with uncertainty that was prevalent in these caregivers' narratives involved maintaining hope. Indeed, the maintenance of hope is critical to positive well-being during chronic illness. Hope helps sustain a sense of challenge and a reason for continuing to fight for life. Without it, as Lazarus (1999) noted, there is only despair.

Hope is important for both the caregiver and the ill person. However, the maintenance and the expression of hope that are beneficial for both parties require skill. This was stated succinctly by one caregiver: "The thing was to walk this fine line . . . to try to be up and positive but at the same time not to bullshit him." Formulaic, but unrealistic expressions of hope have a false ring. Rather than comforting the ill person, such expressions make the person feel even more alone; because they are not credible, they are unlikely to be comforting for the caregiver either. The key is that the hope be credible.

The fine line that distinguishes credible hope from hope that is not credible is difficult to walk. To do so well requires that the person who is offering the statement of hope come to terms with what is actually happening. It can be realistic to hope for a good response to a treatment, or for some time off between infections, or even a new drug or treatment that might help control the disease, but it may be unrealistic to hope for the restoration of full immune functioning.

Coming to terms with what is actually happening can often be more difficult for the caregiver than it is for the person who is ill, who may have been living with "the truth" for some time. Many people with AIDS, as well as people with other life-threatening illnesses, have a very realistic appraisal of their chances for improvement or survival, or they have what Weisman (1972) calls "middle knowledge" about their disease—a vague sense of the truth.

The emotions surrounding hope are complex. The process of revising what is hoped for so that hope remains credible involves giving up hope for outcomes that are no longer realistic. This means that credible hope is likely to be preceded or accompanied by sadness or even anger over the loss of what is no longer realistic or even possible to hope for. In this study, the interplay between the positive feelings that accompany newly formed hope and the negative feelings that accompany the loss of earlier hope was often reflected in the mixture of positive and negative emotions that caregivers experienced.

Hope is based on a probability estimate, often a subjective estimate that differs from information coming from knowledgeable others about the objective odds. The fact that hope implies some probability of an unwanted outcome, no matter how much that probability is discounted or ignored, means that hope is also likely to be mixed with worry, fear, or anxiety (see also Lazarus, 1999). The cognitive coping that goes into maintaining an optimistic appraisal of the odds involves positive reappraisal or cognitive reframing that keeps the person focused on the positive, combined with some denial-like coping to help tamp down fear and anxiety.

Regardless of the difficulty of maintaining a hope that is credible and the negative emotions that may surround it, hope should be seen as a necessary, though perhaps not sufficient, condition for psychological well-being in the midst of the distress associated with a chronic and deteriorating condition.

THE UNEXPECTED

As noted above, until recently AIDS was notorious for its unpredictable, complex, and clinically devastating course. Here is one caregiver's account of what his partner had been through during the previous two years:

> In less than 2 years, my lover has had lymphoma and three rounds of chemo, a brain infection that has partially paralyzed one hand and caused multiple grand mal seizures, pneumonia six times, disseminated TB, which damaged his liver and heart, an infection of the eyes that left him partially blind and

continues to threaten his sight, and a gastrointestinal problem of undetermined origin which makes it impossible for him to eat. . . . At the least, one result is the feeling that you can't escape this thing. You get through one crisis and, BAM, you're hit with another.

The only thing that was certain in the lives of this couple was that something unexpected was bound to happen sometime soon. Often the unexpected events precipitated immediate problem-focused instrumental action, such as getting the patient cleaned up, taking care of a wound, changing a medication, or going to the clinic. Once instrumental needs were taken care of, there was often a delayed but strong emotional response on the part of the caregiver. Here, the unexpected finding I want to highlight was that caregivers turned to their ill partners for emotional support.

We often assume that support flows one way in a caregiving relationship—from the caregiver to the care recipient. This is an incorrect assumption. In over half our interviews about stressful events related to caregiving, the response to our question Who was most helpful in this event? was "My partner." This simple finding has very important implications. Even though the partner was ill and the stressful event had to do with his care, the partner was still the most frequently cited source of support. One of the most frequent ways in which this support was elicited was as a response to admitted distress.

Bill and his partner, Ted, were among those who spoke openly with one another about their own distress when they were thrown off balance by an unexpected and unwanted event—in this case, a sudden drop in Ted's CD4 cells from a count of 225 to 83. Bill said:

> I have heard of swings, but not this dramatic. It was frightening. I expected bad news, but nothing this bad. His doctor is rather honest and direct, and he warned Ted that the DDI [Didanosina] may not help him now. His weight loss is severe. Three weeks ago he lost 3 pounds in a weekend. He is also having severe cramps and uncontrollable diarrhea. We were both in tears. It was like hitting the wall. Later we talked, just talked. The talking helped me.

Although most caregivers let their distress be known, some did not. People have many reasons for not sharing their distress. We are often uncomfortable about revealing our true feelings about another person's bad news. We argue that the other person needs us to be strong and this is no time to show our own concern. We also argue that if we register intense distress, we will confirm the ill person's fears and in that way make him feel worse. Some of us also realize that to acknowledge concern out loud confirms our own worst fears. As long as we do not acknowledge out loud what is going on, we can deny or minimize the significance of what we have learned.

Sometimes arguments in favor of not sharing one's own distress in response to another person's bad news are valid. It depends on the people and the relationship between them. In general, however, sharing fears and worries seems more mutually beneficial than not sharing. Distress may be heightened, especially at first, as each person recognizes the other's anguish; at the same time, this type of sharing increases intimacy, which can be an important source of strength and psychological well-being, especially over the long haul.

The finding that caregivers and their ill partners provided support to each other has important implications for interventions. When we reviewed the literature on caregiver and patient psychosocial interventions, we found that, for the most part, caregivers were sent off to their own groups for support, and patients were sent to theirs. In the few instances in which interventions were designed for the couple, the setting was a couples group. My colleagues and I are now involved in trying to develop an intervention for caregivers and their care recipients that builds on the strengths of the relationship between the two.

WHEN THE UNEXPECTED YIELDS TO THE EXPECTED— DYING AND DEATH

For most patients in this study, the treatment arsenal eventually was exhausted and there was nothing the person with HIV, the physician, or the caregiver could do to slow the course of the disease. Uncertainty and the unexpected yielded to the realization that death was inevitable and imminent.

Ultimately, the caregiver had to make the very painful shift from helping the partner live to helping him let go of life and die. He had to adjust to the loss of hope and begin preparing for the partner's death. Both members of the dyad often experienced complex emotions during this phase. There was sadness and a sense of loss that the battle had been lost, there was relief that a losing battle would come to an end, and, importantly from the perspective of well-being, there was a renewed sense of purpose directed at helping the partner live well while dying and ultimately die well.

Matt said:

> He has gone into the actual situation of dying. For the last 2 weeks he has been talking about it. He wanted the doctor to put him in the hospital for IVs to make him stronger. And the doctor refused and said nothing would

help. When we got home it only took him about 4 hours to realize this is the end. "There is no hope," he said. "This almost makes it easier," he added. "There's no hope. Now I can start letting go." The comforting part is he's at peace with that decision. He wasn't resigned . . . it was just finally okay. That makes it a lot easier for me. He's comfortable with his decision to let go and not in a lot of emotional turmoil. That would be hard to deal with.

Dying is rarely a peaceful, dignified process, as Nuland (1995) so eloquently observes in his book *How We Die.* Death, he says, is "all too frequently a series of destructive events that involve by their very nature the disintegration of the dying person's humanity" (p. xvii). The conditions that characterize the terminal phases of AIDS certainly stack the deck against the possibility of a peaceful and dignified dying process.

The bereavement narratives provided by these caregivers shortly after their partners' deaths, usually within days, offer a glimpse of the emotions caregivers experienced in this moment of profound loss. As in every aspect of the caregiving process, from its earliest stages through the final moments of the ill partner's life, the emotions at the time of death were intense and complicated. Anger, sadness, and despair resided alongside the more comforting emotions of love and relief. There is nothing easy about seeing a loved one die.

Each of the bereavement narratives from these caregivers was unique, not only because of differences in the details of how the ill partner died, but also because of the unique qualities of each caregiver who told his story. Caregivers viewed the experience through their own individual perceptual lenses. No two people watching the same patient die would tell the same story. Nevertheless, several features were common to many of the narratives:

- The caregiver assured his partner of his love.
- The caregiver told his partner that it was all right to die.
- The caregiver felt relief when death finally came and the partner's suffering was ended.
- The caregiver took comfort in the deceased partner's peaceful appearance.

These features speak to the theme of maintaining positive well-being in the presence of severe stress.

The following narrative is one of my favorites. The things this caregiver said to his dying partner served the dual function of reassuring and comforting both the caregiver and his dying partner. In part this was done through the use of spiritual metaphors. Indeed, spirituality was salient in many of the narratives and seemed especially comforting at the time of the partner's death. Finally, a gentle and loving humor is obvious in this story. This type of humor was found in many of the narratives, and I find it particularly moving.

Jeff (age 43):

> I came over and said, "Gordon, are you asleep?" He started to twitch and shake, his eyes were moving. I put my arms around him and said, "Just relax. If there's anything you need me to do, you put that thought in my head." I sat there for a while, and I started crying and said, "Honey, I'm not crying because I want you to stay. I'm crying because I am going to miss you. I have never been one to hold you back from what you wanted to do. If this is what you want to do, need to do, have to do, then I will try to make it as easy as possible for you to do." . . . I put some music on and came over and talked to him, touched and held him and told him things about people he was going to see up there. I told him his friend was probably in line waiting for his wings and maybe he will bump [him] up. I asked one thing: "Please don't ask them for extra fluffy wings. Don't ask for them with black trim. Just take what they give you and make the best of it." I was playing Sylvester's *Immortal* album. Gordon was one of his biggest fans, and I told him that Sylvester was up there too. I told him to reach out and he would help him up. I said, "Just don't be prettier than he is, or he's going to put you at the end of the line." I said, "There are a lot of people up there, so you go up there. But save me space, and you will know when I am coming because there will be a bright pink glow." I would laugh and go out of the room and cry. I could tell by the way he was reacting that I was saying all the right things. He seemed much more relaxed. I said that I didn't want him to go, but it was okay. I would miss him for a while, but I wouldn't have to miss him because he would always be here; he had become part of me. It was great, and I'm glad we had a chance to tell each other and really know what we were saying and why. Some people don't get that. I am at peace. I know that I did my best, and he did too. He went very peacefully at 3:00 in the morning.

By no means were all the deaths as peaceful as the one described by this man, but the narrative illustrates the extraordinary human capacity for experiencing positive well-being in the midst of excruciating sadness and loss.

ACKNOWLEDGMENTS

The study reported in this chapter was supported by grants MH49985 and MH52517 from the National Institute of Mental Health, and MH58069 from the National Institute of Mental Health and the National Institute of Nursing Research.

REFERENCES

Folkman, S. (1997). Positive psychological states and coping with severe stress. *Social Science and Medicine, 45,* 1207–1221.

Lazarus, R. S. (1999). *Stress and emotion.* New York: Springer.

Mishel, M. H. (1995). Response to adult uncertainty in illness: A critical review of research. *Scholarly Inquiry for Nursing Practice, 9,* 25–29.

Moskowitz, J., Folkman, S., Collette, L., & Vittinghoff, E. (1996). Coping and mood during AIDS-related caregiving and bereavement. *Annals of Behavioral Medicine, 18,* 49–57.

Nuland, S. (1995). *How we die: Reflections on life's last chapter.* New York: Vintage Books.

Weisman, A. D. (1972). *On dying and denying: A psychiatric study of terminality.* New York: Behavioral Publications.

Wrubel, J., & Folkman, S. (1997). What caregivers actually do: The caregiving skills of partners of men with AIDS. *AIDS Care, 9,* 691–706.

[26]

Effects of an Abilities-focused Program of Morning Care on Residents Who Have Dementia and on Caregivers

Donna L. Wells, Pamela Dawson, Souraya Sidani, Dorothy Craig, and Dorothy Pringle

In long-term care institutions, morning care occurs between 7:00 A.M. and noon as caregivers are engaged with residents in activities related to bathing, grooming, dressing, and toileting. Morning care is difficult for both residents and caregivers; this is the time when touch and close, intimate contact occur between the two and when agitation in residents is most frequent (Aronson, Post, & Guastadisegni, 1993; Bridges-Parlet, Knopman, & Thompson, 1994; Burgener, Jirovec, Murrell, & Barton, 1992; Cohen-Mansfield, Marx, & Rosenthal, 1989; Miller, 1997; Ryden, Bossenmaier, & McLachlan, 1991; Sloane et al., 1995). Agitated behaviors in residents have been associated with anxiety in caregivers, poorer quality of care, and fiscal strain on institutions because of the need for a high caregiver-to-resident ratio and caregivers' loss of time due to injuries (Beck, Baldwin, Modlin, & Lewis, 1990; Cohen-Mansfield et al., 1989; Taft & Cronin-Stubbs, 1995).

Burgener and colleagues (1992) and Hallberg, Holst, Nordmark, and Edberg (1995) note that residents' and caregivers' behaviors in caregiving situations are related. In a controlled repeated-measures study in two long-term care facilities, Burgener et al. (1992) found significant relationships between caregivers' relaxed and smiling behaviors and residents' calm/ functional behaviors during bathing, dressing, and toileting. In their 18-month, observational qualitative study on two units in one long-term care setting, Hallberg et al. (1995) found that in high-quality cooperative situations, where the nurse and patient reciprocally controlled the extent of resident participation in care and the pace of the activity, there was an absence of escaping behavior and aggression by residents. The investigators concluded that resident behaviors may be relational rather than personal or disease-related. This suggests a need to teach caregivers about the influence of their own behavior on the behaviors of residents (Beck & Shue, 1994; Ryden et al., 1991).

Hagen and Sayers (1995) found a reduction in physical aggression following the implementation of a 3-month staff education program that outlined general goals of care and broad strategies to deescalate resident aggression once it had occurred. Similar findings were reported by Maxfield, Lewis, and Cannon (1996) and Hoeffer, Rader, McKenzie, Lavelle, and Stewart (1997), who used general practice concepts to guide the bathing and grooming practices of caregivers. Dawson, Bruce, and Wells (1994) educated caregivers to provide care based on an understanding of the effects of dementia on people's abilities and found an improvement in residents' level of function and morale and a decrease in their agitation. None of these studies, however, were controlled investigations, and no studies have examined systematic programs of morning care designed to optimize institutionalized residents' level of functioning and interactions and to facilitate caregiving.

The study reported here was a controlled investigation of the effects of an abilities-focused educational program on residents' interaction behaviors, level of agitation, and level of function during morning care, and on caregivers' interaction behaviors and perceptions of caregiving. Residents with dementia who received morning care from caregivers trained in the abilities-focused program were expected to demonstrate increased interaction behaviors with caregivers, decreased agitation, and a higher level of function than residents with dementia who received the usual approach to care. Further, caregivers trained in the abilities-focused approach were expected to show more interactions with residents, greater perceived ease of caregiving, and less stress than caregivers who provided usual morning care.

METHODS

Setting

The study was conducted on four cognitive support units for people with dementia in the nursing home section of a large, university-affiliated geriatric center for the care of the elderly. One of the units had 43 beds; the remaining three had 45 beds each. The ratio of caregivers to residents was 1:7 during the morning care period on all of the units. Caregiver assignments to residents were consistent on all units, and the composition of staff was similar across the units.

Design

A quasi-experimental, repeated-measures design was used to evaluate the effects of the abilities-focused program of morning care. Data were collected at three points: before the implementation of the program (baseline), and at 3 (posttest 1) and 6 (posttest 2) months following program delivery.

One of the four participating units was randomly selected as the experimental unit, and the other three served as control units. Caregivers on the experimental unit were taught to provide the abilities-focused program of care, whereas caregivers on the control units provided the usual morning care.

Sample

Inclusion criteria for residents were a medical diagnosis of dementia, a moderate or severe level of cognitive impairment (Mini-Mental State Examination [MMSE] < 19), and a length of stay on the unit of at least 4 weeks. In order to establish initial group equivalence, residents for the control group were recruited if they were of the same gender, their scores on the MMSE were within 5 points, and their ages were within 5 years of the experimental unit residents' values.

Proxy consent from a family member was obtained for participating residents, and informed written consent was obtained from caregivers. A total of 108 residents were approached for the study, 85 (78.7%) of whom consented to participate. Twenty-nine control residents were not able to be matched to residents on the experimental unit and therefore were excluded. Of the 56 residents on whom baseline data were collected, 16 were lost during the study—an attrition rate of 28.5%. Of these 16 residents, 8 were on the experimental unit and 8 on the control units. Resident death resulting from a flu epidemic on the units was the major reason for subject loss. The final sample consisted of 40 residents and 44 caregivers. Of the 40 residents, 20 were in the experimental unit and 20 in the control units. Of the 44 caregivers, 16 were assigned to the experimental unit and 28 to the control units.

Intervention

The researchers gave all participating caregivers on the experimental unit a five-session educational program on abilities-focused morning care. They were informed about the effects of dementia on the social and self-care abilities of people with dementia, taught a standardized method of assessment for abilities remaining or lost (Dawson, Wells, Reid, & Sidani, 1998), and shown various interventions that can maintain abilities or compensate for those that are diminished (Dawson, Wells, & Kline, 1993).

Abilities-focused care is founded on the concept of enabling or assisting an individual to use her or his abilities. It is described in the book *Enhancing the Abilities of Older Persons with Alzheimer's and Related Dementias: A Nursing Perspective* by Dawson et al. (1993), which also details various assessment and caregiving approaches. More recent research was also incorporated into the program used here. We concentrated on the effects of dementia on the social abilities of giving and receiving attention, being socially accessible, and engaging in conversation and on the self-care abilities of spatial orientation, voluntary movements, and purposeful movements. Twelve interventions on social abilities and 17 interventions on self-care abilities were taught to caregivers. For example, the ways in which bathing and dressing an individual with dementia may be affected by the appearance of the grasp reflex were demonstrated based on research about primitive reflexes. The related interventions of avoiding stimulation of the palm during bathing and moving the hand by holding the top of it were taught. One-page summaries were provided for the studies on which the interventions were based.

The feasibility of providing an educational program on a busy nursing unit and encouraging the attendance of caregivers was enhanced by keeping the sessions short (20 to 30 minutes); conducting the sessions on the nursing unit; incorporating an exercise, role play, or game that required the participation of caregivers; and providing refreshments during the sessions. Each session was repeated until all the caregivers on the experimental unit had received all five sessions. To ensure the consistency of the teaching, a manual was developed for the educational program.

Reinforcement sessions lasting 20 to 30 minutes were provided every second week for 3 months, then monthly for an additional 3 months. In these sessions, caregivers were asked to share their experiences in implementing what had been taught in the program. This served to stimulate discussion among the caregivers, and each caregiver's experience served to reinforce the learning of the other caregivers. When appropriate, the researchers reinforced how the research literature supported the observations and experiences of the caregivers.

To check on program implementation, a research assistant used an abilities-focused intervention checklist developed by the researchers to observe 10 randomly selected caregivers. The checks were conducted on three separate occasions during the 6-month intervention phase of the study. The research assistant who collected the data was unaware of the units' assignment to the experimental and control groups at all times during the study period. To avoid spreading information from the experimental to the control units, the experimental unit caregivers were requested not to discuss the program with colleagues outside their assigned unit. At the conclusion of the study, both the research assistant and the nurses on the control units indicated that they had not known about the educational program.

Measures

The outcome variables for residents were measures of their interaction behaviors, level of agitation, and level of function. The outcome variables for caregivers included measures of their interaction behaviors, perceived ease of caregiving, and level of stress.

Residents' Interaction Behaviors

The Modified Interaction Behavior Measure (MIBM; Burgener et al., 1992) was used to measure interaction behaviors and agitation. The MIBM is an observational measure that consists of two subscales using a 7-point semantic-differential rating scale. The subscales measure residents' personal attending and calm/functional behaviors. The items agitated/calm and resistant/cooperative within the calm/functional subscale constitute one measure of agitation. Higher scores indicate more positive behaviors. The internal consistency (> .80) and interrater reliability (estimates > .70) of the MIBM were demonstrated by Burgener et al. (1992) and in this study.

Residents' Level of Agitation

The Pittsburgh Agitation Scale (PAS; Rosen et al., 1994) was an additional observational measure of residents' agitation. Higher scores on this scale indicate greater agitation. The PAS has demonstrated interrater and internal consistency reliability (estimates > .80 in Rosen et al. [1994] and in this study).

Residents' Level of Function

The London Psychogeriatric Rating Scale (LPRS; Hersch, Kral, & Palmer, 1978), a 36-item rating scale, was used to measure the level of residents' functioning during morning care. The scale was completed by caregivers. The LPRS consists of four subscales reflecting mental, social, physical, and disengagement dimensions of function. Each item is rated as occurring *never* (0), *occasionally/sometimes* (1), or *often/frequently* (2). Higher scores indicate greater disability. The LPRS has an established interrater reliability of .92 and a concurrent validity of .79 (Hersch et al., 1978; Merskey et al., 1980; Reid, Tierney, Zorzitto, Snow, & Fisher, 1991). All subscales demonstrated acceptable internal consistency reliability in this study.

Caregivers' Interaction Behaviors

The Interaction Behavior Measure (IBM; McCrosky & Wright, 1971) was used to examine caregivers' interaction behaviors. This is an observational, 7-point semantic-differential rating scale, which consists of four subscales measuring the following behaviors: (1) relevance, (2) personal attending, (3) relaxed, and (4) social/flexible. Higher scores reflect more positive caregiver behaviors. Internal consistency estimates between .64 and .92 (> .80 in this study) and interrater reliability coefficients between .89 and .95 (> .80 in this study) have been reported for the subscales (Burgener et al., 1992; Burgoon & Aho, 1982; McCrosky & Wright, 1971).

Caregivers' Perceived Ease of Caregiving

A visual analogue scale (VAS) consisting of a 100-mm line was used to determine caregivers' perceptions of ease of caregiving. A VAS was used because it has been found to be valid in capturing subjective perceptions of phenomena (Waltz, Strickland, & Lenz, 1991). The VAS anchors were *giving care to the residents is very difficult* (0) and *giving care to the residents is very easy* (100).

Caregivers' Level of Stress

Caregivers' stress was measured with the 41-item Hassles subscale of the Nurses' Hassles and Uplifts Scale (NHUS; Craig, Khan, & Williams, 1995). Higher scores reflect greater stress. The Hassles subscale has demonstrated internal consistency (> .80) and test-retest reliability (coefficient ≥ .70) and initial concurrent validity ($r = 0.77$, $p = .0001$) (Craig et al., 1995). Caregivers completed the measure at baseline and at posttest 2.

A research assistant who was blind to the study design was trained to collect data during observations of morning care using the MIBM, PAS, and IBM. Later on the same day, the same research assistant collected information about caregivers' perceptions of the residents' level of function (LPRS), caregivers' perceptions of caregiving (VAS), and their level of stress (NHUS). Interrater reliability checks on the observational measures were conducted prior to study start-up by a research assistant and two of the investigators, who used videotapes of morning care sessions in long-term care. Further, for every 10th subject, interrater reliability of the measures was checked at the three data collection points—baseline and at 3 (posttest 1) and 6 months (posttest 2) following program implementation—by the same research assistant and one of the investigators. Internal consistency of the observational measures was also evaluated.

RESULTS

Characteristics of the Experimental and Control Groups

Over 80% of the residents in both groups were female; the mean age in each group was between 88 and 89 years, and the majority of residents were diagnosed with dementia (70% in each group) or alzheimer's disease (25% to 30% of each group). Chi-square tests and independent sample *t*-tests were performed to examine differences between the experimental and control groups at baseline. No significant ($p = .05$) differences were observed between the two groups of residents on any of the variables, suggesting that the experimental and control groups were initially equivalent.

The vast majority of caregivers were females (over 90% of each group) in their mid forties (mean ages of the groups were between 44 and 45). On average, they had more than 10 years of long-term care experience and had worked on the unit for more than 5 years. Almost half of the caregivers were health care aides, with the remainder being split fairly evenly between registered nurses and registered practical nurses. Significant (p = .05) differences were found in the education and employment status of caregivers in the two groups. More nurses in the experimental group than in the control group had completed a baccalaureate degree (χ^2 = 15.1, df = 5, p = .01), and more were employed on a full-time basis (81% vs. 15%; χ^2 = 8.23, df = 2, p = .016).

Effects of the Abilities-focused Program on Residents' Outcomes

As expected, residents who received morning care from caregivers trained in the abilities-focused program demonstrated increased interaction behaviors with caregivers, decreased agitation, and a higher level of function. When a repeated measures analysis of variance (RM-ANOVA) was used to compare residents in the experimental and control groups on change from baseline to time 2 (6 months postintervention), a significant group × time interaction effect was found for residents' personal-attending, calm-functional, and agitation behaviors (see Table 26.1). Residents in the experimental group showed a moderate increase in their scores on the calm-functional and agitation subscales of the MIBM, whereas residents in the control group showed a decrease in these scores. Residents in both groups declined on the personal-attending subscale; however, the drop in the scores on this subscale was greater for those in the control than in the experimental group. The mean scores on the three subscales were significantly different at posttest 2 (p < .05), indicating that the interactions of the residents receiving abilities-focused morning care were more positive and appropriate than the interactions of the residents who received usual care.

Residents in both groups had relatively low levels of agitation on the PAS throughout the study period (means in the lower one third of the possible .01–1.0 range). However, the residents who received morning care from caregivers trained in the abilities-focused approach demonstrated a steady decline in agitation over time, whereas by posttest 2 the control group exhibited greater agitation than they had at baseline. At posttest 2, agitation was significantly lower in experimental group residents than in control group residents (t (38) = −2.12, p = .041). The results suggested that agitation during morning care was reduced for those residents receiving abilities-focused care.

Residents in both groups were moderately disabled. However, as shown in Table 26.1, total scores on the LPRS decreased for experimental residents, indicating improvement in their overall level of function compared to residents in the control group. The difference between the two groups was significant at posttest 2 (t (38) = 2.37, p = .023).

TABLE 26.1 Mean Scores and Standard Deviations on Residents' Outcome Measures

Variable	Group[1]	Baseline		Posttest 1		Posttest 2		Group × time effect		
		Mean	(SD)	Mean	(SD)	Mean	(SD)	F	df	p
Modified Interaction Behavior Measure (MIBM)[2]										
Personal attending	Control	4.02	(.95)	3.09	(1.11)	3.08	(.78)	3.36	2,76	.040
	Experimental	4.07	(.98)	3.82	(1.06)	3.73	(1.15)			
Calm/ functional	Control	4.09	(.91)	4.25	(.94)	3.92	(1.16)	3.94	2,76	.023
	Experimental	4.11	(.82)	4.43	(.97)	4.68	(1.06)			
Agitation	Control	4.55	(1.23)	4.91	(1.28)	4.11	(1.48)	4.06	2,76	.021
	Experimental	4.50	(1.06)	4.94	(1.14)	5.02	(1.21)			
Pittsburgh Agitation Scale (PAS)[3]	Control	.29	(.38)	.16	(.31)	.33	(.38)	4.43	2,37	.019
	Experimental	.35	(.33)	.25	(.29)	.17	(.24)			
London Psychogeriatric Rating Scale (LPRS)[4]	Control	1.16	(.25)	1.15	(.17)	1.20	(.15)	3.84	3,37	.030
	Experimental	1.18	(.18)	1.09	(.26)	1.04	(.25)			
Subscales:										
Mental	Control	1.23	(.31)	1.21	(.23)	1.24	(.16)	1.25	2,37	.293
	Experimental	1.57	(.26)	1.11	(.37)	1.04	(.24)			
Physical	Control	1.35	(.40)	1.25	(.31)	1.42	(.33)	1.74	2,37	.183
	Experimental	1.37	(.28)	1.22	(.35)	1.28	(.38)			
Social	Control	0.61	(.40)	0.59	(.45)	0.57	(.42)	4.47	2,37	.015
	Experimental	0.83	(.48)	0.60	(.38)	0.45	(.32)			
Disengagement	Control	.48	(.25)	1.60	(.13)	1.61	(.10)	.36	2,37	.694
	Experimental	1.41	(.33)	1.50	(.30)	1.46	(.36)			

[1]Control (n = 20); experimental (n = 20).
[2]A 7-point semantic-differential rating scale; higher score indicates more positive resident behaviors.
[3]Higher scores indicate greater agitation.
[4]Items score from 0 to 2, with higher scores indicating greater disability.

For the subscales of the LPRS, a significant group × time interaction effect was found only for the social function subscale. The control group began with a lower level of socially inappropriate behavior than the experimental group, but they did not change throughout the study period. In contrast, the residents who received abilities-focused care showed a constant decrease in socially inappropriate behavior. The differences in the groups' mean scores on the LPRS and social subscale were significant at posttest 2 ($p < .05$), indicating that residents in the experimental group had improved their overall and social function, unlike those in the control group.

Effects of the Abilities-focused Program on Caregivers' Outcomes

Caregivers trained in the abilities-focused approach showed increased interactive behaviors with residents; caregivers who provided usual morning care did not. When RM-ANOVA was used to compare caregivers in the experimental and control groups on change from baseline to time 2 (6 months postintervention), there were significant group × time interaction effects on caregivers' verbal relevance, personal-attending, relaxed, and social/flexible behaviors (see Table 26.2).

On the subscales of verbal relevance, personal-attending, and relaxed behaviors, experimental caregivers' scores consistently increased throughout the study period, whereas the caregivers in the control group declined from their baseline scores on these subscales. Thus, caregivers who received the abilities-focused educational program were interacting with the residents in a more personal and relevant way than caregivers who did not receive the program.

Social/flexible behaviors of caregivers improved slightly but not significantly between baseline and posttest 2 in the experimental group (paired t (19) = 3.10, $p = .006$), while they decreased in the control group. The significant difference between the two groups at posttest 2 (t (38) = −3.08, $p = .005$) indicated that caregivers in the experimental group demonstrated more social/flexible behaviors than control caregivers when interacting with residents during morning care. However, caregivers trained in the abilities-focused approach did not perceive a greater ease of caregiving or a lower level of stress than those providing usual morning care.

DISCUSSION

The abilities-focused educational program for caregivers enhanced the interaction behaviors of residents as well as their social and overall function.

TABLE 26.2 Mean Scores and Standard Deviations on Caregivers' Outcome Measures

Variable	Group[1]	Baseline Mean	(SD)	Posttest 1 Mean	(SD)	Posttest 2 Mean	(SD)	Group × time effect F	df	p
Interaction Behavior Measure (IBM)[2]										
Verbal	Control	5.38	(.83)	5.13	(.81)	5.29	(.99)	6.30	3,37	.003
	Experimental	5.53	(.54)	5.89	(.71)	6.10	(.74)			
Personal attending	Control	3.43	(1.36)	2.83	(1.57)	2.80	(1.62)	4.08	3,37	.021
	Experimental	3.69	(1.11)	3.93	(1.40)	4.12	(1.42)			
Relaxed	Control	4.93	(1.06)	4.52	(1.20)	4.57	(1.25)	3.85	3,37	.026
	Experimental	5.37	(.83)	5.58	(.73)	5.92	(.98)			
Social/ flexible	Control	3.42	(.70)	3.12	(.49)	2.97	(.46)	4.94	3,37	.010
	Experimental	3.53	(.57)	3.71	(.56)	3.68	(.91)			
Ease of caregiving[3]	Control	32.9	(27.2)	26.8	(22.7)	32.1	(23.4)	.97	2,37	.382
	Experimental	37.6	(27.2)	29.6	(25.7)	44.7	(27.6)			
Stress[4]	Control	1.88	(.66)			2.25	(.75)	.210	1,17	.650
	Experimental	1.54	(.85)			1.91	(1.16)			

[1]Control ($n = 28$); experimental ($n = 16$).
[2]A seven-point semantic-differential rating scale; higher score indicates more positive caregiver behaviors.
[3]A visual analogue scale; anchors are *giving care to residents is very difficult* (0) and *giving care to residents is very easy* (100).
[4]Higher scores indicate greater stress.

Residents in the experimental group were more personal, interested, and involved, and more relaxed than those in the control group. This finding is consistent with the work of Burgener et al. (1992) and Hallberg et al. (1995), who found a significant relationship between positive caregiver and resident behaviors.

Also, residents who received the abilities-focused program showed a decline in agitation and were calmer and more cooperative. The focus on abilities may thus prevent the emergence of excess disability.

The program improved caregivers' interaction behaviors. The effects were most evident at 6 months, suggesting that it may take some time for caregivers to internalize new knowledge and adjust their practices. Also, it should be noted that caregivers in the experimental group had a higher educational level, and more caregivers in this group than in the control group were employed full-time. Educational preparation and employment status might have moderated the effects of the educational program.

The lack of effect on perceived ease of caregiving and caregivers' level of stress is not surprising. All caregivers found caregiving difficult, which is consistent with other descriptions of caring for residents with dementia (Hagen & Sayers, 1995; Hallberg et al., 1995). It has been suggested that advanced understanding of dementia may be associated with more positive perceptions of caregiving (Feldt & Ryden, 1992), but that was not the case in this study. Although more nurses in the experimental group had completed a university degree, they did not perceive caregiving as easier or less stressful than the control caregivers.

Caring for people who have dementia is an arduous task. Nonetheless, this study provides evidence of the positive effects that an abilities-focused educational program for caregivers can have on both caregivers and residents, despite the progressive nature of dementia. No changes or additions to staff were required to implement the abilities-focused program. These promising results suggest that caregiving practices should be oriented toward the abilities of people with dementia because of their positive effects on residents' interaction behaviors, agitation, and function, and on caregivers' interaction behaviors.

ACKNOWLEDGMENTS

This research was supported by a grant from the Alzheimer's Societies of Canada and Ontario (#96-23), which the authors gratefully acknowledge. Also, the editorial support of Barbara Bauer from the Faculty of Nursing, University of Toronto, was very much appreciated. This chapter is adapted from Wells, D. L., Dawson, P., Sidani, S., Craig, D., & Pringle, D. (2000). Effects of morning care on residents who have dementia and on caregivers. *Journal of the American Geriatrics Society, 48*(4). Copyright by Lippincott, Williams & Wilkins, 1999. Printed with permission.

REFERENCES

Aronson, M. K., Post, D. C., & Guastadisegni, P. (1993). Dementia, agitation, and care in the nursing home. *Journal of the American Geriatrics Society, 41*, 507–512.

Beck, C., Baldwin, B., Modlin, T., & Lewis, S. (1990). Caregivers' perception of aggressive behaviour in cognitively impaired nursing home residents. *Journal of Neuroscience Nursing, 22,* 169–172.

Beck, C. K., & Shue, V. M. (1994). Interventions for treating disruptive behaviour in demented elderly people. *Nursing Clinics of North America, 29,* 143–153.

Bridges-Parlet, S., Knopman, D., & Thompson, T. (1994). A descriptive study of physically aggressive behaviour in dementia by direct observation. *Journal of the American Geriatrics Society, 42,* 192–197.

Burgener, S. C., Jirovec, M., Murrell, L., & Barton, D. (1992). Caregiver and environmental variables related to difficult behaviors in institutionalized, demented elderly persons. *Journal of Gerontology (Psychological Sciences), 47,* P242–P249.

Burgoon, J. K., & Aho, L. (1982). Violations of conversational distance. *Communication Monographs, 49,* 71–79.

Cohen-Mansfield, J., Marx, M., & Rosenthal, A. (1989). A description of agitation in a nursing home. *Journal of Gerontology (Medical Sciences), 44,* M77–M84.

Craig, D., Kahn, P., & Williams, J. (1995). *Nurses Hassles and Uplifts Scale.* Unpublished report.

Dawson, P., Bruce, B., & Wells, D. (1994, November). *Evaluation of a clinical program for elderly people with cognitive impairment.* Paper presented at the 47th Annual Gerontological Society of America Meeting, Atlanta.

Dawson, P., Wells, D. L., & Kline, K. (1993). *Enhancing the abilities of older persons with Alzheimer's and related dementias: A nursing perspective.* New York: Springer.

Dawson, P., Wells, D. L., Reid, D., & Sidani, S. (1998). An abilities assessment instrument for elderly persons with cognitive impairment: Psychometric properties and clinical utility. *Journal of Nursing Measurement, 6,* 35–54.

Feldt, K. S., & Ryden, M. B. (1992). Aggressive behaviour: Educating nursing assistants. *Journal of Gerontological Nursing, 18,* 3–12.

Hagen, B. F., & Sayers, D. (1995). When caring leaves bruises: The effects of staff education on resident aggression. *Journal of Gerontological Nursing, 21,* 7–16.

Hallberg, I. R., Holst, G., Nordmark, A., & Edberg, A. (1995). Cooperation during morning care between nurses and severely demented institutionalized patients. *Clinical Nursing Research, 4,* 78–104.

Hersch, E. L., Kral, V. A., & Palmer, R. B. (1978). Clinical value of the London Psychogeriatric Rating Scale. *Journal of the American Geriatrics Society, 26,* 348–354.

Hoeffer, B., Rader, J., McKenzie, D., Lavelle, M., & Stewart, B. (1997). Reducing aggressive behavior during bathing cognitively impaired nursing home residents. *Journal of Gerontological Nursing, 23,* 16–23.

Maxfield, M., Lewis, R. E., & Cannon, S. (1996). Training staff to prevent aggressive behavior of cognitively impaired elderly patients during bathing and grooming. *Journal of Gerontological Nursing, 22,* 37–43.

McCrosky, J. C., & Wright, D. W. (1971). The development of an instrument for measuring interaction behaviour for groups. *Speech Monographs, 38,* 25–131.

Merskey, H., Ball, M., Blume, W., Fox. A., Hersch, E., Kral, V., & Palmer, R. (1980). Relationships between psychological measurements and cerebral organic changes in Alzheimer's disease. *Canadian Journal of Neurological Science, 7,* 45–49.

Miller, M. F. (1997). Physically aggressive resident behaviour during hygienic care. *Journal of Gerontological Nursing, 23,* 24–39.

Reid, D. W., Tierney, M. C., Zorzitto, M. I., Snow, G., & Fisher, R. H. (1991). On the clinical value of the London Psychogeriatric Rating Scale. *Journal of the American Geriatrics Society, 39,* 368–371.

Rosen, M. D., Burgio, L., Koller, M., Cain, M., Allison, M., Fogleman, M., Micheal, M., & Zubenko, G. S. (1994). The Pittsburgh Agitation Scale: A user friendly instrument for rating agitation in patients. *American Journal of Geriatric Psychiatry, 2,* 52–58.

Ryden, M. B., Bossenmaier, M., & McLachlan, C. (1991). Aggressive behaviour in cognitively impaired nursing home residents. *Research in Nursing and Health, 14,* 87–95.

Sloane, P. D., Rader, J., Barrick, A.-L., Hoeffer, B., Dwyer, S., McKenzie, D., Lavelle, M., Buckwalter, K., Arrington, L., & Pruitt, T. (1995). Bathing persons with dementia. *The Gerontologist, 35,* 672–678.

Taft, L. B., & Cronin-Stubbs, D. (1995). Behavioural symptoms in dementia: An update. *Research in Nursing and Health, 18,* 143–163.

Waltz, C. F., Strickland, O. L., & Lenz, E. R. (1991). *Measurement in nursing research* (2nd ed.). Philadelphia: F. A. Davis.

[27]

Family Involvement in Care: Negotiated Family-Staff Partnerships in Special Care Units for Persons with Dementia

Meridean L. Maas, David Reed, Janet P. Specht, Elizabeth Swanson, Toni Tripp-Reimer, Kathleen C. Buckwalter, Debra Schutte, and Lisa S. Kelley

Dementia, of which there are several types, is a common and very serious health problem for elders. Prevalence rates of 8.4% of persons age 65 and older and 30% of persons older than 85 were recently reported (Hendrie, 1997); approximately 4 million persons in the United States are afflicted (Agency for Health Care Policy and Research, 1996). Although the speed of progression and the manifestations of deterioration vary, all dementias share a similar deteriorating course. Subtle memory impairments in the early stages are followed by losses in judgment, logic, concentration, orientation, and functional abilities. As the disorder progresses, secondary behavioral symptoms such as emotional outbursts, catastrophic reactions, and wandering occur. In the late stages, the person deteriorates markedly and may become mute, incontinent, and incapable of ambulation or self-care (Kane, Ouslander, & Abrass, 1994).

A family member is typically the caregiver for the person with dementia. As the disease progresses, caring for the demented person at home becomes a heavy burden for the family member. Eventually, the burden of care forces most family caregivers to place the relative in a nursing home (Reisberg & Ferris, 1982); the result is that approximately two thirds of nursing home residents are persons with dementia (Hing, 1987).

Relocation relieves many problems for the family caregiver but does not necessarily mean an end to caregiver stress (Ade-Ridder & Kaplan, 1993; Dellasega, 1991; George & Gwyther, 1986; Pratt, Jones, Shin, & Walker, 1989; Stephens, Kinney, & Ogrocki, 1991; Zarit & Whitlatch, 1992). Stress often continues and may even be exacerbated (Collins, Stommel, Wang, & Given, 1994; Stephens et al., 1991; Zarit & Whitlatch, 1992). Following institutionalization, family caregivers must develop a different role in the care of their relatives, one that inevitably has some new and different aspects. The stress of caregiving often increases due to loss of a positive relationship with the care recipient, guilt for removing the care recipient to a nursing home, and feelings of captivity because of restrictions imposed by the obligation to provide or oversee care. In extreme cases, the caregiver experiences a change from complete responsibility for caregiving to nearly complete exclusion from caregiving, yet continues to feel an obligation for caregiving (Maas, Buckwalter, Kelley, & Stolley, 1991).

Relocation of the relative also offers opportunities (Fink & Picot, 1995). Without the need to devote full time to meeting basic needs of the relative with dementia, there is more time to devote to the relationship and to focus on enhancing the relative's quality of life. Unfortunately, family members usually do not know how to go about changing from direct care tasks to a more indirect, supportive interpersonal role and they may receive little or no assistance in going about it from nursing home staff (Peters et al., in review). Further, family members are usually not encouraged to continue direct caregiving even if they desire to do so.

Indeed, family members may meet resistance from staff in attempting to carry out decision making, protective care, or other aspects of a new role. Once a resident is admitted to a nursing home, many staff members view the family as "visitors" and are not open to family member participation in care. Attempts by family members to continue participating in caregiving are resented by staff, who feel that only they are in control of residents' care. When family members try to participate or control aspects of care received by the residents, staff members may perceive them as disruptive outsiders rather than as clients. This staff perspective often results in family-staff role conflicts (Buckwalter, Maas, & Reed, 1997), which are stressful not only for families but also for staff, depriving them of the benefits of cooperation, personal information about residents, and coordination of caregiving. Conflicts with family members add to the task burdens and feelings of inadequacy that are often experienced by staff caring for persons with dementia (Dellasega & Mastrian, 1995; Hare & Skinner, 1990). Thus, there is a need for interventions to help family members form a new caregiving partnership with staff when a person with dementia is relocated to a nursing home. This chapter reports some findings from a study that tested the effects of the intervention, Family Involvement in Care, on family and staff caregivers of persons with dementia in nursing home special dementia care units.

The Family Involvement in Care (FIC) intervention was developed to improve family, staff, and resident outcomes through the establishment of family-staff partnerships in caregiving. The intervention is based on theoretical models of person-environment fit and interaction (Kahana, 1975; Lawton, 1975; Parr, 1980), the Progressively Lowered Threshold Model (Hall & Buckwalter, 1987), and role theory (Hardy & Conway, 1978; O'Neill & Ross, 1991). Figure 27.1 depicts the relationships among major concepts and the hypothesized effects of the FIC intervention. Person-environment fit and interaction are conceptualized along a trajectory of

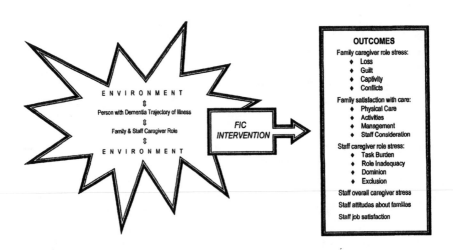

FIGURE 27.1 Theoretical framework for Family Involvement in Care (FIC) intervention and outcomes.

change over time for residents with dementia, family members, and staff caregivers. This theoretical framework helps to guide awareness of the increasingly compromised ability of persons with dementia to cope with environmental cues and stimuli, understand the stressors for family and staff caregivers along the trajectory of the deteriorating illness, and suggest nursing interventions to relieve the stress and increase positive attitudes. The need for new role expectations and behaviors for family and staff as partners in care and the expected outcomes are clarified. As partners with staff, family caregivers' stress resulting from role changes, loss, guilt, obligations to provide care, and conflicts with staff should be reduced and their perceptions of the care received by their relatives should be more positive. Staff who are partners with family caregivers should have more positive attitudes toward families and their jobs and less stress from conflict with family members who seek some participation in the care of their relatives. The partnerships also should relieve some of the task burden and role inadequacy perceived by staff who have limited resources to deal with both persons with dementia and their family members (Maas, Buckwalter, Swanson, Specht, et al., 1994; Mobily, Maas, Buckwalter, & Kelley, 1992).

The FIC intervention protocol is composed of four key elements: (1) orientation of an identified primary family caregiver (and other family caregivers, if they wish to participate) to the facility, the special care unit, and the proposed partnership role; (2) education of family members for involvement in care; (3) negotiation and formation of a partnership agreement; and (4) follow-up family member and staff evaluation and renegotiation of the partnership agreement (Maas, Buckwalter, Swanson, Specht, et al., 1994).

Central to the intervention is a family/staff conference for negotiating the form and extent of family member involvement in care. In negotiating this agreement, the family member and staff begin by discussing goals and approaches to resident care. Then they discuss the activities that each will perform in order to achieve agreed-upon goals. It is made clear to family members that the process is meant to enable them to do those activities they *want* to do, not to require them to participate in care. The partnership agreement is documented on a form, the Family-Staff Partnership Agreement, which details what the family member and staff have agreed to do. The intensity of participation, contact length, and frequency of contact are negotiated, agreed, and documented on this form. In the study evaluating the effects of the FIC intervention, activities that family members agreed to perform ranged from simple provision of information about the resident to active participation in physical care and assistance with psychosocial modalities.

Education of the family caregiver (FC) begins with a brochure that explains the general principles of caregiving and interactions with persons with dementia. The primary nurse or social worker discusses specific ways to make involvement in therapeutic activities and personal care meaningful and enjoyable for both the family caregiver and the resident. To assist with this, the *Education Resource Manual for Families* is available to staff. This manual contains nursing activities and interventions designed for persons with dementia, including art therapy, behavior management, environmental fit, exercise, eating and nutrition, medication management, music therapy, nonrestraint strategies, personal care, and therapeutic recreation. Each activity/intervention section of the manual contains a brief introduction, definition of the activity/intervention, purpose of the activity/intervention, and guidelines for carrying out the activity/intervention. The manual also includes two or three published articles on each activity/intervention so that staff and family caregivers who want additional material to read have it available. All of this information can be used by nursing staff to instruct family members on how to increase their involvement in the care of the resident. In addition, the manual is available for family members/caregivers to review at home.

Renegotiation of the partnership agreement permits adjustment of the agreement to the changing mental and physical condition of the resident and the changing ideas of family members about the role they wish to play. Monthly sessions to reevaluate the terms of the partnership agreement are recommended.

An educational program for staff, with 8 hours of training delivered in three sessions, prepares staff for negotiating sessions with family caregivers. The first session presents information about dementia. The second session discusses the problems faced by family members of residents in a long-term care facility. All staff involved with persons with dementia are expected to attend both of these sessions. The third session discusses how to negotiate the role family members can play in providing care. Only staff members doing the negotiating need to attend this session.

The purpose of the FIC intervention is to decrease family caregivers' stress from loss of the positive aspects of the relationship with the care recipient, guilt, restrictions imposed by the obligations to provide care, and conflicts with staff, and to increase their satisfaction with the care of their relative with dementia. In addition, the intervention is designed to improve staff job satisfaction, increase positive attitudes toward families, and reduce perceived stressors: role inadequacy, task burden, dominion (control of care vis-à-vis family members), and exclusion (resistance to participation in care by family members).

METHODS

A quasi-experimental design with nonequivalent groups and repeated pre-test and posttest measures was used to examine the effects of the FIC intervention on family, staff, and resident outcomes (the outcomes for residents with dementia are not included in this report). Fourteen nursing homes in Iowa and Wisconsin with designated special care units (SUs) for persons with dementia were recruited for the study. Each of the SUs met Iowa standards for licensing special dementia care units. The facility costs and benefits of participation in the study were thoroughly explained to the administrator of each nursing home, and a commitment of administrative support was obtained. The nursing homes were grouped into pairs matched on ownership type (private nonprofit, private for-profit, and public) and unit size. One nursing home in each pair was randomly assigned to be an experimental site and the other to be a control site. All residents with dementia who were residing in or admitted to the SUs during a 2-year period and their family members were eligible to participate. The primary nurse and/or social worker in the SU identified the family caregiver most closely involved with each resident's care and asked that caregiver if he or she was willing to be contacted to participate in the study. If the family member chose to be contacted, a research staff member explained the study and obtained informed consent to participate. Family members or a legal representative provided consent for resident subjects with dementia. All staff assigned to work on the SUs or who had a caseload assignment on the SUs were invited to participate. Assignment of staff was nonrandom and done by the agencies' administrators.

Staff measures were collected at baseline, before staff were trained on how to conduct partnership meetings and implement the FIC intervention, and every 6 months for the 2 years of the study in each nursing home. Once staff training was completed, family members were recruited to partici-pate. A 9-month trial of the FIC intervention was completed for each family member. Family member outcome measures were collected bimonthly, including two pretests and three posttests. Implementation of the FIC intervention protocol began as soon as family member baseline measures were obtained. Interviews were conducted with each family member at baseline and during months 5 and 9.

Family Measures

Family members' outcomes reported here were measured by the Family Perceptions of Care Tool (FPCT), the Family Perceptions of Caregiving

Role (FPCR) instrument, and interviews conducted at baseline, midway, and at the end of the 9-month FIC trial. These measures were developed by the investigators and pretested for reliability and validity (Maas & Buckwalter, 1990). The FPCR tool measures the degree of stress experienced by family members; items measure the dimensions of loss of aspects of the relationship with the person with dementia, guilt from perceived failure in caregiving, captivity resulting from obligations of caregiving, and conflict with staff over caregiving. The higher the score, the more stress is perceived by the family member. Using baseline data, Cronbach's alphas were .73 for the Loss subscale, .70 for the Guilt subscale, .81 for the Captivity subscale, and .84 for the Conflict subscale.

The FPCT has subscales reflecting perceived satisfaction with physical care, activities for residents, unit management, and staff consideration for the resident and family member. Items in the Management subscale evaluate, for example, whether there are adequate resources devoted to care. Items in the Consideration subscale evaluate such issues as whether staff preserve the privacy of the resident and provide emotional support to the family member. Higher satisfaction is reflected in higher scores. For this tool, Cronbach's alphas using baseline data were .97 for Physical Care, .87 for Activities, .88 for Management, and .85 for Consideration.

The semi-structured interview guide queried family members about other responses to the institutionalization of their relatives with dementia, changes in their caregiver roles and relationships with the residents, their perceived stress and satisfaction associated with relocation of the care recipient to a nursing home, and evaluation of care and relationships with staff and other family members. Only the results of analysis of a small number of randomly selected baseline interviews were available for this report (Kelley, Swanson, Maas, & Tripp-Reimer, 1999).

Staff Measures

Staff completed measures of general job satisfaction, caregiver stress, perceptions of caregiving role, and attitudes toward family members. Some of these measures were developed by the investigators and were pretested for reliability and validity in earlier work (Maas & Buckwalter, 1990).

The General Job Satisfaction Index (GJS) measures the satisfaction of staff in their working environment. Reported internal consistency reliability is .77 (Oldham, Hackman, & Stepina, 1978); for this study it was .65. The Staff Perceptions of Caregiving Role (SPCR) examines staff perceptions of family and staff caregiving roles as sources of stress. Many of the items are analogous to items in the Family Perceptions of Caregiving Role (FPCR) instrument and, like the FPCR, high scores reflect high stress. In this study, a factor analysis was completed and four dimensions emerged: task burden, role inadequacy, dominion, and exclusion (Maas & Swanson, 1992). Task burden reflects the costs of caregiving, such as feeling angry or feeling overworked. Role inadequacy is the feeling that there are no benefits from caregiving (i.e., what one does fails to help residents with dementia). Dominion reflects the attitude that staff should be in control of caregiving. (This term was chosen to express the territorial aspect of control, the sense that the "turf" belongs to the staff.) Exclusion reflects the view that family members should not participate in caregiving in the nursing home. Exclusion is conceptually distinct from dominion, because conceivably family members may participate extensively without being involved in decision making regarding care. The total scale of the SPCR correlated significantly in a negative direction with staff job satisfaction ($r = -.28$, $p < .01$). Cronbach's alpha coefficients for the dimensions of the SCPR were .71 (Dominion), .70 (Exclusion), .84 (Task Burden), and .82 (Role Inadequacy).

The Caregiver Stress Inventory (CSI) is designed to measure three dimensions of stress related to resident verbal/physical behavior, resident emotional/social behavior, and staff knowledge, abilities, and resources for providing care to persons with dementia. A high score indicates high stress. Cronbach's alpha using baseline data was .96. The Attitudes toward Families Checklist (AFC) measures general staff attitudes toward family members of the resident with dementia, including family visitation, family requests regarding care of the resident, and family participation in the care of the relative. A high score indicates a positive attitude toward family caregivers. The AFC was pretested using 60 nursing home staff and yielded an internal consistency reliability coefficient of .91 (Cronbach's alpha) (Maas & Buckwalter, 1990); using baseline data from the current study, the reliability coefficient was .74.

RESULTS

Samples

Two hundred family members were initially enrolled in the study. Of these, 185 were subsequently determined to be eligible and completed baseline questionnaires. Their average age was 61 years. The family member sample was predominantly Caucasian (94%), and about three quarters were women. Nearly 60% had more than a high school education. Forty percent were daughters, 21% wives, 7% husbands, 14% sons, 10% other relatives (niece, grandchild, sibling, etc.), and 8% nonrelative friends or guardians. A third were of the same generation as the resident and 67% of a younger generation. The 165 residents to whom they were related had been in the nursing home a median time of approximately 1 1/2 years (565 days), with a range of 23 days to 10.8 years. Fifty-seven of the residents had been in another nursing home previously, for a median time of 6 months, with a range of 30 days to 7 years. Ninety-nine family members completed the entire 9-month trial of the FIC intervention.

There were 845 staff members who agreed to participate in the study. Ninety-three percent were Caucasian and 92% were women. Their average age was 37 years, and the median number of years of work in their occupation was 5 (mean = 8.6 years). Forty-eight percent of the staff were nursing assistants, 5% were medication aides, 13% were registered nurses, 10% were licensed practical nurses, and 10% were housekeeping, laundry, or maintenance personnel. One hundred twelve staff members classified themselves as activities technician/assistant/therapist ($n = 44$), dietitian ($n = 24$), social worker ($n = 18$), administrator ($n = 11$), ward or unit clerk ($n = 4$), occupational therapy technician/assistant ($n = 3$), physical therapy technician/assistant ($n = 2$), speech/language therapist ($n = 2$), music therapist ($n = 2$), or religious activities director ($n = 2$). The average number of months working at the facility by all staff was 53 months, with a range of 0 to 432 months ($SD = 69$ months). The mean number of years in the occupation was 9 years, with a range of 0 to 50 ($SD = 9$).

Qualitative Analysis

Baseline interviews conducted with family caregivers indicated that the decision to put a relative in a nursing home was very distressing (Kelley et al., 1999). Adult child caregivers said of the decision: "The worst time in my life," "[I]t about killed me to do it," "[I]t really bothered me because I knew she would be angry with me," and "[M]y brothers didn't agree with me, and that was a worry." While spouses reported some of these feelings, they tended to be more concerned about the loss of the spouse and the role of caring for the mate. Comments included: "I knew I would miss him," "I hated thinking about not being able to take care of him," and "I kept thinking about how he would probably miss me and the things I do for him."

The majority of children, spouses, and other relatives noted that it was very hard to actually see the relative go to a nursing home. They commented: "I cried all the way home," "[I]t was so empty at home and I felt so lonely," "I knew she would miss her things, so I took as much along as I could, pictures and such. She had so much and then so little, it didn't seem fair," and "[H]e kept saying he wanted to go home and tried to leave with me . . . it was so sad." Many of the family members' comments, however, indicated that they also were relieved, though ambivalent: "[I]t was hard, but I felt like a weight had been lifted," "I feel guilty saying so, but I was so glad it was finally done," "I felt free to do some things for myself again," and "[I]t was hard to do, but I knew it was best for my family."

Themes that emerged from the analysis were the importance of continuing to be "faithful" to their relatives with dementia following placement in the nursing home, the need to be the "eyes and ears" for the relatives to monitor the care received and promote better care, and the need to maintain continuity of the family unit (Kelley et al., 1999). With their changing relationships with the residents with dementia, caregivers also expressed concern about being forgotten, the need to change roles, poor perceptions of nursing homes, and uncertainties about how to relate to the residents and assist with care.

Quantitative Analysis: Family Members

At baseline, family members' scores on the FPCT were most positive on the Consideration subscale ($M = 5.29$; scale = 1 to 7, with 7 being the most positive) and least positive on the Management subscale ($M = 4.38$), with scores on the Physical Care ($M = 5.02$) and Activities subscales ($M = 4.92$) in between. Scores on the FPCR subscales were highest (worst) in regard to loss of the positive aspects of their relationship with the care recipient. The next highest scores were on Captivity ($M = 3.14$), with the Guilt ($M = 2.68$) and Conflict ($M = 2.74$) subscales having the lowest scores. At baseline, there were significant generational differences in scores on the Loss subscale ($M = 4.74$; $F(1,81) = 20.29$, $p < .001$) and the Captivity ($F(1,81) = 5.02$, $p < .05$) subscale, with family members in the same generation having higher (worse) scores than those in a younger generation.

The FIC intervention had positive effects on family caregivers (see Table 27.1). There was, however, an interaction of the intervention with generation. On both the FPCT and the FPCR, positive intervention effects were found only for family caregivers of the same generation as the resident. On the FPCT subscales, there were positive effects for the Physical Care subscale ($F(1,90) = 5.24$, $p < .05$) and the Consideration subscale ($F(1,90) = 6.35$, $p < .05$). No effects were found on the Management or Activities subscales. On the FPCR subscales, a positive intervention effect was found on the Loss subscale ($F(1,81) = 4.96$, $p < .05$) for caregivers of the same

TABLE 27.1 Baseline and Follow-up Means and Standard Deviations for Family Measures that Differed Significantly between the Experimental and Control Groups

Subscale	Generation	Intervention Status	Baseline Mean	(SD)	Follow-up Mean	(SD)
Family Perceptions of Care Tool[a]						
Consideration	Same	Experimental	5.26	(1.45)	5.60	(1.23)
		Control	5.28	(1.05)	4.84	(0.94)
Physical Care	Same	Experimental	4.61	(1.97)	5.37	(1.67)
		Control	5.12	(1.40)	4.81	(1.40)
Family Perceptions of Caregiving Role[b]						
Loss	Same	Experimental	5.58	(0.77)	5.29	(0.88)
		Control	5.39	(0.82)	5.94	(0.55)

[a]Scale from 1 (least positive) to 7 (most positive).
[b]Scale from 1 (least stress) to 7 (most stress).

generation. No intervention effects were found for Captivity (restrictions imposed by the obligation to provide care), Conflict, or Guilt.

Quantitative Analysis: Staff

Overall, staff scores on the General Job Satisfaction instrument were quite high, with a mean score at baseline of 5.6 on a scale of 1 (least satisfaction) to 7 (most satisfaction). Baseline staff scores on the Perceptions of Caregiving Role Instrument were highest (worst; 1 = most desirable, 7 = least desirable) for Role Inadequacy ($M = 4.62$), followed by scores on Dominion (resistance to sharing control of caregiving with family members) ($M = 3.73$) and Exclusion (resistance to participation of family members in caregiving) ($M = 2.82$). Scores were lowest (best) for Task Burden ($M = 2.38$). The mean score on the Caregiver Stress Inventory was 3.6, indicating a moderate stress level for staff. Scores on the Attitudes toward Families Checklist averaged 4.65 (possible range from 1 to 7, most desirable), indicating a moderately favorable attitude toward family members.

There was no intervention effect on general job satisfaction or general stress of staff. A positive intervention effect was found for attitudes toward families ($F(1,125) = 8.66$, $p < .01$). On the SPCR subscales, there was an intervention effect on measures pertaining to relations with family members, but not on those pertaining to providing care for residents (see

TABLE 27.2   Means and Standard Deviations for Staff Measures at Baseline and Follow-up by Intervention Status

Measure	Intervention Status	Baseline Mean (SD)	Follow-up Mean (SD)
Staff Perceptions of Caregiving Role[a]			
Dominion	Control	3.67 (0.96)	3.64 (0.95)
	Experimental	3.81 (0.94)	3.38 (0.80)
Exclusion	Control	2.77 (0.76)	2.84 (0.82)
	Experimental	2.90 (0.66)	2.76 (0.71)
Task Burden	Control	2.43 (0.81)	2.53 (0.81)
	Experimental	2.32 (0.82)	2.30 (0.74)
Role Inadequacy	Control	4.67 (1.01)	4.52 (1.04)
	Experimental	4.56 (0.94)	4.30 (1.02)
Attitudes toward Families[b]	Control	4.76 (0.73)	4.10 (0.45)
	Experimental	4.49 (0.73)	4.22 (0.40)

[a]Scale from 1 (most desirable response) to 7 (least desirable response).
[b]Scale from 1 (least desirable response) to 7 (most desirable response).

Table 27.2). That is, staff at intervention sites improved their scores on the Dominion ($F(1,188) = 9.19$, $p < .01$) and Exclusion ($F(1,188) = 4.43$, $p < .05$) subscales, but there was not a significant intervention effect on either the Task Burden or Role Inadequacy subscales. In both control and intervention sites, there was improvement over the course of the study in Role Inadequacy scores ($F(1,188) = 9.49$, $p < .01$). It may be that participation in research provided staff at both types of sites a sense that they were doing something worthwhile.

CONCLUSIONS AND IMPLICATIONS

With an ever growing number of persons with dementia, primarily Alzheimer's disease, and fewer family members willing and able to devote themselves to full-time caregiving, the numbers of persons with dementia in nursing homes and other types of long-term care facilities will continue to increase. Thus, increasing numbers of family members will need to develop a satisfying role in long-term care facilities, a role that minimizes the stress of continued caregiving for their relatives with dementia. This study indicates that meaningful partnerships with staff that clearly delineate cooperative role behaviors, eliminate role ambiguity, and resolve or prevent conflicts are effective. The FIC intervention had positive effects for both family and staff caregivers.

Baseline interviews revealed that the transition to the nursing home is a particularly difficult time for family members. Persons with dementia who are placed in nursing homes may be highly resistant and fearful of the change. Given their diminished capacity for reasoning, it may be impossible to convince them that they require institutionalization. Constant requests to be taken home are especially stressful to families. Because of these circumstances, relationships with residents are difficult for family caregivers; they feel guilty and uncertain about how to perform their changing roles. In this study the FIC intervention ameliorated feelings of loss and guilt for family caregivers who were of the same generation as the care recipient, most of whom were spouses. Relationships of family caregivers with residents and staff also became more positive after implementation of the intervention. Finding ways to achieve greater staff compliance with the intervention may increase its positive effects on family members' stress and increase their satisfaction with management and provision of care for residents.

It is especially important for family members to implement the FIC intervention as soon as, or even before, the resident with dementia is admitted to the nursing home. Because nearly all of the family members participating in this study had relatives who had been residing in a nursing home for at least 6 months, it was not possible to determine whether there were differential effects for family members with newly admitted relatives and those with relatives who were long-term residents. However, the interviews indicated that family members often had concerns about care but were reluctant to express those concerns to staff. This implies that the intervention might be more effective if it were implemented before family members established a pattern of deference to staff in decision making.

Although the intervention did not significantly reduce staff stress associated with caregiving task burden or role inadequacy, staff attitudes toward families were positively affected. These changes in attitudes will assist staff in their caregiving by maximizing the exchange of information about residents and enabling greater family assistance with agreed-upon care activities.

Throughout the study, the master clinicians who implemented the FIC protocol felt that many of the nursing home staff failed to accept "ownership" of the intervention, seeing it as something done for the research staff, not for themselves. Positive results were achieved, but even better results could be achieved if the nursing staff were more committed to the intervention. If nursing homes wish to realize the benefits of increasing family involvement through the FIC intervention, leaders must demonstrate full and active commitment to the intervention. Leaders need to define family-staff partnerships as desirable and provide support for staff to implement the intervention. It seems likely that staff who learn to work with families as partners and as clients will feel greater role adequacy through the achievement of positive outcomes for families and residents.

To successfully implement the FIC partnerships, registered nurses (RNs) need to provide leadership for other staff. Partnerships cannot be realized without the active involvement of nursing assistants, who make up the greatest part of the nursing staff and have most direct contacts with residents and families. The role of the RN is to lead other staff to ensure quality of care. Not surprisingly, RNs in this study had the lowest dominion scores (i.e., were least resistive to sharing control with families). This suggests that RNs are inclined to welcome family involvement in care, which should enable them to help other staff increase their comfort in partnering with families.

The positive results of the FIC intervention in nursing home SUs suggest that it may be useful for family and staff caregivers of other patient populations in other settings. To facilitate the use and evaluation of the intervention with other populations in other settings, a research-based protocol is available from the Iowa Gerontological Nursing Intervention Research Center, Research Development and Dissemination Core.[1]

ACKNOWLEDGMENTS

This research was supported by NIH NINR funded grant, "Interventions for Alzheimer's: Family Role Trials," R01 NR01869, Meridean Maas and Elizabeth Swanson, co-principal investigators.

NOTE

1. The FIC Intervention protocol is available from Marita Titler, PhD, RN, FAAN, Department of Nursing—RDDC, University of IA Hospitals and Clinics, 200 Hawkins Drive T152 GH, Iowa City, IA 52242-1009 (319-353-7589); e-mail: donna-valiga@uiowa.edu.

REFERENCES

Ade-Ridder, L., & Kaplan, L. (1993). Marriage, spousal caregiving, and a husband's move to a nursing home: A changing role for the wife. *Journal of Gerontological Nursing, 19*(10), 13–23.

Agency for Health Care Policy and Research. (1996). *Early Alzheimer's disease: Recognition and assessment* (Guideline Overview No. 19 AHCPR Publication No. 97-R123). Rockville, MD: U.S. Department of Health and Human Services.

Buckwalter, K., Maas, M., & Reed, D. (1997). Assessing family and staff caregiver outcomes in Alzheimer disease research. *Alzheimer Disease and Associated Disorders, 11*(Suppl. 6), 105–116.

Collins, C., Stommel, M., Wang, S., & Given, C. (1994). Caregiving transitions: Changes in depression among family caregivers of relatives with dementia. *Nursing Research, 43*(4), 220–225.

Dellasega, C. (1991). Caregiving stress among community caregivers for the elderly: Does institutionalization make a difference? *Journal of Community Health Nursing, 8*(4), 197–205.

Dellasega, C., & Mastrian, K. (1995). The process and consequences of institutionalizing an elder. *Western Journal of Nursing Research, 17*(2), 123–140.

Fink, S., & Picot, S. (1995). Nursing home placement decisions and post placement experiences of African American and European American caregivers. *Journal of Gerontological Nursing, 21*(12), 35–42.

George, L., & Gwyther, K. (1986). Caregiver wellbeing: A multidimensional examination of family caregivers of demented adults. *The Gerontologist, 26,* 253–259.

Hall, G. R., & Buckwalter, K. C. (1987). Progressively lowered stress threshold: A conceptual model for care of adults with Alzheimer's disease. *Archives of Psychiatric Nursing, 1*(6), 399–406.

Hardy, M. E., & Conway, M. (1978). *Role therapy: Perspectives for health professionals.* New York: Appleton-Century-Crofts.

Hare, J., & Skinner, D. A. (1990, Fall). The relationship between work environment and burnout in nursing home employees. *Journal of Long Term Care Administration, 19,* 9–12.

Hendrie, H. (1997). *Epidemiology: Prevalence, risk factors, and genetics.* Paper presented at the Consensus Conference on the Treatment of Alzheimer's Disease and Related Dementias, Washington, DC.

Hing, E. (1987, June/July). Use of nursing homes by the elderly: Preliminary data from the 1985 National Nursing Home Survey. *National Gerontological Nursing Association Newsletter.*

Kahana, E. (1975). A congruence model of person-environment interaction. In P. Windleyu, T. Byerts, & F. Ernst (Eds.), *Theory development in environment and aging.* Washington, DC: Gerontological Society of America.

Kane, R. L., Ouslander, J. G., & Abrass, I. B. (1994). *Essentials of clinical geriatrics* (3rd ed.). New York: McGraw-Hill.

Kelley, L., Swanson, E., Maas, M., & Tripp-Reimer, T. (1999). Family visitation on special care units. *Journal of Gerontological Nursing, 25*(2), 14–21.

Lawton, M. (1975). Competence, environmental press and the adaptation of older people. In P. Windleyu, T. Byerts, & F. Ernst (Eds.), *Theory development in environment and aging.* Washington, DC: Gerontological Society of America.

Maas, M., & Buckwalter, K. (1990). Final report: Phase II nursing Evaluation Research: Alzheimer's Care Unit [R01 NR01689—NCNR]. Rockville, MD: National Institutes of Health.

Maas, M., Buckwalter, K., Kelley, L., & Stolley, J. (1991). Family members' perceptions: How they view care of Alzheimer's patients in a nursing home. *Journal of Long Term Care Administration, 19*(1), 21–25.

Maas, M., Buckwalter, K., Swanson, E., & Mobily, P. (1994). Training key to job satisfaction. *Journal of Long Term Care Administration, 22*(1), 23–26.

Maas, M., Buckwalter, K., Swanson, E., Specht, J., Hardy, M., & Tripp-Reimer, T. (1994, November/December). The caring partnership: Staff and families of persons institutionalized with Alzheimer's disease. *Journal of Alzheimer's Disease and Related Disorders*, 21–30.

Maas, M., & Swanson, E. (1992). *Nursing Interventions for Alzheimer's: Family Role Trials* (Research Grant, National Institute of Nursing Research RO1-NRO1689). Rockville, MD: National Institutes of Health.

Mobily, P., Maas, M., Buckwalter, K., & Kelley, S. (1992). Taking care of the caregivers: Staff stress and burnout on a special Alzheimer's unit. *Journal of Psychosocial Nursing, 30*(9), 25–31.

Oldham, G. R., Hackman, J. R., & Stepina, L. P. (1978). *Norms for the Job Diagnostic Survey*. New Haven, CT: Yale University Department of Organization and Management.

O'Neill, G., & Ross, M. M. (1991). Burden of care: An important concept for nurses. *Health Care for Women International, 12*, 111–122.

Parr, J. (1980). The interaction of persons and living environments. In L. W. Poon (Ed.), *Aging in the 1980s: Psychological issues* (pp. 393–406). Washington, DC: American Psychological Association.

Peters, J., Specht, J., Brenneman, D., Maas, M., Swanson, L., & Tripp-Reimer, T. (in review). Caregiving partnerships: Family perspectives on involvement in dementia care in the nursing home. *Journal of Gerontological Nursing*.

Pratt, C., Jones, L., Shin, H., & Walker, A. (1989). Autonomy and decision making between single older women and their caregiving daughters. *The Gerontologist, 29*, 792–797.

Reisberg, B., & Ferris, S. H. (1982). Diagnosis and treatment of the older patient. *Hospital and Community Psychiatry, 33*(2), 104–110.

Stephens, M. A. P., Kinney, J. M., & Ogrocki, P. K. (1991). Stressors and well-being among caregivers to older adults with dementia: The in-home versus nursing home experience. *The Gerontologist, 31*, 217–224.

Zarit, S., & Whitlatch, C. (1992). Institutional placement: Phases of the transition. *The Gerontologist, 32*(5), 665–672.

[28]

Limiting Developmental Regression in Hospitalized Children with Chronic Conditions by Supporting Parents

Sharon Ogden Burke, Elizabeth Kauffmann, Margaret B. Harrison, Carol Wong, and Jennifer D. Lowe

Despite advances in control of some infectious diseases (e.g., polio and rheumatic fever), the prevalence of childhood chronic conditions is not decreasing, and severity is increasing. Thus the proportion of children with chronic conditions in hospitals has increased. An estimated 5% to 10% of children have a severe or serious chronic health condition or disability, and most often, it is these children who are hospitalized (Newacheck & Taylor, 1992).

Hospitalizations can cause developmental delays in children, especially those with chronic conditions (Thompson, 1986). Educational and psychosocial support interventions have been shown to be effective in alleviating transient developmental and behavioral problems among healthy children who are briefly hospitalized (McClowry, 1988; Melamed & Ridley-

Johnson, 1988). However, hospitalization concerns for children with chronic conditions are very different from those for children who are hospitalized once with the expectation of a good outcome.

Preparing children with chronic health conditions for hospitalization and supporting children and their families are especially challenging because many of these children and families have already had negative experiences with hospitalization, and some children have developmental delays, learning problems, and physical difficulties.

Although these families might be considered veterans, hospitalizations continue to be very stressful events (Association for the Care of Children's Health, 1982; Burke, Costello, & Handley-Derry, 1989; Curley & Wallace, 1992). Poorer mental health, for example, has been reported among mothers of children with chronic conditions than among mothers of other ill children (Thomlinson, Harbaugh, Kotchevar, & Swanson, 1995). Particular issues for parents of hospitalized children with chronic conditions include (1) maintaining or modifying procedures and routines related to the child's condition (e.g., exercises, administration of medications), (2) protecting and maintaining the child's fragile and complex activities of daily living (e.g., feeding, toileting, mobility), (3) developing and maintaining long-term relationships and communicating with health care professionals, and (4) accommodating family life during hospitalizations (Burke et al., 1989; Robinson, 1987; Webster & Moss, 1986).

Parents know their child's history and idiosyncrasies, and they are in the best position to support their child before, during, and after hospitalization. Therefore, our approach is to work with parents, focusing on the family's own issues and concerns surrounding the hospitalization. We call this Stress-Point Intervention by Nurses (SPIN) (Kauffmann, Harrison, Burke, & Wong, 1998). A study by Burke, Costello, Handley-Derry, Kauffmann, and Dillon (1997) showed that SPIN was effective in enhancing parent coping, improving family functioning, and limiting hospital-induced developmental regression in children. The study was carried out under ideal conditions in a single setting with well-prepared research nurses who worked primarily in the family home. The study reported here was a test of the effectiveness of SPIN when used by staff nurses in the busy, natural setting of ambulatory clinics. Using a family focus, nurses worked with parents to deal with current stress points surrounding repeated hospitalizations of their child with a chronic health condition. Parents who received SPIN, compared to those with usual care, were expected to have better family functioning and better parent coping after their children's repeated hospitalizations. It was also expected that children whose parents received SPIN would show less developmental regression and fewer behavioral problems 3 months after a hospitalization than children receiving usual care.

METHODS

Using a three-site, pretest-posttest design, the study randomly assigned ambulatory care nurses and their respective child patients and families to the experimental SPIN group or usual care control group.

Clinic Sites and Study Nurses

Twenty-two nurses in three pediatric ambulatory clinic settings in large to midsize Ontario, Canada, health science centers participated in the study. Participating nurses' primary clinics were orthopedics, myelodysplasia, nephrology/urology, oncology, cerebral palsy/neuromuscular, and cystic fibrosis. Clinic nurses were grouped by similar clinic populations and were then randomly assigned to either the experimental group (12 SPIN nurses) or the control group (10 usual care nurses).

SPIN and usual care nurses were similar to each other. They had an average of 19 years in pediatric nursing and 12 years in ambulatory clinics. The majority worked full time (57%). About one third were baccalaureate prepared (31%), and a few were master's prepared (9%). All were blind to the study's expected outcomes and the child and family measures. Usual care nurses were not aware of the SPIN content. All of the nurses possessed good clinical knowledge of chronic conditions and related medical and surgical treatments.

Study Children and Families

One hundred and thirty-nine families agreed to participate, and 115 (83%) of those met study criteria and completed the study (46 in SPIN and 69 in usual care). All study children had a chronic condition but were in no immediate danger of dying from their health problems. Primary medical diagnoses were cerebral palsy ($n = 23$), spina bifida ($n = 16$), congenital genitourinary defects ($n = 15$), cancer responding to treatment ($n = 14$), chronic renal disease ($n = 12$), cystic fibrosis ($n = 6$), congenital hip defects ($n = 4$), other orthopedic conditions (e.g., osteogenesis imperfecta, scoliosis) ($n = 8$), cardiac defects ($n = 3$), gastrointestinal conditions ($n = 3$), muscular dystrophy ($n = 3$), cleft palate ($n = 2$), diabetes ($n = 2$), epilepsy ($n = 2$), and other ($n = 2$).

The children's average age was 7 years; ages ranged up to 15 years. For children over 12 years, developmental age was 11 years or less. About one fourth of the children had learning problems and/or mental health problems. Many had visible handicaps, using wheelchairs, prescribed foot-wear, other types of braces, and/or hearing aids. All children had been hospitalized in the past, an average of nine times. Reasons for hospitaliza-tions included treatment of the primary condition and complications re-lated to the primary condition, as well as infections (e.g., tonsillitis) and procedures (e.g., dental extraction) that required hospitalization because of the child's chronic condition. Seventy-eight percent of the children had a surgical procedure during the study hospitalization, which lasted an average of 7 days with a range of 1 day to over 3 months.

Most families had two adults in the home, but 16% were single-parent families, and 8% had three or four adults in the home. Parents' mean education was 13.6 years, with a range from 8 to 19 years. Income varied widely, with a mean of approximately US$31,000 and a standard deviation of US$23,000. Parent age averaged 35 years, with a range of 25 to 56 years. Parents spent an average of 3 nights in their child's hospital room (range from 0 to 17 nights).

Stress-Point Intervention by Nurses (SPIN)[1]

SPIN is a psychosocial and educational support intervention that focuses on parent-identified issues and concerns surrounding a child's hospitaliza-tions. Nurses who use SPIN draw on their broad clinical knowledge and their knowledge of particular families. The SPIN process (1) identifies stressful issues surrounding the expected or anticipated hospitalization, (2) develops and implements a plan with the parent to handle these issues, and (3) evaluates the success of the intervention through follow-up. The approach uses assessment tools, including the Burke Assessment Guide to Stressors and Tasks in Families with a Child with a Chronic Condition (Burke, Kauffmann, Harrison, & Wiskin, 1999) and aspects of the Calgary Family Assessment Model and Intervention Model (Wright & Leahey, 1994) to identify family processes and resources and to review past hospitalization stressors and anticipated new problems.

Intervention strategies include working with parents to (1) customize preparation and support during a procedure for a child who is developmen-tally delayed and has had distressing reactions to the same procedure in the past, (2) rethink the need to room-in the entire stay, (3) anticipate sibling reactions and plan possible parental responses, and (4) identify realistic sources of support among family and friends.

The strategies used to deal with current problems are highly individual-ized, since SPIN addresses the parent's self-identified issues and problem-solving processes for the family and the child. SPIN does not use predefined content or a highly structured teaching program, like programs for first-time hospitalizations of essentially well children with elective procedures. However, aspects of such programs or other teaching programs are incorporated into SPIN as the parent and nurse see fit.

SPIN aims to alter parents' ways of thinking about their stress points and encourages them to find ways of dealing with the current hospital-related issues. SPIN is designed to have direct and indirect effects on the child. For example, when a stressor is child preparation or management, the experienced nurse can assist parents to find better ways of helping their child. The child also benefits indirectly when parents cope more effectively with broader family issues, since parents then have more time and energy to prepare and support their child during and following hospitalization.

SPIN is unique in that (1) only parent-identified stressful issues guide the process and (2) the nurse is cued to take steps to prompt the parent to action. SPIN is oriented to issues involved with most chronic conditions, and it has a range of content options. Although the context and experience of the nurse may lie with a specific medical diagnosis, the focus of SPIN is more on family issues and problem-solving processes.

In the study reported here, SPIN (see Figure 28.1) began with an initial assessment at the clinic or occasionally at a home visit. To enhance the depth and range of the assessment, a genogram (Wright & Leahey, 1994) was used along with the Burke Assessment Guide to Stressors and Tasks in Families with a Child with a Chronic Condition (Burke et al., 1999; Burke, Kauffmann, Costello, Wiskin, & Harrison, 1998). These assessment data, with a discussion with the parent, made it possible to identify current family issues and concerns (typically 2 to 4 points). The nurse and parent then problem-solved together to deal with the most urgent concerns, and interventions were begun. The nurse followed up the initial interview with a letter commending the parent on his or her strengths and outlining the plans made together to help the family deal with its issues over the course of the child's hospitalization. At this and other contact points, the nurse made herself available to the families by phone. At least one follow-up call was made to the family before the child's admission to the hospital. The nurse made visits on the unit during the hospitalization. After discharge, follow-up was done by telephone and at clinic visits. The assessments, interventions, and evaluations the nurse chose for each family were tracked in a specially designed Nursing Intervention Record.

Each nurse in the intervention group completed a SPIN self-directed learning program on the protocol (see Kauffmann et al., 1998, for details). Content on chronic conditions was not included, since all the nurses were

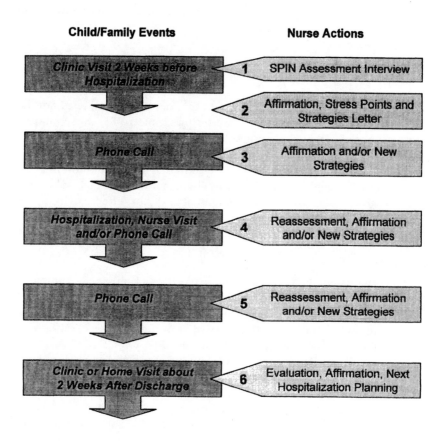

FIGURE 28.1   A typical Stress-Point Intervention by Nurses (SPIN) process.

experienced pediatric nurses. Learning to use SPIN took an average of 8 hours, with a range of 4 to 12 hours.

SPIN began about 2 weeks before hospitalization, included hospitalization, and concluded about 2 weeks after the child's discharge from hospital. Nurse contact time varied widely for both SPIN and usual care groups, ranging from only a few minutes to 8.5 hours. Usual care nurses averaged 1.5 hours, and SPIN nurses averaged 3.3 hours of contact time per family, or about 1.8 hours more than usual care nurses. Both SPIN and usual care nurses spent about the same amount of time doing treatments and procedures with the children. However, SPIN nurses spent more time helping families to problem-solve.

Outcome Measures

Parent coping, family functioning, and child developmental level and behavior were measured 2 weeks before hospitalization (T1) and 3 months after discharge (T3). Sociodemographic and economic data were collected about 10 days after the child's discharge from the hospital (T2). T3 was designed to avoid the period of about 1 month that it takes for most negative effects to fade among essentially healthy children with brief hospitalizations (Lende, 1971). This allowed documentation of the effects of repeated hospitalizations and SPIN on longer-term child and family reactions.

Feetham Family Functioning Survey (FFFS)

The 25-item revised FFFS (Feetham & Carroll, 1988; Feetham & Humenick, 1982), designed for families in which there is a child with a chronic health condition, measures parents' satisfaction with the functioning of their families. Test-retest reliability of .85 has been shown after 2 weeks (Roberts, 1979). Internal consistency has been strong for samples of 25 or more parents of children with health problems or at risk for such problems, ranging from .77 (Youngblut & Schiao, 1993) to .89 (Roberts, 1979). Parents rate both "what is" and "what should be" on a 7-point scale. Higher scores indicate less satisfaction and have been interpreted as less "optimal" family functioning (Mercer & Ferketich, 1990). Changes of 1/2 standard deviation (SD) or more in FFFS scores were considered clinically significant in this study.

Coping Health Inventory for Parents (CHIP)

CHIP (McCubbin et al., 1983) was used to measure parental coping. CHIP assesses coping by parents caring for a child with a chronic condition on a scale of 0 (not helpful) to 3 (always helpful). Three scales measure family coping (maintaining family integration, cooperation, and an optimistic view of the situation), parents' personal coping (maintaining social support, self-esteem, and psychological stability), and health care communication coping (understanding the medical situation through communicating with other parents and consulting with health care professionals). The authors added one item to the latter scale, "talking with the nurse about my concerns about my child." CHIP has shown differences between parents with generally low stress and those with usually high stress from repeated hospitalizations of their physically disabled child (Burke et al., 1989). In this study, internal consistency for pretest scores was high (.92).

Scales of Independent Behavior (SIB)

Changes in study children's developmental level were measured with the SIB (Bruininks, Woodcock, Weatherman, & Hill, 1985), which assesses independent functioning within the home, social, and community settings. Each task was rated by the parent on a 4-point scale from never or rarely to always/almost always or does very well. Motor skills, social, and communication skills, and personal living skills scale scores yielded developmental ages (DA), from which developmental quotients (DQ) were calculated (DA/chronological age × 100). Summing motor, personal, and social DQ scores and dividing by 3 yielded an overall mean DQ. Children whose DQ increased by 7.5 were considered to have experienced a developmental gain, whereas those with a drop of 7.5 or more were considered to have regressed developmentally over the course of the study hospitalization. Children with DQ changes between +7.5 and −7.5 were considered clinically unchanged.

Parenting Stress Index (PSI)

The child scales of the PSI (Abidin, 1986) were used to measure changes in child behavior from the perspective of the parent. The PSI has been shown to have a strong linear relationship with the Child Behavior Checklist (Achenbach & Edelbrock, 1983; Meyer & Vadsay, 1994). The scales, each with 5 to 11 items, are child distractibility/hyperactivity, reinforcing parents, mood, acceptability, demandingness, and adaptability. Each of the 47 items is rated by parents on a 5-point scale from strongly agree to strongly disagree. Higher scores indicate more child behavior problems. In this study each child was classified as behaviorally unchanged, behaviorally worse, or behaviorally improved based on calculated difference scores (posttest-pretest) for each of the scales.

Study Procedures

Children were identified by the study nurses and each site's nurse coordinator. The study was explained to parents, and informed consent was obtained. Before SPIN began at T1, parental coping (CHIP) and satisfaction with family (FFFS) data, along with child developmental and behavioral data from the SIB and PSI, were obtained from the parent (usually the mother) by a research assistant who was unaware of group membership and SPIN. Sociodemographic and hospitalization data were collected about 10 days after discharge in a phone interview (T2). Three months after discharge, FFFS, CHIP, SIB, and PSI were readministered to parents (T3). T1 and T3 data were collected at the family home or another site convenient to the parent.

RESULTS

Effects of SPIN on Family Functioning and Parental Coping

Family functioning (FFFS) and parent coping (CHIP) before hospitalization were similar for both the SPIN and usual care groups. At 3 months after hospitalization, parents in the experimental SPIN group had significantly greater satisfaction with their family's functioning than usual care parents (see Tables 28.1 and 28.2). Overall, parental perceptions of family functioning were better for the SPIN families. Only 4% of SPIN parents reported poorer family functioning 3 months after discharge, compared to 38% of the usual care group. Conversely, 32% of the SPIN families had better family functioning compared to only 18% of the usual care families. Among SPIN families, there was also significantly less discrepancy between the ideal and real views of the family. In contrast, 3 months after hospitalization, among usual care families there was a larger discrepancy between real and ideal. Therefore, SPIN played a small but significant role in improvement in satisfaction with family functioning.

Family problems, individual relationships, and family support were explored to gain a better understanding of SPIN's effects on the families.

TABLE 28.1 Changes in Family Functioning by Study Group

Feetham Family Functioning Survey Discrepancy Score Changes	SPIN	Usual Care
More discrepancy (worse)	4%	38%
Same	64%	44%
Less discrepancy (better)	32%	18%
Totals	100%	100%

TABLE 28.2   Comparison of SPIN and Usual Care Groups[a]

	Before Hospitalization		After Hospitalization		Changes (After–Before)		Analysis of Covariance Effect of SPIN		
	M	SD	M	SD	M	SD	F	df	p
Family Functioning (FFFS)[b,c]									
SPIN	30.7	18.1	25.8	16.3	−4.9	11.5	8.05	2,110	.005
Usual Care	28.9	17.8	33.5	20.3	4.6	14.8			
Parental Coping (CHIP)[b,c]									
SPIN	95.7	23.8	100.0	18.4	4.3	17.5	5.74	2,111	.014
Usual Care	97.1	19.7	97.4	22.7	0.3	17.7			
Developmental Level (SIB)[d]									
SPIN	65.1	44.0	70.8	45.6	5.7	22.9	6.2	2,399	.014
Usual Care	98.5	46.0	87.2	37.9	−11.3	20.5			

[a]Parenting Stress Index (PSI) not significant.
[b]No significant differences between groups at pretesting.
[c]Nurse contact time removed as covariate.
[d]Effects of pretest developmental age and nurse conduct time removed.

Neither family problems (problems with children, parent illness, and lost spouse work time) nor individual relationships (time alone, discussing concerns, emotional support and sexual relationships with spouse, help from spouse with children and housework, time with children, disagreements with spouse, and satisfaction with the marriage) differed significantly from usual care families. However, family support (discussing concerns, emotional support and help with children and housework from friends and relatives, time with neighbors, and time for housework) improved for the SPIN families and worsened among the usual care families.

Changes in Parent Coping

Better coping was seen among SPIN parents than among usual care parents after the effect of nurse contact time was removed (see Table 28.2). Parent coping by maintaining social support, self-esteem, and psychological stability was similar between the SPIN and usual care groups. Family coping by maintaining family integration, cooperation, and an optimistic definition of the situation, and health care communication coping by understanding the medical situation through communication and consultation were greater in the SPIN group. However, only scores on the health care communication scale differed significantly between the SPIN and usual care groups.

Effects of SPIN on Child Development and Behavior

The children's average prehospitalization developmental levels were well below the norm in all areas of development, although the range was from very delayed to advanced for the child's age. The SPIN children were more likely than usual care children to maintain their overall developmental level or make developmental gains after hospitalization (see Table 28.2). The usual care children were more apt to have developmental regression following hospitalization.

The pattern of improved developmental progress among the SPIN children was seen both overall and in the children's motor skills (fine and gross), social and communication skills (comprehension, expression, social interaction), and personal living skills (eating, toileting, dressing, personal self care). Clinically important differences between the SPIN and usual care groups were seen both overall and in motor, personal living, and social and communication skills. SPIN's effect on overall developmental reactions was thus to limit regression and enhance developmental maintenance and gains over repeated hospitalizations. Overall, only 17% of the SPIN children regressed developmentally, compared to 56% of the usual care group.

The effect of SPIN on motor skills was to limit regression and maintain skill level. In the usual care group, most children (61%) showed motor skill regression. In contrast, most children in the SPIN group (67%) maintained their motor developmental level after hospitalization.

In personal living skill development (e.g., eating, toileting, dressing, and personal self-care), there were important differences between children in the SPIN and usual care groups. Skill enhancements occurred slightly more often in the SPIN group (35% SPIN vs. 25% usual care), but such skills were also more apt to be maintained for SPIN children than usual care children (48% vs. 32%). The usual care children were much more apt to show developmental regression than SPIN children (44% vs. 17%).

A large enhancement in social and communication skills was found for the SPIN children, with 37% showing gains, compared to only 14% of the usual care children. Fewer SPIN children than usual care children had social and communication skill regression (22% vs. 46%).

Children in both the SPIN and usual care groups had many behaviors that were distressing to parents, reflected in the very high Parent Stress

Index (PSI) scores on the child scales at both pretest and posttest. The percentage of children with high pretest scores ranged from 14% to 41% (only 10% of the general population would be expected to have such high scores, above the 90th percentile). The highest proportions of difficult behaviors were in child acceptability to the parent and child demandingness/degree of bother. Parents reported essentially the same behaviors 3 months after discharge. In both study groups, there was little change in behaviors that were distressing to parents. However, children who were more demanding before hospitalization and less demanding after hospitalization tended to have had more nurse-parent contact time over the course of the study.

DISCUSSION

Stress-point intervention by ambulatory clinic nurses was effective in enhancing parents' coping with the hospitalization of their child with a chronic health condition. Particular improvements were seen in coping through communicating with people in the health care system, maintaining family cooperation, and developing an optimistic view of the family's situation. SPIN was also effective in enhancing satisfaction with family interactions, including help with family tasks from friends, neighbors, and relatives. In addition, SPIN was effective in reducing hospital-induced developmental regression among children with chronic conditions.

All types of families and children benefited from SPIN. The child's and family's medical, hospitalization, and sociodemographic characteristics did not appear to determine who would benefit most from SPIN; however, the fewer adults involved in the care of the child, the more apt SPIN was to positively affect family functioning. It could be that these families were most in need of what SPIN offered.

The lack of difference in the effects of SPIN by child's diagnostic group suggests that SPIN is a generic intervention, with utility across many settings and with a wide range of children with chronic conditions. Our results point to the need for communication, support, and problem-solving strategies for families with children with a wide range of chronic conditions.

SPIN encourages parental identification of family stressors and difficult tasks and enhances the likelihood that families will assess their situation as amenable to change. With the help of the nurse, parents are more apt to believe their problems can be solved. In turn, with an optimistic appraisal, families are more apt to employ problem-focused coping strategies (Lazarus & Folkman, 1984) and actively engage in coping with their current problems (Austin & McDermott, 1988).

SPIN also helps parents to reshape their view of the situation, enhances and adds to parents' ideas about dealing with their current problems, and helps them identify new coping strategies if coping attempts do not bring about desired responses.

NOTES

1. A self-directed learning package for SPIN and a list of additional video-tapes and reading materials are available from the authors. Please write Elizabeth Kauffmann for details and cost.

REFERENCES

Abidin, R. R. (1986). *Parenting Stress Index.* Charlottesville, VA: Pediatric Psychology Press.

Achenbach, T. M., & Edelbrock, C. (1983). *Child Behavior Checklist.* Burlington, VT: University Medical Education Associates.

Association for the Care of Children's Health. (1982). *Preparing your child for repeated or extended hospitalization.* Washington, DC: Author.

Austin, J. K., & McDermott, N. (1988). Parental attitude and coping behaviors in families of children with epilepsy. *Journal of Neuroscience Nursing, 20,* 174–179.

Bruininks, R. H., Woodcock, R. W., Weatherman, R. F., & Hill, B. K. (1985). *Development and standardization of the Scales of Independent Behavior.* Allen, TX: DLM Teaching Resources.

Burke, S. O., Costello, E. A., & Handley-Derry, M. (1989). Maternal stress and repeated hospitalizations of children who are physically disabled. *Children's Health Care, 18*(2), 82–90.

Burke, S. O., Costello, E. A., Handley-Derry, M., Kauffmann, E., & Dillon, M. (1997). Stress-point preparation for parents of repeatedly hospitalized children with chronic conditions. *Research in Nursing and Health, 20*(6), 475–485.

Burke, S. O., Kauffmann, E., Costello, E. A., Wiskin, N., & Harrison, M. B. (1998). Stressors in families with a child with a chronic condition: An analysis of qualitative studies and a framework. *Canadian Journal of Nursing Research, 30*(1), 71–95.

Burke, S. O., Kauffmann, E., Harrison, M. B., & Wiskin, N. (1999). Assessment of stressors in families with a child who has a chronic condition. *MCN: The Journal of Maternal Child Nursing, 24,* 98–106.

Curley, M. Q., & Wallace, J. (1992). Effects of the Nursing Mutual Participation Model of Care on parental stress in the pediatric intensive care unit—a replication. *Journal of Pediatric Nursing, 7,* 377–385.

Feetham, S. L., & Carroll, R. B. (1988). Further development of reliability and validity of the Feetham Family Functioning Survey. *International Family Nursing Conference Proceedings*. Calgary, Alberta. (Abstract).

Feetham, S. L., & Humenick, S. S. (1982). The Feetham Family Functioning survey. In S. S. Humenick (Ed.), *Analysis of current assessment strategies in the health care of young children and childbearing families* (pp. 249–268). East Norwalk, CT: Appleton-Century-Crofts.

Kauffmann, E., Harrison, M. B., Burke, S. O., & Wong, C. (1998). Family matters: Stress-point intervention for parents of children hospitalized with chronic conditions. *Pediatric Nursing, 24*(4), 362–366.

Lazarus, R. S., & Folkman, S. (1984). *Stress, appraisal, coping*. New York: Springer.

Lende, E. W. (1971). The effect of preparation on children's response to tonsillectomy and adenoidectomy surgery. *Dissertation Abstracts International, 32*, 3642B.

McClowry, S. G. (1988). A review of the literature pertaining to the psychosocial responses of school-aged children to hospitalization. *Journal of Pediatric Nursing, 3*, 296–311.

McCubbin, H. I., McCubbin, M. A., Patterson, J. M., Cauble, A. E., Wilson, L. R., & Warwick, W. (1983). CHIP—Coping Health Inventory for Parents: An assessment of parental coping patterns in the care of the chronically ill child. *Journal of Marriage and the Family*, 359–370.

Melamed, B. G., & Ridley-Johnson, R. (1988). Psychological preparation of families for hospitalization. *Developmental and Behavioral Pediatrics, 9*, 96–102.

Mercer, R. T., & Ferketich, S. L. (1990). Predictors of family functioning eight months following birth. *Nursing Research, 39*(2), 76–82.

Meyer, D. J., & Vadsay, P. F. (1994). *Sibshops: Workshops for siblings of children with special needs*. Baltimore: Paul H. Brookes.

Newacheck, P. W., & Taylor, W. R. (1992). Childhood chronic illness: prevalence, severity, and impact. *American Journal of Public Health, 82*(3), 364–371.

Roberts, C. A. (1979). *The relationship of family functioning to the habilitation of children born with myelodysplasia*. Unpublished doctoral dissertation, Wayne State University, Detroit.

Robinson, C. A. (1987). Roadblocks to family centered care when a chronically ill child is hospitalized. *Maternal Child Nursing Journal, 16*, 181–193.

Thompson, R. H. (1986). Where we stand: Twenty years of research on pediatric hospitalization and health care. *Children's Health Care, 14*, 200–210.

Tomlinson, P. S., Harbaugh, B. L., Kotchevar, J., & Swanson, L. (1995). Caregiver mental health and family health outcomes following critical hospitalization of a child. *Issues in Mental Health Nursing, 16*(6), 533–545.

Webster, J. A., & Moss, V. A. (1986). Caring for special people: Perioperative nursing of handicapped children. *American Operating Room Nurses Journal, 44*, 252–260.

Wright, L. M., & Leahey, M. (1994). *Nurses and families: A guide to family assessment and intervention*. Philadelphia: Davis.

Youngblut, J. M., & Shiao, S. P. (1993). Child and family reactions during and after pediatric ICU hospitalization: A pilot study. *Heart and Lung, 22*(1), 46–54.

[29]

The Effects of a Parent Education Program on the Coping and Stress Levels of Parents of Children with Chronic Conditions

Connie J. Canam

Families of children with chronic health conditions face many similar issues, regardless of the child's diagnosis (Burke, Kauffmann, Wiskin, & Harrison, 1995; Canam, 1993; Stein & Jessop, 1989). Further, the majority of these issues are psychosocial rather than medical (Canam, 1993; Hobbs, Perrin, & Ireys, 1985). However, providing support for families to manage psychosocial issues related to a child's chronic condition poses a major challenge for health professionals. Traditionally, they have undertaken interventions only after a problem has been identified, rather than helping parents anticipate and develop resources to cope with their child's care. Patterson and Geber (1991) suggest that one way to help families manage the demands facing them is to assist them in increasing their skills in coping with disease-related stress.

Group programs, based on education or counseling models, have shown promise in helping families manage the demands of their child's condition. Parents who participated in these programs have shown a more positive attitude toward their children (Omizo, Williams, & Omizo, 1986), more confidence in their ability to parent (Hornby & Murray, 1983), increased knowledge (Duffy & Halloran, 1987; Lewis, Hatton, Salas, Leake, & Chiofalo, 1991), decreased anxiety (Lewis et al., 1991), and better physician-parent communications (Bywater, 1984). However, to date most programs and groups have been organized around specific disease conditions (Duffy & Halloran, 1987; Lewis et al., 1991), and their effectiveness has not been systematically evaluated (Bartholomew et al., 1991; Heiney, Wells, Coleman, Swygert, & Ruffin, 1990).

The study reported here evaluated a group educational program designed to enhance coping and decrease stress of parents of children with a variety of chronic conditions. The program focused on helping parents to develop the knowledge and skills needed to manage the adaptive tasks of parenting a child with any chronic condition (Canam, 1993). Parents who participated in the program were expected to report a greater increase in the use of effective coping strategies and a greater decrease in stress after completion of the program than a control group of similar parents who did not participate. Further, the improvements shown by participants in the program were expected to be maintained at the 3-month follow-up.

METHODS

Study Design

A pretest/posttest, control group design (Campbell & Stanley, 1963) with an additional 3-month follow-up for the experimental group was used.

Sample

Brochures describing the program were sent, along with a cover letter outlining the study, to community health centers, pediatricians' and family physicians' offices, social service agencies, community centers, libraries, and the ambulatory clinics and inpatient units of a large metropolitan pediatric hospital. Local newspapers also ran information on the program. If parents were interested, they contacted the researchers for more information and were screened by a research assistant to determine if they met the study criteria. To be admitted to the study, parents were required to have a child with a chronic health condition who had been diagnosed for a minimum of 6 months, have a good command of written and spoken

English, and not be currently receiving any individual or family counseling. Parents also had to agree to attend all classes. To include as many families as possible, only one parent was included from a family.

Intervention

The intervention was a group program based on McCubbin and Patterson's (1982) Double ABCX Model of Adjustment and Adaptation and designed to help parents develop new coping strategies to deal with the demands facing them. These demands were presented to families as adaptive tasks in order to communicate the view that a chronic condition poses not hardships to be endured or demands to be met, but challenges or tasks that can be mastered by acquiring specific knowledge and skills.

The program consisted of eight 2-hour group sessions based on the common adaptive tasks facing parents whose child has a chronic condition (Canam, 1993). The tasks include accepting the child's health condition, managing the child's condition on a day-to-day basis, meeting the child's developmental needs, meeting the needs of other family members, coping with ongoing stress and periodic crises, helping family members deal with their feelings, educating others about the child's health condition, and developing and utilizing resources. Each of these tasks was presented in a separate session. The program was reviewed by a panel of eight experts in the field of childhood chronic illness, including two parents of children with chronic conditions, and revisions were made based on feedback from the panel.

The program offered a minimum of lecturing and a maximum of parental involvement. A brief introduction to the topic was followed by group activities such as dividing into pairs, role playing, and completing pencil-and-paper exercises. The main goals of each session were to provide information while also using parents' own experience with the adaptive task being presented, and to give parents opportunities to practice related skills. Although each session had a focus, it was the parents' own experience with that particular topic that provided the learning. Parents were also asked to do homework activities, which gave them an opportunity to practice skills related to particular adaptive tasks.

The program was facilitated by two nurses who had experience in leading groups and in working with families of chronically ill or handicapped children. Two manuals were used in conjunction with the program. One was a facilitator's manual or curriculum guide outlining the structure of each session and including the objectives for the session, preclass preparation, and session plans, with instructions for all exercises. The other manual was a parent's manual; this included detailed content on each of the session topics, so that parents could use it as a reference during and after the program.

Instruments

Parental coping strategies and stress levels were measured by the Coping Health Inventory for Parents (McCubbin, McCubbin, & Cauble, 1979) and the Parenting Stress Index (Abidin, 1986). A demographic information form was also completed by subjects. The Coping Health Inventory for Parents (CHIP) is a 45-item self-report checklist of specific coping strategies used by parents in the management of family life and the care of a chronically ill child. Coping behaviors such as "having my child with the medical condition seen at the clinic/hospital on a regular basis" and "allowing myself to get angry" are listed, and parents are asked to record on a scale of 0 to 3 how helpful the behaviors are to them in their particular family situation. The 45 items are divided into three coping patterns. Coping Pattern I consists of 19 behavioral items that focus on family dynamics and parents' outlook on life and the illness. It is labeled "Maintaining Family Integration, Cooperation, and an Optimistic Definition of the Situation (FAM)." Coping Pattern II consists of 18 behavioral items that focus on parents' efforts to maintain a sense of their own well-being through social relationships, involvement in activities that enhance their self-esteem, and management of psychological tensions. It is labeled "Maintaining Social Support, Self-Esteem, and Psychological Stability (SUP)." Coping Pattern III consists of 8 behavioral items that focus on parents' efforts to understand the medical situation and master the information needed to care for their child at home through communication with other parents and consultation with medical staff. The coping pattern is labeled "Understanding the Medical Situation through Communication with other Parents and Consultation with Medical Staff (MED)." These three coping patterns were derived from factor analysis and accounted for 71% of the variance in the items. Chronbach's alpha, computed for the items on each coping pattern, indicated reliabilities of .79, .79, and .71, respectively (McCubbin et al., 1983).

The Parenting Stress Index (PSI) is a 120-item self-report questionnaire that identifies specific characteristics of the child and parent as stressors. A numerical value is given to the stressors to indicate the relative amount of stress they impose on the parent-child dyad. Items include such statements as "My child is not able to do as much as I expected" and "I feel capable and on top of things when I am caring for my child," and parents are asked to rate their agreement with such statements on a scale from 1 (strongly agree) to 5 (strongly disagree). The items are divided into three main sources of stress: (1) child characteristics, such as demandingness, mood, and adaptability; (2) parent characteristics, such as depression, sense of competence, social isolation, relationship with spouse, and health; and (3) life stress, or the amount of stress the parent is experiencing outside the parent-child relationship. The reliability coefficients for the child and parent domains are .89 and .93, respectively. A total stress score is obtained by adding the scores from the child and parent domains. The reliability coefficient for this score is .95.

Procedures

Randomization into groups was done at the time of recruitment, which was 2 to 4 months before the program began. Parents assigned to the experimental group (group 1) were enrolled in the first program held in the fall, and parents assigned to the control group (group 2) were enrolled in a second program held in the spring. The program was offered to all parents because it was considered unethical to withhold a treatment that was desired by parents and had the potential for producing positive results. The fact that all of the parents recruited for the study wanted to participate in the program speaks to the need for this type of intervention.

All participants were assessed three times: prior to the beginning of the first program, 1 week after the experimental group had completed the program, and 1 week after the control group completed the second program. For the experimental group, the third assessment occurred 3 months after completion of the program and served to identify lasting effects of the program. Although the control group was assessed at the same times as the experimental group, they did not receive the intervention until just before the third assessment point. Thus, for the control group, the third assessment was used to assess the effects of the program and to compare these to the experimental group's preprogram/postprogram measures.

RESULTS

Fifty-one parents of children with chronic health conditions participated in the study, 27 in the control group and 24 in the experimental group. Forty-seven subjects were mothers, 3 were fathers, and 1 was a grandmother. Subjects were predominantly Caucasian (91.6%) and middle class, with

60% having a college/university degree or some college/university courses, and 45% earning over $40,000 a year. Eighty-one percent were married, and the average number of children per family was two. Forty-eight percent of the subjects were employed, although the majority of these (65%) worked part-time. Fifty-six percent of the children with a chronic condition were female; their ages ranged from 7 months to 18 years, with a mean age of 8.3 years. The children had a wide variety of chronic conditions, including asthma, cerebral palsy, congenital heart disease, cystic fibrosis, cancer, diabetes, hearing impairment, and juvenile rheumatoid arthritis. Fifty-six percent had been diagnosed for at least 2 years.

The experimental and control groups were similar in age, education, marital status, income, age of the child with the chronic condition, and number of children in the family. The two groups differed in employment status and time since diagnosis of the child. Sixty-five percent of the experimental subjects worked either part-time or full-time, as compared to only 36% of the control subjects. In 41% of the experimental group, the child had been diagnosed less than a year, as compared to 11% of the control group. In 41% of the control group, the child had been diagnosed 2 to 4 years, as compared to 13% of the experimental group.

Parental Coping

The pretest and posttest 1 means and standard deviations for the CHIP subscales, along with p values for changes in mean scores, are presented in Table 29.1 for the experimental and control groups. The experimental group scores on all subscales increased from the pretest to posttest 1, suggesting an intervention effect. For two of the three subscale scores, this increase was significant (support [$p = .0006$] and medical [$p = .040$]), and the increases were maintained from the pretest to posttest 2 (support [$p = .018$] and medical [$p = .035$]), demonstrating an intervention effect that was maintained at 3 months. In sum, parents who participated in the program showed a significant increase in the use of effective coping strategies in two of three areas and the increase was maintained 3 months after completion of the program. The control group showed a decrease in two of the three CHIP subscales from pretest to posttest 1 and only a slight increase in the third subscale, indicating no real change.

The change in the experimental group mean from pretest to posttest 1 was significantly higher than that of the control group for all three subscales of CHIP (family [$p = .037$], support [$p = .014$], and medical [$p = .040$]), demonstrating that the intervention worked; that is, participation in the

TABLE 29.1 Means and Standard Deviations for CHIP Coping Variables for Experimental and Control Groups

	Experimental (n = 24)		Control (n = 27)	
Coping Variable	Mean	SD	Mean	SD
Family				
Pretest	36.2	8.1	38.6	7.7
Posttest 1	39.1	6.4	36.4	7.7
Posttest 2	38.3	7.6	36.9	8.3
Support				
Pretest	26.6	8.7	27.6	7.9
Posttest 1	30.9[a]	7.1	28.2	8.6
Posttest 2	31.1[b]	10.0	29.0	8.6
Medical				
Pretest	15.0	4.9	17.6	4.8
Posttest 1	17.0[a]	4.7	17.0	4.6
Posttest 2	17.1[b]	3.3	17.0	4.0

[a]Posttest 1 significantly different from pretest (support $p = .0006$, medical $p = .04$).
[b]Posttest 2 significantly different from pretest (support $p = .018$, medical $p = .035$).

program resulted in a significant increase in the use of effective coping strategies when compared to the control group.

To determine if the effect of the intervention on the experimental group was replicated when the control group received the delayed intervention, the p values for changes in means from pretest to posttest 1 for the experimental group and from posttest 1 to posttest 2 for the control group were compared. These time points were chosen to represent the immediate pre- and postintervention assessments for each group. As noted above, within the experimental group two of the three subscale scores increased significantly from the pretest to posttest 1. However, in the control group, there were no significant increases on any of the subscales from posttest 1 to posttest 2. This indicates that there was no significant intervention effect for this group.

The means and standard deviations for the PSI subscales are presented in Table 29.2 for the experimental and control groups. While the experimental group's stress scores decreased more than the control group's scores from pretest to posttest 2, the difference was not significant. This indicates that there was no intervention effect on the stress levels of parents who participated in the program.

TABLE 29.2   Means and Standard Deviations for PSI Stress Variables for Experimental and Control Groups

Stress Variable	Experimental (n = 24)		Control (n = 26)	
	Mean	SD	Mean	SD
Total stress				
Pretest	235.8	52.4	241.8	48.2
Posttest 1	233.0	51.0	238.3	45.7
Posttest 2	215.2	59.5	235.4	55.5
Parent domain				
Pretest	107.6	25.0	113.6	30.3
Posttest 1	103.9	28.0	111.3	29.1
Posttest 2	96.7	30.0	110.6	33.5
Child domain				
Pretest	128.2	32.1	128.2	25.2
Posttest 1	129.1	29.8	126.9	22.2
Posttest 2	118.5	33.0	124.9	26.4

DISCUSSION

Parents who participated in the first educational program reported a significant increase in the use of effective coping strategies after completion of the program, as compared to the control group of parents who did not participate in the program. In two of the three coping patterns measured, parents maintained this improvement to the 3-month follow-up.

The greatest improvement occurred on the Support subscale of the CHIP, which taps social support, self-esteem, and psychological stability. This suggests that, as a result of their participation in the program, parents felt better about themselves and more supported. The support that parents gain from interacting with parents in similar situations has also been documented by others (Bentz, Unger, Frager, Test, & Smith, 1990; Yoak & Chesler, 1985). What is unique about this study is that the parents had children with different diseases. The finding here suggests that parents can identify with other parents whose child has a chronic condition even though the diseases the children have are different. It also lends support to an approach that emphasizes similar experiences in parenting children with chronic conditions such as disciplining the child and interacting with health care professionals.

One component of the program focused on helping parents understand the importance of taking care of themselves and their other relationships because of the tendency, particularly for mothers, to become overinvolved with the ill child at the expense of other relationships. After participation in the program, parents reported that they were taking time for themselves and realizing the importance of this for coping effectively with their child's condition.

Parents also improved their scores on the Medical subscale of the CHIP, which focuses on parents' efforts to understand the medical situation and master the information needed to care for their child at home. Two aspects of coping addressed by the parent program were getting accurate and complete information about their child's condition and interacting with health care professionals. The program emphasized being proactive in acquiring information and helped parents to understand their right to full information about their child's condition. Communication and assertiveness skills were also taught so that parents could effectively interact with health care professionals. The improvement in parents' scores on the Medical subscale suggests that an important component of coping is having the skills to acquire the information needed to manage the child's condition.

The Family subscale of CHIP showed the least change. This subscale focuses on family dynamics and the individual parent's outlook on life and the illness. It is possible that coping changed less in this area because only one parent attended the program. Although family dynamics were addressed, it would no doubt have been more central if both parents had attended the program together; thus, the potential for change in this variable would have been greater.

The failure of the control group to demonstrate a significant increase in coping scores after receiving the intervention may be explained by the time since diagnosis of the child's condition. In 41% of this group the child had been diagnosed 2 to 4 years, as compared to 13% of the experimental group. The optimal time for parents to learn coping skills may be early; beyond this time an educational intervention may become ineffective because parents have learned and become comfortable with particular coping behaviors. In discussions with the group facilitators, parents noted that it was important to wait at least 6 months after the diagnosis before taking the program because they would not have been able to "take anything in" during the time immediately following diagnosis. The best timing of interventions for parents may be between 6 months and a year after diagnosis, but this will need to be examined further.

There was no significant difference in the stress levels of the experimental group before and after they completed the program or between the experimental and the control group. We expected that when individuals improved their ability to cope with a stressful situation, their stress would decrease. The findings did not support this; there was no correlation between coping scores and stress scores. Because they are dealing with multiple ongoing stressors, parents' stress levels may remain high even if they perceive themselves as coping better (Burke, Costello, & Handley-Derry, 1989; Cameron, Dobson, & Day, 1991; Holroyd & Gutherie, 1986). This is an area that warrants further investigation. It is also possible that the PSI tool used in this study may not have been the most sensitive tool to use with this population. The PSI explores a broad range of stressful events experienced by parents during the child's younger years. An instrument that explores specific stressors in parenting a child with a chronic condition might be more sensitive to stress levels in this population.

Nurses who work with families of children with chronic conditions in the hospital or the community are aware of the demands confronting these parents. This study suggests that nurses can strengthen parental coping by helping parents develop the knowledge, skills, and support to master the common tasks facing them. The findings also suggest that parents of children with a wide variety of chronic conditions may benefit from a group program in which they acquire knowledge and skills and gain support from other parents.

Stein and colleagues (1989) concluded from their study of health care services received by children with chronic illnesses that we must provide broader and more effective services for these children and their families. Recent societal and health care trends support these conclusions. The pressure to contain health care costs means that hospital-based services are becoming increasingly unavailable, particularly to those who are not in an acute illness situation. In addition, the trend toward early discharge from acute care hospitals is placing greater demands on families and community resources. An educational group program based on common issues facing families of children with chronic conditions is one cost-effective, comprehensive way of providing services for this population.

REFERENCES

Abidin, R. R. (1986). *Parenting Stress Index manual.* Charlottesville, VA: Pediatric Psychology Press.

Bartholomew, L. K., Parcel, G. S., Seilheimer, D. K., Czyzewski, D., Spinelli, S. H., & Congdon, B. (1991). Development of a health education program to promote self-management of cystic fibrosis. *Health Education Quarterly, 18*(4), 429–443.

Bentz, C., Unger, O., Frager, B., Test, L., & Smith, C. (1990). A survey of self-help groups in California for parents of children with chronic conditions. *Pediatric Nursing, 16*(3), 293–296.

Burke, S. O., Costello, E. A., & Handley-Derry, M. H. (1989). Maternal stress and repeated hospitalizations of children who are physically disabled. *Children's Health Care, 18*(2), 82–90.

Burke, S. O., Kauffmann, E., Wiskin, N., & Harrison, M. (1995). Children with chronic illnesses and their parents in the community. In M. Stewart (Ed.), *Community nursing: Promoting Canadians' health* (pp. 284–313). Toronto: W. B. Saunders.

Bywater, E. (1984). Coping with a life-threatening illness: An experiment in parents' groups. *British Journal of Social Work, 14,* 117–127.

Cameron, S. J., Dobson, L. A., & Day, D. M. (1991, March). Stress in parents of developmentally delayed and non-delayed preschool children. *Canada's Mental Health,* 13–17.

Campbell, D. T., & Stanley, J. C. (1963). *Experimental and quasi experimental design for research.* Chicago: Rand McNally.

Canam, C. (1993). Common adaptive tasks facing parents of children with chronic conditions. *Journal of Advanced Nursing, 18,* 46–53.

Duffy, D. M., & Halloran, M. C. (1987). Effect of an educational program on parents of children with asthma. *Childrens Health Care, 16*(2), 76–81.

Heiney, S. P., Wells, L. M., Coleman, B., Swygert, E., & Ruffin, J. (1990). Lasting impressions: A psychosocial support program for adolescents with cancer and their parents. *Cancer Nursing, 13*(1), 13–20.

Hobbs, N., Perrin, J. M., & Ireys, H. T. (1985). Effects of chronic illness on children, families, and communities. In N. Hobbs, J. M. Perrin, & H. T. Ireys (Eds.), *Chronically ill children and their families* (pp. 62–101). London: Jossey-Bass.

Holroyd, J., & Gutherie, D. (1986). Family stress with chronic childhood illness: Cystic fibrosis, neuromuscular diseases, and renal disease. *Journal of Clinical Psychology, 42*(4), 522–561.

Hornby, G., & Murray, R. (1983). Group programmes for parents of children with various handicaps. *Child: Care, Health, and Development, 9*(4), 185–198.

Lewis, M. A., Hatton, C. L., Salas, I., Leake, B., & Chiofalo, N. (1991). Impact of the Children's Epilepsy Program on parents. *Epilepsia, 32*(3), 365–374.

McCubbin, H. I., McCubbin, M. A., & Cauble, E. (1979). *CHIP: Coping Health Inventory for Parents (Form A).* Available from Family Social Science, University of Minnesota, St. Paul, MN 55108.

McCubbin, H. I., & Patterson, J. M. (1982). Family adaptation to crises. In H. I. McCubbin, A. E. Cauble, & J. M. Patterson (Eds.), *Family stress, coping, and social support* (pp. 26–47). Springfield, IL: Charles C. Thomas.

McCubbin, H. I., McCubbin, M. A., Patterson, J. M., Cauble, A. E., Wilson, L. R., & Warwick, W. (1983, May). CHIP—Coping Health Inventory for Parents: An assessment of parental coping patterns in the care of the chronically ill child. *Journal of Marriage and the Family,* 359–370.

Omizo, M. M., Williams, R. E., & Omizo, S. A. (1986). The effects of participation in parent group sessions on child-rearing attitudes among parents of learning disabled children. *The Exceptional Child, 33*(2), 134–139.

Patterson, J., & Geber, G. (1991). Preventing mental health problems in children with chronic illness or disability. *Children's Health Care, 20*(3), 150–161.

Stein, R. E. K., & Jessop, D. J. (1989). What diagnosis does not tell: The case for a noncategorical approach to chronic illness in childhood. *Social Science and Medicine, 29*(6), 769–778.

Yoak, M., & Chesler, M. (1985). Alternative professional roles in health care delivery: Leadership patterns in self-help groups. *Journal of Applied Behavioral Science, 21*(4), 427–441.

Part VI

APPLYING RESEARCH TO PRACTICE

[30]

Strategies for Using Research to Improve Care

Linda R. Cronenwett and Jennifer Leeman

This book has provided clinicians with information on some of the latest research on interventions for the prevention and management of chronic illness. The question is, to what extent will these interventions actually be implemented in practice settings and translated into improved care for the chronically ill? Evidence is a necessary but not a sufficient condition for change, and many research findings continue to fail to reach clinical practice.

These are particularly challenging times for those who seek to introduce new interventions into health care. Recently, there has been a tremendous growth in managed care plans in which physician practices have contracts with multiple health plans (Bodenheimer, 1999); this reduces the potential for the integration that is critical to the effective management of chronic illness (Christianson, Taylor, & Knutson, 1998; Wagner, Austin, & Von Korff, 1996). Further, the majority of managed care plans are for-profit organizations (Gabel, 1997), and with cost as the primary basis for competition, there are few incentives to implement new interventions to improve quality (Bailit, 1997; Kuttner, 1996; Malloy, 1997). As plans compete by reducing costs, they are reducing staff and increasing the ratio of patients to providers. Thus, clinicians have ever-growing demands on their time and fewer opportunities to either learn or implement the latest findings from research.

Recognizing these challenges, this chapter offers some beginning strate-gies for effectively using interventions from the literature to improve prac-tice. The strategies include (1) adapting research to the practice setting, (2) winning organizational support for change, (3) getting clinicians to adopt new interventions, (4) extending change beyond traditional health care settings, and (5) influencing the research agenda.

ADAPTING RESEARCH TO THE PRACTICE SETTING

Published research findings rarely fit neatly in the practice setting. Indeed, nurses' use of research has been hindered by its lack of relevance to practice (Funk, Champagne, Wiese, & Tornquist, 1991). One writer has described the challenge as follows:

> In general, research questions are defined by researchers and investigated with atypical populations in settings that differ from practice, and the resulting answers are often difficult to translate into clinically useful information. Re-searchers themselves are the major consumers of research; much medical research has simply not been useful in guiding practice. (Nutting & Green, 1994, p. 152)

Numerous factors contribute to the publication of research findings that cannot be easily translated into practice. As Nutting and Green note, researchers tend to study interventions with very controlled patient popula-tions, which are very different from those encountered by clinicians in practice. In order to control variation in the effect of the intervention, the researcher selects subjects who are as uniform as possible. The experience of the practicing clinician is in direct contrast to that of the researcher. In clinical practice, patients may share a diagnosis and yet vary with respect to age, culture, ethnicity, financial resources, and health status. The inter-vention may require adaptation for use with these different patient popula-tions, yet research publications rarely provide information about implementation with groups other than the one included in the study. One area of particular concern for those working with the chronically ill is variation in comorbidities. Most research restricts its focus to subjects with only one condition, but many people, particularly older people, are living with multiple chronic illnesses (Hoffman, Rice, & Sung, 1996).

Further, researchers tend to study interventions in settings that are incon-gruent with the realities of clinical practice. For example, using research funding to hire a full-time intervention nurse is very different from adding responsibility for a new intervention to an already very busy nursing staff.

Researchers have the freedom to configure space, staff, and other resources to fit the intervention. In clinical practice, nurses generally need to configure the intervention to fit the setting.

Because of the way that most new interventions are designed, tested, and reported in the literature, clinicians face the task of adapting the research to their own local conditions, to patient preferences and values, and to the cultural context of care (Brown, Shye, & McFarland, 1995). Implementing a new intervention requires an up-front investment of time and energy to adapt that intervention to the setting. All relevant disciplines need to be involved in the process of adaptation, which should consider the requirements of the intervention as it compares to current resources and practice in the clinical setting. Adaptation also needs to accommodate the intervention to the resources and culture of the patient population.

As nurses look for new interventions that may improve care for chronically ill patients, they need to expand the search to research outside a particular practice area. The chapters in this book offer insights into common issues in developing healthy lifestyles, the commonalities of different chronic conditions, common symptom clusters, common behavior management issues, and common issues in adapting interventions to the individual in the context of his or her life. Clinicians tend to identify with information that relates to a specific patient population or specific techniques or procedures. Clinicians identify with AIDS, they identify with cardiac care, they identify with critical care; they do not identify with chronic illness. As nurses look for interventions that may work with a particular patient population, it is important to consider interventions proven effective with other types of chronic illness and determine whether the commonalities across illnesses are greater than the differences, providing opportunities to borrow and combine interventions from a broader base of literature.

WINNING ORGANIZATIONAL SUPPORT FOR CHANGE

Only rarely do we have the opportunity to implement change in the absence of some level of support from the organizational hierarchy. Most significant change requires additional resources or permission to change the present system of care. In order to have the knowledge necessary to strategically guide change and also to have input into decision making, it is helpful to be at the table when the organization makes decisions about future directions and the reallocation of resources. Sitting on committees and actively participating in organizational decision making provide opportunities for input while also yielding information about barriers and opportunities for change.

Efforts to gain support are most successful if they incorporate an understanding of the organization's capacity and incentives. Each organization has a defined capacity—resources that are available for the fulfillment of its objectives. Change strategies are more effective when they incorporate an understanding of resource availability and limitations. In our present environment of limited resources, any shift in resources will require compelling evidence that a problem exists and that it is of sufficient significance to merit a shift in the organization's resources. Sometimes clinicians and administrators do not recognize that there is a problem. They do not realize that a group of patients suffers fatigue or that another group is depressed. It is crucial to collect data that demonstrates the need for change and learn how to interpret and present the data collected.

Even if an organization is not prepared to fully back a new program, it may be willing to support a pilot study. Pilot studies can be a valuable beginning for something new and possibly threatening. A pilot study provides an opportunity for the organization to try the intervention on a small scale and to collect data on how well it works and whether it is feasible. If the pilot goes well and generates compelling data, it is hard for the organization to say no to the new program.

In addition to organizational capacity, it is helpful to be aware of the incentives driving organizational decision making. Those seeking to gain support for change can make effective use of organizational incentives such as attracting new patients, making a profit, fulfilling the requirements of accrediting agencies, and maintaining good public relations.

Maintaining financial solvency is an important consideration for both for-profit and nonprofit organizations. Given the present health care environment, we need to be able to document the difference our interventions make. This documentation needs to include analyses of what it costs to deliver the intervention and the health benefits achieved for each dollar spent. These are the kinds of questions that are often ignored in nursing research but are important in the administration of health care. Cost analysis answers the question of interest to the people who control the resources, What will be the additional benefit gained for each extra dollar it will cost to implement the proposed intervention?

The bottom line is not the only incentive driving organizational decision making. Requirements established by accrediting bodies can be used to motivate positive change. Nurses need to be aware of the demands of accrediting bodies and learn to use them to bolster their requests for resources and other support. As an example, chapter 24 of this book discusses disease management programs. Purchasers and accreditors of health plans are asking for inclusion of these programs, and provider organizations and health plans are responding. Incorporating an intervention into a broader disease management plan may be one effective way of gaining organizational support. Incentives change over time, and successful change leaders monitor the broader environment for new opportunities. For example, if the First Lady is diagnosed with breast cancer, that may be the ideal time to present an organization's leadership with a breast cancer management program, along with a plan for publicizing it.

GETTING CLINICIANS TO ADOPT NEW INTERVENTIONS

As health care systems become less integrated, nurses are expected to impose coordination and integration. In their roles as case manager and team leader, nurses have the opportunity to step outside their usual roles, to span the boundaries across different levels of care, and to look beyond the needs of the patient to the wider needs of the patient population. In the present "nonsystem," nurses working at hospital, unit, and clinic levels are critical players in ensuring that comprehensive prevention and management are provided for their patients. Nurses can take these opportunities and make the most of them to improve chronic illness prevention and management.

What are strategies for getting clinicians to adopt new interventions? A recent review of strategies for changing physician behavior emphasizes the importance of incorporating education, reinforcement, participation, and administrative supports in efforts to get clinicians to adopt new interventions (Greco & Eisenberg, 1993). Education alone tends to have a limited impact on behavior change. However, there are strategies to strengthen the effectiveness of education. One strategy involves identifying and enlisting clinicians whose opinions are respected by their peers. These opinion leaders can be trained to teach the intervention to other clinicians. Clinicians experience tension between desire to adopt a potentially beneficial intervention and confidence with what is already familiar. To resolve this tension, clinicians look to the accepted practices and expectations of other clinicians within their organizations and professions (Greer, 1994; Kaluzny et al., 1991). Interventions that incorporate clinicians as disseminators effectively use opinion leaders to build momentum for practice changes (Lomas et al., 1991). Interpersonal contact between members of the potential adopting group and those who have direct knowledge of the innovation can also strengthen the education effort. Ideally, clinicians will be provided an opportunity to talk to other clinicians who have used the intervention, not to a researcher who has never tried to put it into practice. How the information is communicated is also critical to determining the effectiveness of education. Effective education should be as simple, brief, and clear as possible (Gorton, Cranford, Golden, Walls, & Pawelak, 1995).

Once clinicians are educated, reinforcement encourages and maintains behavior change. Reinforcement is most effective when it provides clinicians with data about their behavior by auditing individual performance and providing feedback (Buntinx, Winkens, Grol, & Knottnerus, 1993). Sometimes people think they are doing more than they actually are. Audit and feedback without punishment can be a powerful way to get people to change practice. When clinicians learn how they look with respect to their peers, they will work to change. Computers offer one effective means of providing feedback. We are building systems now that can provide data to the practitioner when the practitioner is actually making the decision about what to do next.

Active participation in the planning and implementation of an intervention facilitates users' adoption. If other disciplines are to be involved in the innovation, their buy-in and input must be sought early on. Chronic care interventions, in particular, can rarely be implemented by a single clinician, but require change across an interdisciplinary team of providers and across a continuum of care (Corbin & Strauss, 1992; Von Korff, Gruman, Schaefer, Curry, & Wagner, 1997). It is important to involve as many people as possible in the change process, especially the resistors. The information should be user-oriented so that the key points are understood by the users, and potential users should be involved so that everyone who has to live with this change is a part of the process.

Finally, implementation needs to include consideration of administrative and organizational processes that may need to be changed. "The assumption that research implementation is the province of the researcher or the individual practitioner, at the clinical or managerial level, rather than being part of an organizational process, involving people at all levels is increasingly being discounted" (Closs & Cheater, 1994, p. 770). Unfortunately, the literature on models for chronic illness treatment suggests that, in their design and implementation, relatively little attention has been paid to organizational issues (Christianson et al., 1998). Chapter 24 points to the importance of attending to organizational factors in the design of programs for the chronically ill. That chapter outlines the characteristics of successful programs and stresses the importance of attention to delivery system design. Reorganization of practice may include redefinition of the roles of different disciplines on the care team, changes in the length and timing of patient visits, and prompts to ensure attention to established protocols. Implementation will often require the reshaping of work actually performed within the practice, beyond simply changing the knowledge and attitudes of providers (Kaluzny et al., 1991). Forms may need to be redesigned, reimbursement agreements renegotiated, and staffing and space reassigned. The prevailing sense is that health care work is too urgent and workers are too busy for evaluating and redesigning the organizational system in which care occurs. Learning is often viewed as personal: Do I, as a clinician, know what to do? We need to move beyond this perspective and increase our understanding of what systems do and how they can be improved to better serve both clinicians and patients.

EXTENDING CHANGE BEYOND TRADITIONAL HEALTH CARE SETTINGS

The management of chronic illness is, by its very nature, a process that involves multiple players over an extended period of time. Because many health problems involve multiple, intertwined medical and social causes, efforts to prevent and manage chronic illness will require change at the level of families, social networks, organizations, and communities (Richard, Potvin, Kishchuk, Prlic, & Green, 1996; Sallis & Owen, 1997). An optimal chronic care delivery system requires integration of medical care with home- and community-based services, as well as integration of both patient and family perspectives into the care process (Lewis & Gibson, 1996). Achieving this level of integration will require moving beyond traditional practice settings in order to work with people in the context of their families, social networks, and community organizations. As evidenced in this book, nurses' efforts to improve the management and prevention of chronic illness are moving out of health care settings and into elementary schools, senior centers, homes, and the community.

INFLUENCING THE RESEARCH AGENDA

One of the most important things we can do is to actively participate in identifying and setting scientific priorities and strategies. We need to become active in influencing the scientific agenda of universities, research institutes, and the health care system. Input from clinicians can help researchers design studies and interventions that address health problems of high priority to society, patients, and health care providers. Clinicians can also increase researchers' awareness of the organizational structures and processes within which clinical care is provided (Kaluzny et al., 1991). This awareness is key to the design of clinically feasible interventions. Researchers need clinicians' input on whether the intervention is appropriate for the desired change in practice, how the intervention will be perceived, and whether clinicians and administrators are likely to support the proposed change in practice (Greco & Eisenberg, 1993). Influencing the scientific agenda requires that we be at the table to help define the questions to be asked and the variables to be studied.

CONCLUSION

As the health care system devolves into less integrated models of managed care, the system is losing its ability to initiate innovations from the top down. The organization has few incentives and limited capacity to implement improvements from the highest level down to the level of clinical practice. Within this environment, practicing clinicians may be the persons with the greatest potential to introduce new interventions. A health services researcher studying innovation in managed care plans recently noted that the most promising innovations are those that are percolating upward (Savitz, personal communication, October 1998). New ways of caring for patients are being devised and piloted at the level of patient care, and, after successful implementation, they are coming to the attention of the organizational hierarchy and being considered for system-wide implementation.

In the present health care environment we face many challenges to our efforts to improve the prevention and management of chronic illness. We need to remember that we also face many opportunities. By working together as clinicians, administrators, and researchers, we can implement the latest findings from research and improve the prevention and management of chronic illness. If we are to be successful, we must be prepared to partner with other disciplines and other organizations to work for change in both the research and the practice environments. To realize improvements, we must be leaders in advocating for change in clinical practice, in health care organizations, and in research.

REFERENCES

Bailit, M. (1997). Ominous signs and portents: A purchaser's view of health care market trends. *Health Affairs, 16*(6), 85–88.

Bodenheimer, T. (1999). The American health care system—Physicians and the changing medical marketplace. *New England Journal of Medicine, 340,* 584–588.

Brown, J. B., Shye, D., & McFarland, B. (1995). The paradox of guideline implementation: How AHCPR's depression guideline was adapted at Kaiser-Permanente Northwest Region. *Journal of Quality Improvement, 21,* 5–21.

Buntinx, F., Winkens, R., Grol, R., & Knottnerus, J. A. (1993). Influencing diagnostic and preventive performance in ambulatory care by feedback and reminders: A review. *Family Practice—An International Journal, 10*(2), 219–230.

Christianson, J., Taylor, R., & Knutson, D. (1998). *Restructuring chronic illness management*. San Francisco: Jossey-Bass.

Closs, S. J., & Cheater, F. (1994). Utilization of nursing research: Culture, interest and support. *Journal of Advanced Nursing, 19*, 762–773.

Corbin, J., & Strauss, A. (1992). A nursing model for chronic illness management based upon the trajectory framework. In P. Woog (Ed.), *The chronic illness trajectory framework* (pp. 9–28). New York: Springer.

Funk, S. G., Champagne, M. T., Wiese, R. A., & Tornquist, E. M. (1991). Barriers to using research findings in practice: The clinician's perspective. *Applied Nursing Research, 4*, 90–95.

Gabel, J. (1997). Ten ways HMOs have changed during the 1990s. *Health Affairs, 16*(3), 134–145.

Gorton, T. A., Cranford, C. O., Golden, W. E., Walls, R. C., & Pawelak, J. E. (1995). Primary care physicians' response to dissemination of practice guidelines. *Archives of Family Medicine, 4*(2), 135–142.

Greco, P. J., & Eisenberg, J. M. (1993). Changing physicians' practices. *New England Journal of Medicine, 329*, 1271–1273.

Greer, A. L. (1994). *"You can always tell a doctor . . . ": Effective dissemination of clinical and health information* (Pub. No. 95-0015). Silver Spring, MD: Agency for Health Care Policy and Research.

Hoffman, C., Rice, D., & Sung, H. Y. (1996). Persons with chronic conditions: Their prevalence and costs. *Journal of the American Medical Association, 276*(18), 1473–1479.

Kaluzny, A. D., Harris, R. P., Strecher, V. J., Stearns, S., Qaqish, B., & Leininger, L. (1991). Prevention and early detection activities in primary care: New directions for implementation. *Cancer Detection and Prevention, 15*(6), 459–464.

Kuttner, R. (1996). Columbia/HCA and the resurgence of the for-profit hospital business. *New England Journal of Medicine, 335*(5, 6), 362–367, 446–451.

Lewis, S., & Gibson, R. (1996). Managed care and chronic care: Challenges and opportunities. *Managed Care Quarterly, 4*(2), 5–11.

Lomas, J., Enkin, M., Anderson, G., Hanna, W., Vayda, E., & Singer, J. (1991). Opinion leaders vs. audit and feedback to implement practice guidelines. *Archives of Internal Medicine, 155*, 625–632.

Malloy, C. (1997). Managed care—What is its impact on nursing education and practice. *Journal of Gerontological Nursing*, 26–31.

Nutting, P. A., & Green, L. A. (1994). From research to policy to practice: Closing the loop in clinical policy development for primary care. In E. V. Dunn, P. G. Norton, M. Stewart, F. Tudiver, & M. J. Bass (Eds.), *Disseminating research/Changing practice* (pp. 151–161). Thousand Oaks, CA: Sage.

Richard, L., Potvin, L., Kishchuk, N., Prlic, H., & Green, L., (1996). Assessment of the integration of the ecological approach in health promotion programs. *American Journal of Health Promotion, 10*(4), 318–328.

Sallis, J. F., & Owen, N. (1997). Ecological models. In K. Glanz, F. M. Lewis, & B.
    K. Reiner (Eds.), *Health behavior and health education: Theory, research, and practice*
    (pp. 403–424). San Francisco: Jossey-Bass.
Von Korff, M., Gruman, J., Schaefer, J., Curry, S., & Wagner, E. (1997). Collaborative
    management of chronic illness. *Annals of Internal Medicine, 127*(12), 1097–1102.
Wagner, E., Austin, B. T., & Von Korff, M. (1996). Organizing care for patients
    with chronic illness. *Milbank Quarterly, 74*(4), 511–544.

Index